D1256873

Pediatric Rheumatology

Guest Editors

RONALD M. LAXER, MDCM, FRCPC
DAVID D. SHERRY, MD

PEDIATRIC CLINICS OF NORTH AMERICA

www.pediatric.theclinics.com

April 2012 • Volume 59 • Number 2

SAUNDERS an imprint of ELSEVIER, Inc.

W.B. SAUNDERS COMPANY
A Division of Elsevier Inc.

1600 John F. Kennedy Boulevard • Suite 1800 • Philadelphia, Pennsylvania 19103-2899

http://www.theclinics.com

THE PEDIATRIC CLINICS OF NORTH AMERICA Volume 59, Number 2
April 2012 ISSN 0031-3955, ISBN-13: 978-1-4557-3909-7

Editor: Kerry Holland
Developmental Editor: Donald Mumford

The Pediatric Clinics of North America (ISSN 0031-3955) is published bimonthly by Elsevier Inc., 360 Park Avenue South, New York, NY 10010-1710. Months of issue are February, April, June, August, October, and December. Periodicals postage paid at New York, NY and additional mailing offices. Subscription prices are $191.00 per year (US individuals), $444.00 per year (US institutions), $259.00 per year (Canadian individuals), $591.00 per year (Canadian institutions), $308.00 per year (international individuals), $591.00 per year (international institutions), $93.00 per year (US students and residents), and $159.00 per year (international and Canadian residents and students). To receive students/resident rare, orders must be accompanied by name of affiliated institution, date of term, and the signature of program/residency coordinator on institution letterhead. Orders will be billed at individual rate until proof of status is received. Foreign air speed delivery is included in all *Clinics* subscription prices. All prices are subject to change without notice. **POSTMASTER:** Send address changes to *The Pediatric Clinics of North America*, Elsevier Health Sciences Division, Subscription Customer Service, 3251 Riverport Lane, Maryland Heights, MO 63043. **Customer Service: 1-800-654-2452 (US and Canada). From outside of the US and Canada: 1-314-447-8871. Fax: 1-314-447-8029. For print support, E-mail: JournalsCustomerService-usa@elsevier.com. For online support, E-mail: JournalsOnlineSupport-usa@elsevier.com.**

Reprints. For copies of 100 or more, of articles in this publication, please contact the Commercial Reprints Department, Elsevier Inc., 360 Park Avenue South, New York, NY 10010-1710. Tel.: 212-633-3812; Fax: 212-462-1935; E-mail: reprints@elsevier.com.

The Pediatric Clinics of North America is also published in Spanish by McGraw-Hill Inter-americana Editores S.A., Mexico City, Mexico; in Portuguese by Riechmann and Affonso Editores, Rua Comandante Coelho 1085, CEP 21250, Rio de Janeiro, Brazil; and in Greek by Althayia SA, Athens, Greece.

The Pediatric Clinics of North America is covered in *MEDLINE/PubMed (Index Medicus), Excerpta Medica, Current Contents, Current Contents/Clinical Medicine, Science Citation Index, ASCA, ISI/BIOMED,* and *BIOSIS.*

Printed in the United States of America.

GOAL STATEMENT

The goal of the *Pediatric Clinics of North America* is to keep practicing physicians and residents up to date with current clinical practice in pediatrics by providing timely articles reviewing the state-of-the-art in patient care.

ACCREDITATION

The *Pediatric Clinics of North America* is planned and implemented in accordance with the Essential Areas and Policies of the Accreditation Council for Continuing Medical Education (ACCME) through the joint sponsorship of the University Of Virginia School Of Medicine and Elsevier. The University Of Virginia School of Medicine is accredited by the ACCME to provide continuing medical education for physicians.

The University of Virginia School of Medicine designates this enduring material activity for a maximum of 15 *AMA PRA Category 1 Credit(s)*™ for each issue, 90 credits per year. Physicians should only claim credit commensurate with the extent of their participation in the activity.

The American Medical Association has determined that physicians not licensed in the US who participate in this CME enduring material activity are eligible for a maximum of 15 *AMA PRA Category 1 Credit(s)*™ for each issue, 90 credits per year.

Credit can be earned by reading the text material, taking the CME examination online at http://www.theclinics.com/home/cme, and completing the evaluation. After taking the test, you will be required to review any and all incorrect answers. Following completion of the test and evaluation, your credit will be awarded and you may print your certificate.

FACULTY DISCLOSURE/CONFLICT OF INTEREST

The University of Virginia School of Medicine, as an ACCME accredited provider, endorses and strives to comply with the Accreditation Council for Continuing Medical Education (ACCME) Standards of Commercial Support, Commonwealth of Virginia statutes, University of Virginia policies and procedures, and associated federal and private regulations and guidelines on the need for disclosure and monitoring of proprietary and financial interests that may affect the scientific integrity and balance of content delivered in continuing medical education activities under our auspices.

The University of Virginia School of Medicine requires that all CME activities accredited through this institution be developed independently and be scientifically rigorous, balanced and objective in the presentation/discussion of its content, theories and practices.

All authors/editors participating in an accredited CME activity are expected to disclose to the readers relevant financial relationships with commercial entities occurring within the past 12 months (such as grants or research support, employee, consultant, stock holder, member of speakers bureau, etc.). The University of Virginia School of Medicine will employ appropriate mechanisms to resolve potential conflicts of interest to maintain the standards of fair and balanced education to the reader. Questions about specific strategies can be directed to the Office of Continuing Medical Education, University of Virginia School of Medicine, Charlottesville, Virginia.

The faculty and staff of the University of Virginia Office of Continuing Medical Education have no financial affiliations to disclose.

The authors/editors listed below have identified no financial or professional relationships for themselves or their spouse/partner:
Roberta Berard, MD, MSc, FRCPC; Scott W. Canna, MD; Sabrina Chiesa, PhD; Marco Gattorno, MD; Peter J. Gowdie, MBBS, FRACP; Kerry Holland, (Acquisitions Editor); Adam M. Huber, MSc, MD; Sylvia Kamphuis, MD, PhD; Ronald M. Laxer, MDCM, FRCPC (Guest Editor); Jay Mehta, MD, MS; Alessia Omenetti, MD, PhD; Karen Rheuban, MD (Test Author); Rosie Scuccimarri, MD, FRCPC; David D. Sherry, MD (Guest Editor); Ori Toker, MD; Kathryn S. Torok, MD; Shirley M.L. Tse, MD, FRCPC; Peter Weiser, MD; and Pamela F. Weiss, MD, MSCE.

The authors/editors listed below identified the following professional or financial affiliations for themselves or their spouse/partner:
Jonathan D. Akikusa, MBBS is an industry funded research/investigator for Pfizer, Inc.
Edward M. Behrens, MD is a consultant for Genentech.
Philip J. Hashkes, MD, MSc is an industry funded research/investigator and is on the Speakers' Bureau for Novartis, and is an industry funded research/investigator and a consultant for UrlPharma.
Deborah M. Levy, MD, MS, FRCPC is on the Advisory Board for Pfizer, Inc.
Troy R. Torgeson, MD, PhD is an industry supported research/investigator for Baxter Biosciences and CSL Behring, and is on the Advisory Board for Baxter Biosciences.

Disclosure of Discussion of Non-FDA Approved Uses for Pharmaceutical Products and/or Medical Devices
The University of Virginia School of Medicine, as an ACCME provider, requires that all faculty presenters identify and disclose any off-label uses for pharmaceutical and medical device products. The University of Virginia School of Medicine recommends that each physician fully review all the available data on new products or procedures prior to clinical use.

TO ENROLL

To enroll in the Pediatric Clinics of North America Continuing Medical Education program, call customer service at 1-800-654-2452 or visit us online at www.theclinics.com/home/cme. The CME program is available to subscribers for an additional fee of $223.00.

Contributors

GUEST EDITORS

RONALD M. LAXER, MDCM, FRCPC
Staff Rheumatologist, Division of Rheumatology, The Hospital for Sick Children, Professor of Paediatrics and Medicine, University of Toronto, Toronto, Ontario, Canada

DAVID D. SHERRY, MD
Chief, Rheumatology Section, The Children's Hospital of Philadelphia, Philadelphia, Pennslylvania

AUTHORS

JONATHAN D. AKIKUSA, MBBS, FRACP
Rheumatology Service, Department of General Medicine; Murdoch Childrens Research Institute, Royal Children's Hospital, Parkville, Melbourne, Australia

EDWARD M. BEHRENS, MD
Assistant Professor of Pediatrics, Division of Rheumatology, The Children's Hospital of Philadelphia, Philadelphia, Pennsylvania

ROBERTA BERARD, MD, MSc, FAAP, FRCPC
Assistant Professor of Pediatrics, Western University; Pediatric Rheumatology, Children's Hospital, London Health Sciences Centre, London, Ontario, Canada

SCOTT W. CANNA, MD
Division of Rheumatology, The Children's Hospital of Philadelphia, Philadelphia, Pennsylvania

SABRINA CHIESA, PhD
UO Pediatria II, G. Gaslini Institute, Genova, Italy

MARCO GATTORNO, MD
UO Pediatria II, G. Gaslini Institute, Genova, Italy

PETER J. GOWDIE, MBBS, FRACP
Division of Rheumatology, The Hospital for Sick Children, University of Toronto, Toronto, Ontario, Canada

PHILIP J. HASHKES, MD, MSc
Head, Pediatric Rheumatology Unit, Department of Pediatrics, Shaare Zedek Medical Center, Jerusalem, Israel; Associate Professor of Medicine and Pediatrics, Department of Rheumatic Diseases, Cleveland Clinic Lerner School of Medicine, Cleveland, Ohio

ADAM M. HUBER, MSc, MD
Division of Pediatric Rheumatology, IWK Health Centre and Dalhousie University, Halifax, Nova Scotia, Canada

SYLVIA KAMPHUIS, MD, PhD
Assistant Professor, Pediatric Rheumatologist/Immunologist, Sophia Children's Hospital, Erasmus University Medical Center, Rotterdam, The Netherlands

DEBORAH M. LEVY, MD, MS, FRCPC
Assistant Professor of Pediatrics, Division of Rheumatology, Hospital for Sick Children, University of Toronto, Toronto, Ontario, Canada

JAY MEHTA, MD, MS
Division of Pediatric Rheumatology, Albert Einstein College of Medicine, Children's Hospital at Montefiore, Bronx, New York

ALESSIA OMENETTI, MD, PhD
UO Pediatria II, G. Gaslini Institute, Genova, Italy

ROSIE SCUCCIMARRI, MD, FRCPC
Assistant Professor, Pediatric Rheumatologist, Program Director, Division of Pediatric Rheumatology, Department of Pediatrics, Montreal Children's Hospital, McGill University, Montreal, Quebec, Canada

ORI TOKER, MD
Fellow, Allergy and Clinical Immunology Unit, Hadassah Medical Center, Jerusalem, Israel

TROY R. TORGERSON, MD, PhD
Assistant Professor of Pediatrics, Divisions of Immunology and Rheumatology, Department of Pediatrics, University of Washington and Seattle Children's Hospital, Seattle, Washington

KATHRYN S. TOROK, MD
Assistant Professor, University of Pittsburgh Scleroderma Center, Division of Rheumatology, Department of Pediatrics, Children's Hospital of Pittsburgh of the University of Pittsburgh Medical Center, Pittsburgh, Pennsylvania

SHIRLEY M.L. TSE, MD, FRCPC
Division of Rheumatology, The Hospital for Sick Children, University of Toronto, Toronto, Ontario, Canada

PETER WEISER, MD
Assistant Professor, Division of Pediatric Rheumatology, Department of Pediatrics, Children's of Alabama, University of Alabama at Birmingham, Birmingham, Alabama

PAMELA F. WEISS, MD, MSCE
Assistant Professor, Division of Rheumatology, Department of Pediatrics, Center for Pediatric Clinical Effectiveness, Perelman School of Medicine at the University of Pennsylvania, Children's Hospital of Philadelphia; Center for Clinical Epidemiology and Biostatistics, University of Pennsylvania, Philadelphia, Pennsylvania

Contents

The immune system consists of 2 branches: *innate* and *adaptive*. The former represents the first line of host defense during infection and plays a key role in the early recognition and protection against invading pathogens. The latter orchestrates elimination of pathogens in the late phase of infection and leads to the generation of immunologic memory. Innate and adaptive immunity should not be considered separate compartments. Innate and adaptive immune responses represent an integrated system of host defense. The authors review the mechanisms driving the induction and perpetuation of the inflammatory responses observed during pathogen-associated, autoimmune, and autoinflammatory diseases.

Arthritis is manifested as a swollen joint having at least 2 of the following conditions: limited range of motion, pain on movement, or warmth overlying the joint. This article discusses an approach to the evaluation of a child with arthritis of one (mono) or several (poly) joints.

In children, laboratory evaluations can assist in the screening of patients for inflammatory disorders, confirm diagnoses, allow for monitoring of disease activity and response to therapy, and suggest prognoses and risk of morbidities associated with rheumatic diseases. This review provides an overview of the usefulness and interpretation of both the commonly ordered tests ordered by the general pediatrician as well as those frequently used in the pediatric rheumatology clinic for diagnosis and disease monitoring. Studies discussed include the complete blood count, acute phase reactants, autoantibodies, serum complement, urinalysis, streptococcal antibody tests, and commonly used genetic studies.

This article presents five clinical scenarios in which the initial manifestations of pediatric rheumatic diseases constitute life-threatening medical emergencies. It is intended as a problem-oriented guide for pediatricians to assist in the recognition of rheumatologic differentials in children presenting with critical illness and provides an approach to their initial investigation and management.

Contents

patients showing extracutaneous disease manifestations such as arthritis and uveitis. Vascular, cutaneous, gastrointestinal, pulmonary, and musculoskeletal involvement are most commonly seen in children with SSc. Treatment of both forms targets the active inflammatory stage and halts disease progression; however, progress needs to be made toward the development of more effective antifibrotic therapy to help reverse disease damage.

Childhood vasculitis is a challenging and complex group of conditions that are multisystem in nature and often require integrated care from multiple subspecialties, including rheumatology, dermatology, cardiology, nephrology, neurology, and gastroenterology. Vasculitis is defined as the presence of inflammation in the blood vessel wall. The site of vessel involvement, size of the affected vessels, extent of vascular injury, and underlying pathology determine the disease phenotype and severity. This article explores the classification and general features of pediatric vasculitis, as well as the clinical presentation, diagnostic evaluation, and therapeutic options for the most common vasculitides.

Kawasaki disease is a systemic vasculitis and the leading cause of acquired heart disease in North American and Japanese children. The epidemiology, cause, and clinical characteristics of this disease are reviewed. The diagnostic challenge of Kawasaki disease and its implications for coronary artery outcomes are discussed, as are the recommended treatment, ongoing treatment controversies, concerns associated with treatment resistance, and the importance of ongoing follow up.

There has been an expansion of the autoinflammatory syndromes due to the discovery of new diseases related to mutations in genes regulating the innate immune system and the knowledge gained from these diseases as applied to more common nongenetic inflammatory conditions. Autoinflammatory syndromes are characterized by unprovoked (or triggered by minor events) recurrent episodes of systemic inflammation involving various body systems, which are often accompanied by fever. Inflammation is mediated by polymorphonuclear and macrophage cells through cytokines, particularly interleukin-1. This article reviews the clinical approach to patients with suspected autoinflammatory syndromes, several of the main and new (mostly genetics) syndromes, advances in treatment, and prognosis.

Musculoskeletal pain is one of the most common presenting symptoms at the pediatrician's office. Etiology ranges from benign conditions to serious ones requiring prompt attention. This article addresses entities that present as musculoskeletal pain but are not associated with arthritis. The most common nonarthritic conditions are benign limb pain of childhood (growing pains), hypermobility, overuse syndromes with or without skeletal abnormalities, malignancies, and pain amplification syndromes. The| initial decision process, diagnosis, and treatment options for each of these conditions are discussed.

Troy R. Torgerson

Most clinicians associate primary immunodeficiency disorders (PIDDs) with susceptibility to frequent or severe infections. It is less commonly recognized, however, that PIDDs are frequently associated with autoimmune or rheumatologic manifestations. This review provides a synopsis of the rheumatic manifestations associated with immunodeficiencies in each of the major compartments of the immune system.

PEDIATRIC CLINICS OF NORTH AMERICA

Preface

Pediatric Rheumatology

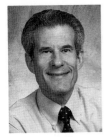 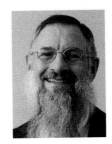

Ronald M. Laxer, MDCM, FRCPC   David D. Sherry, MD
Guest Editors

The pediatric rheumatic diseases comprise a diverse group of disorders that range from mild and self-limited (eg, transient synovitis) to devastating and fatal (eg, macrophage activation syndrome). They can be extremely well-localized (eg, oligoarthritis affecting only one joint) or involve multiple systems (eg, systemic lupus erythematosus). A solid knowledge of the basic sciences such as biochemistry, immunology, and genetics is central to their understanding, and a very careful and thorough clinical approach is required to make a diagnosis. Tremendous advances in the basic sciences have allowed clinicians to understand and therefore manage patients with rheumatic diseases better.

It is with great pleasure that we present this issue of *Pediatric Clinics of North America* on the rheumatic diseases that afflict children. As we considered the brave new world of pediatric rheumatology, we enlisted the help of a new generation of pediatric rheumatologists to bring fresh insights and vitality to his or her topic. Each author has kept the front-line pediatrician in mind to address the problems that occur generally in the children under one's care as well as a framework to evaluate those rare patients who present with problems that bespeak a significant rheumatic condition.

The broad scope of this volume makes it, like so many other *Pediatric Clinics of North America*, a valuable reference that will serve the pediatrician for many years as a readable and useful resource for pediatric rheumatology. Each author took care to address the practical problems faced in sorting out laboratory tests, picking out pertinent symptoms and signs to help establishing diagnoses, as well as initiating treatment.

Pediatr Clin N Am 59 (2012) xiii–xiv
doi:10.1016/j.pcl.2012.03.015

As editors, we want to thank all the authors for their skill and expertise, which has made our jobs quite easy. Additionally, we are grateful for the help and support provided by Kerry Holland at Elsevier in making this volume possible and the editorial process painless.

Ronald M. Laxer, MDCM, FRCPC
Division of Rheumatology
The Hospital for Sick Children
University of Toronto
Toronto, Ontario, Canada

David D. Sherry, MD
The Children's Hospital of Philadelphia
10th Floor Colket
34th and Civic Center Boulevard
Philadelphia, PA 19104, USA

E-mail addresses:
Ronald.laxer@sickkids.ca (R.M. Laxer)
sherry@email.chop.edu (D.D. Sherry)

Principles of Inflammation for the Pediatrician

Alessia Omenetti, MD, PhD, Sabrina Chiesa, PhD,
Marco Gattorno, MD*

KEYWORDS

- Inflammation • Innate immunity • Adaptive immunity
- Cytokines • Inflammasome • Interleukin 1
- Pathogen-associated molecular patterns
- Pattern recognition receptors

THE IMMUNE SYSTEM: INNATE AND ADAPTIVE IMMUNITY

The innate immune system is phylogenetically ancient compared with the more evolved form of host defense existing only in vertebrates. The cellular effectors of the innate immune system consist of neutrophils, monocytes, macrophages, and natural killer (NK) cells, which are all characterized by specific phagocytic and killing activities, whereas complement components and cytokines represent the circulating effector proteins of the innate system.

Surface receptors on phagocytes are able to specifically recognize and interact with highly conserved structures of microbial pathogens that are not present in mammalian cells. The binding of microbial structures to these receptors triggers the cell to phagocytize the pathogen and cause the activated cells to produce several proinflammatory molecules. Thus, innate immunity not only represents an early effective defense mechanism against infection but also provides the alert to the presence of an infection against which a subsequent adaptive immune response has to be built up.[1]

The main features of the adaptive immune system are (1) the ability to interface with microbes in the presence of a high level of molecular specificity, (2) to remember this interaction, and (3) to be able to respond more promptly and powerfully to subsequent exposures to the same microbe (ie, immunologic memory). In this regard, any element capable of being recognized by the adaptive immune system is called an *antigen*.

The cellular effectors are represented by lymphocytes, a heterogeneous cell group that consists of various subsets that are morphologically similar but functionally different.

UO Pediatria II, G. Gaslini Institute, Largo G. Gaslini 5, 16147 Genova, Italy
* Corresponding author.
E-mail address: marcogattorno@ospedale-gaslini.ge.it

Pediatr Clin N Am 59 (2012) 225–243
doi:10.1016/j.pcl.2012.03.004
0031-3955/12/$ – see front matter © 2012 Elsevier Inc. All rights reserved.

pediatric.theclinics.com

Based on the presence of specific antigen receptors, lymphocytes are capable of recognizing either soluble or membrane-bound antigenic determinants by specific antigen receptors.

There are 2 main types of lymphocytes: (1) those that mature in the thymus, known as T (thymus) lymphocytes and (2) those that undergo their maturation in the bone marrow and are, therefore, known as B (bone marrow) lymphocytes. The latter produce antibodies and are responsible for humoral immunity. Their antigen receptors are membrane-bound antibodies that can recognize soluble antigens.

INDUCTION OF THE IMMUNE RESPONSE: HOW CELLS OF THE INNATE SYSTEM RECOGNIZE NONSELF PROTEINS AND BECOME ACTIVATED

The innate immune response relies on the recognition of evolutionarily conserved structures on pathogens, termed *pathogen-associated molecular patterns* (PAMPs), through a limited number of germ line–encoded *pattern recognition receptors* (PRRs).[2] Among them, the family of Toll-like receptors (TLRs) has been studied most extensively.[3,4] The peculiarity of PAMPs is being tightly conserved among classes of pathogens and distinctly discernible from self. This feature allows the immune system to detect the presence of different microbial infections through a limited number of germ line–encoded PRRs. The surface of cells of the innate immune system (eg, macrophages and dendritic cells) present different classes of PPRs, which act as tissue sentinels through the continuous monitoring of peripheral tissues for the possible invasion of microbial pathogens. TLRs are recognized by having an extracellular leucine-rich repeat (LRR) domain and an intracellular Toll/interleukin 1 (IL-1) receptor (TIR) domain (**Fig. 1**). To date, 10 TLRs have been identified in humans and each recognize distinct PAMPs derived from various microbial pathogens, including viruses, bacteria, fungi, and protozoa (**Table 1**).[2,5] Some TLRs (TLR-1, -2, -4, -5, -6, and -10) are expressed on the cell surface, whereas others (TLR-3, -7, -8, and -9) are located in intracellular compartments, including endosomes and lysosomes (see **Fig. 1**). Given their position, the former mainly recognize bacterial products unique to bacteria and not produced by the host, whereas the latter are specialized in recognition of nucleic acids.[3,4] The PAMP binding to TLRs through the PAMP-TLR interaction causes receptor oligomerization, which triggers intracellular signal transduction, ultimately resulting in the generation of an antimicrobial proinflammatory response, which is also capable of involving and driving the adaptive branch of the immune system (see later discussion).

In addition to the transmembrane receptors on the cell surface and in endosomal compartments, cells of the innate immune system also contain intracellular (cytosolic) receptors that function in the pattern recognition of viral and bacterial pathogens. These receptors include nucleotide-binding oligomerization domain (NOD)-like receptors (NLRs)[6] and the intracellular sensors of viral nucleic acids, such as retinoic-acid-inducible gene I (RIG-I) or melanoma differentiation–associated gene 5, grouped under the term RIG-I-like receptors (RLRs) (see **Fig. 1**).[7] NLRs are a large family of intracellular proteins with a common protein-domain organization but diversified functions.[7] NOD and subfamilies are the most characterized among NLRs. The proteins of the NOD subfamily, NOD1 and NOD2, are both involved in sensing bacterial molecules derived from the synthesis and degradation of peptidoglycan.[8] NOD1 recognizes diaminopimelic acid produced primarily by gram-negative bacteria,[9] whereas NOD2 is activated by muramyl dipeptide (MDP), a component of both gram-positive and gram-negative bacteria.[10]

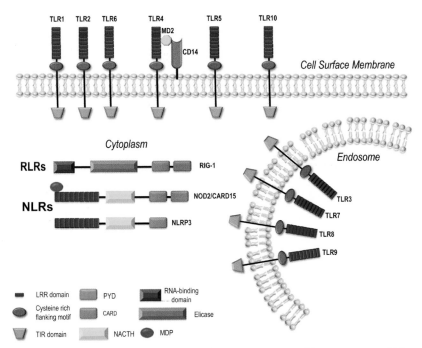

Fig. 1. Localization and structure of cellular pattern recognition receptors. TLRs are membrane-bound receptors localized at the cellular or endosomal membranes. In addition, there are intracellular (cytosolic) receptors that function in the pattern recognition of bacterial and viral pathogens. Nucleotide-binding oligomerization domain (NOD)2/CARD15 and NALP3 belong to the NOD-like receptors (NLR) family. Most NLRs contain a LRR domain for PAMPs recognition, such as muramyl dipeptide (MDP) for NOD2/CARD15. Retinoic-acid-inducible gene I (RIG-I) represents an example of a class of intracellular sensors of viral nucleic acids grouped under the term of RIG-I–like receptors (RLRs). Thanks to its C-terminal helicase domain, RIG-I bind to viral RNA and become activated to transduce CARD-dependent signaling, ultimately resulting in an antiviral response mediated by type I interferon production.

The Nucleotide-binding oligomerization domain, Leucine rich Repeat and Pyrin domain containing family (NLRP) subfamily of NLRs consists of 14 members. Some of them are involved in the induction of the inflammatory response mediated by the IL-1 family of cytokines, which includes IL-1β and IL-18.[11] These cytokines are synthesized as inactive precursors that need to be cleaved by proinflammatory caspases (ie, caspases 1, 4, and 5). These caspases are activated through a multiprotein complex known as the inflammasome (see later discussion). Most of the aforementioned PRRs are capable of sensing not only pathogens (namely through PAMPS) but also get activated/alerted by misfolded/glycated proteins or exposed hydrophobic portions of molecules released at high levels by injured cells, the so-called *damage-associated molecular pattern* (DAMP).[12]

Dendritic cells (DCs) belong to the cell machinery driving innate immunity and are specialized in the processing and presentation of exogenous pathogen-derived antigens to T cells during the adaptive immune response at the level of secondary lymphoid organs.[13,14] Thus, DCs should be considered as key players in bridging innate and adaptive immunity.

Table 1
TLR

TLR	Localization	Expression	Ligand	Origin of Ligand
TLR1	Plasma membrane	MOs, MPs, B cells, T cells, DCs, PMN, nonimmune cells[a]	Triacetylated lipopeptides, porins	Bacteria
TLR2	Plasma membrane	MOs, MPs, DCs, PMN, nonimmune cells[a]	Zymosan Peptidoglycans Lipoteichoic acids Lipoarabinomannan Porins Envelope glycoproteins	Fungi Gram-positive bacteria Gram-positive bacteria Mycobacteria Neisseria Viruses (eg, measles, HSV, CMV)
TLR3	Endosome	DCs, MPs, mast cells, NK cells, nonimmune cells[a]	dsRNA	Viruses
TLR4	Plasma membrane	MOs, MPs, DCs, PMN, nonimmune cells[a]	LPS Lipoprotein Hsp60, Hsp70, HMGB1 Fusion protein	Gram-negative bacteria Many pathogens Chlamydia pneumoniae RSV
TLR5	Plasma membrane	MOs, MPs, T cells, DCs, PMN, nonimmune cells[a]	Flagellin	Flagellated Bacteria
TLR6	Plasma membrane	MOs, MPs, B cells, T cells, DCs, PMN, NK cells, nonimmune cells[a]	Diacyl lipopeptides, Lipoteichoic acid	Mycoplasma Gram-positive bacteria
TLR7	Endolysosome	B cells, plasmacytoid DCs	ssRNA, purine analogue compounds (imidazoquinolines)	Viruses, bacteria from group B streptococcus
TLR8	Endolysosome	MOs, myeloid DCs	ssRNA, purine analogue compounds (imidazoquinolines)	Viruses
TLR9	Endolysosome	B cells, plasmacytoid DCs, GI epithelial cells, Keratinocytes	CpG DNA, DNA containing immunocomplexes	Bacteria, viruses (eg, HSV, CMV), protozoa
TLR10	Endolysosome	B cells, plasmacytoid DCs	Unknown	Unknown

Abbreviations: CMV, cytomegalovirus; DCs, dendritic cells; GI, gastrointestinal; HSV, herpes simplex virus; MOs, monocytes; MPs, macrophages; PMN, polymorphonuclear leukocytes.

[a] Nonimmune cells: astrocytes, fibroblasts, keratinocytes, endothelial, and epithelial cells.

The recognition of microbial or viral products through the same PRR that are present on the surface of phagocytes triggers the migration of DCs to lymph nodes where they undergo functional maturation and start to express costimulatory molecules (eg, CD80, CD86, CD40, and antigen-presenting major histocompatibility complex [MHC] molecules) that enable them to function as antigen-presenting cells to T cells.[13] DCs control many T-cell responses. For example, under the control of DCs, helper T cells (Th) acquire the capability to produce powerful cytokines that differentially regulate their tasks, defining functionally different subsets. Th1 cells mainly secrete interferon-γ (IFNγ) and activate macrophages to resist infection by facultative and obligate intracellular microbes; Th2 cells produce IL-4, IL-5, and IL-13 to mobilize white cells against helminths; and Th17 cells make IL-17 to mobilize phagocytes at the site of invasion of extracellular bacilli (see later discussion).

B lymphocytes constitute an interesting cell population sharing functional features common to both innate (ie, same PRR expression and antigen presenting function for T cells) and adaptive (ie, specific response to antigens and immunologic memory) immunity. B cells develop in the bone marrow, express cell surface immunoglobulins functioning as antigen receptors,[15] and localize to secondary lymphoid organs and in low number in the circulation.[15]

In order for B cells to become activated, a second signal is required in addition to the binding of the antigen receptor to its specific ligand. The second signal may be provided by the pathogen itself (thymus-independent [TI] antigens) or be delivered by an already-primed T cell (for thymus-dependent [TD] antigens). The so-called TI antigens[16] are nonprotein antigens that elicit antibody production in athymic individuals. The most important TI antigens are polymeric polysaccharides or glycolipids present in the bacterial cell wall. These antigens induce maximal cross-linking of membrane immunoglobulins, resulting in B-cell activation without the necessity of T-cell help.

The functional interplay between T and B cells takes place in peripheral lymphoid organs (lymph nodes, spleen, mucosal immune system). In lymphoid organs, naïve B and T cells are anatomically compartmentalized and separated but, following an antigen-induced activation, are elicited to migrate toward one another. The recognition of the specific peptide-MHC complex on the surface of B cells cause Th cells to become activated and express the cell surface molecule CD40L, resulting in cytokine secretion. The link between CD40L (expressed on activated Th cells) and CD40 (constitutively expressed on B cells) leads to further activation of B cells, with the same mechanisms already described for DC.

ROLE OF THE INNATE SYSTEM IN THE INITIATION OF THE INFLAMMATORY RESPONSE

On engagement of PRRs by individual PAMPs, several different signaling pathways are elicited in the cells of the innate system. Initially, signal transduction is mediated by adaptor molecules, which, at least in part, determine the specificity of the response.[17] Recruitment of one or more adaptor molecules to a given PRR is followed by the activation of downstream signal transduction pathways through different processing, such as phosphorylation, ubiquitination, or protein-protein interactions, which eventually culminate in the activation of transcription factors that ultimately orchestrate the expression of gene patterns regulating inflammation and antimicrobial host defense (**Fig. 2**).[18] TLR-elicited signaling pathways can be broadly classified by their use of different adaptor molecules (ie, dependent on or independent of the adaptor MyD88 or the TIR domain–containing adaptor inducing IFN-γ [TRIF] and their respective activation of individual kinases and transcription factors).[17] Three major

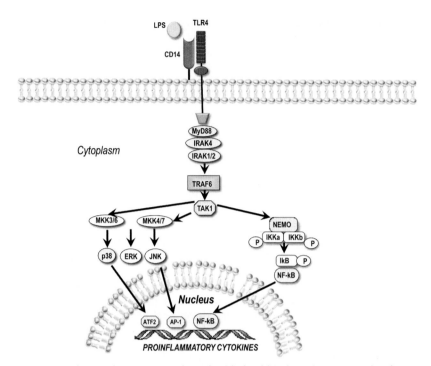

Fig. 2. TLR signaling pathways. Lipopolysaccharide (LPS) binds to the CD14 molecule present on phagocyte surface. Then, the LPS-CD14 complex associates to TLR4 for the subsequent intracellular signaling. The lipopolysaccharide-binding protein is a circulating protein that binds to LPS in the blood or extracellular fluid forming a complex that facilitates LPS binding to CD14. The MyD88-dependent signaling pathway is responsible for the early phase NF-κB and mitogen-activated protein kinases activation, which control the induction of proinflammatory cytokines.

signaling pathways engaged in TLR-induced responses consist of (1) Nuclear Factor kappa-light-chain-enhancer of activated B cells (NF-κB), (2) mitogen-activated protein kinases (MAPKs), and (3) IFN regulatory factors (IRFs).[19] NF-κB and MAPKs play a key role in driving a proinflammatory response, whereas IRFs are essential to stimulate IFN production.[18] Following ligand binding, TLRs dimerize and undergo conformational changes required for the subsequent recruitment of cytosolic TIR domain-containing adaptor molecules (see **Fig. 2**).

NF-κB exists in an inactive form in the cytoplasm physically associated with its inhibitory protein, inhibitor of NF-κB (IκB). Once an inflammatory stimulus occurs, IκB gets degraded through phosphorylation processing by a kinase complex called IκB kinase (IKK), releasing NF-κB from its inhibition. Thus, NF-κB gets activated and translocates from the cytosol to the nucleus. NF-κB is, hence, enable to interact with nuclear target gene promoters or enhancers, leading to the increased transcription and expression of several proinflammatory proteins, such as cytokines, chemokines, and other soluble mediators.[5,20]

MAPKs constitute a major kinase family driving a rapid downstream inflammatory signal transduction, which results in the induction of several nuclear proteins and transcription factors.[21] MAPK pathways undergo a complex activation process through sequential phosphorylation, starting with the activation of MAPK kinase kinase (MAPKKK), which phosphorylates and activates MAPK kinase (MAPKK). The latter, in turn, activates MAPK through phosphorylation. MAPK pathways include p38, c-Jun N-terminal kinase, and extracellular-signal-regulated kinase that induce activation of some transcription factors, such as ATF-2 and AP-1, known to be necessary for the upregulation of several proinflammatory molecules.[21]

In some cases, the complete inflammatory response is achieved by the combined action of cytosolic PRRs and that played by membrane-bound TLRs. A paradigmatic example is represented by the NLRP protein role in the activation and secretion of one of the most potent proinflammatory cytokines of innate immunity, IL-1β.

Unlike most cytokines and proinflammatory proteins, IL-1β (together with IL-18 and IL-33) lacks a secretory signal peptide and is externalized by monocytic cells through a nonclassical pathway, arranged in 2 steps.[22,23] First, TLR ligands, such as lipopolysaccharides (LPS), induce gene expression and synthesis of the inactive IL-1β precursor (pro–IL-1β). The activation of caspase-1 later catalyzes the cleavage of the IL-1 precursor pro–IL-1β in the 17kd active form.[11,24] A protein complex responsible for this catalytic activity has been identified and termed the inflammasome.[25] The inflammasome is a multiprotein complex, which consists of the adaptor apoptosis-associated specklike protein containing a caspase activation and recruitment domains (ASC), procaspase-1, and an NLR family member, such as NLRP1 or NLRP3.[25] The oligomerization of these proteins results in the activation of caspase-1, which subsequently cleaves the accumulated IL-1β precursor and eventually results in the secretion of biologically active IL-1β (**Fig. 3**).[11]

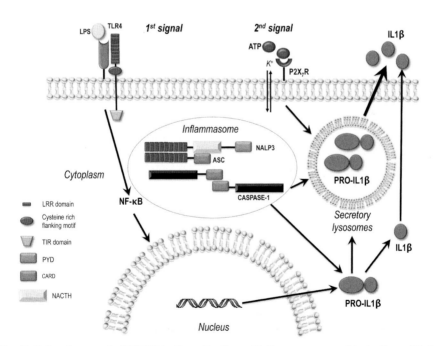

Fig. 3. Role of cryopyrin (NLRP3) in the activation of Inflammasome and induction of IL-1β secretion. TLR ligands, such as lipopolysaccharide (LPS), are the first signal for gene expression and synthesis of the inactive IL-1β precursor (pro-IL-1β). Following LPS stimulation, NLRP3 oligomerizes and becomes available for the binding of the adaptor protein ASC (apoptosis-associated specklike protein containing CARD). This association activates directly 2 molecules of caspase-1 that, in turn, converts pro–IL-1β to the mature, active 17 kDa form. A second stimulus, such as exogenous ATP, strongly enhances proteolytic maturation and secretion of IL-1β.

NLRP3 plays a role in the recognition of ATP,[24] uric acid crystals,[26] viral RNA,[27] and bacterial DNA.[28] These stimuli represent a crucial second hit leading to the secretion of active IL1β (see **Fig. 3**).

As described previously, pathogen recognition elicits the activation of cells belonging to the innate immune system resulting in the production of several proinflammatory proteins and molecules. In this phase of the immune response, the 2 major goals are (1) to recruit other cells with phagocytic activity into the site of invasion of the pathogens (acute inflammation) and (2) to alert cells of the adaptive immune system in lymphoid organs to build a more specialized response toward the invading pathogen, achieving an appropriate host response.

ACUTE INFLAMMATION

The acute phase of the inflammatory response elicited by infection or tissue injury involves the coordinated delivery of blood components (plasma and leukocytes) to the site of infection or injury. At first, tissue resident macrophages and mast cells carry out the recognition of pathogens and lead to the local production of vasoactive amines, cytokines, chemokines, eicosanoids, and other products of proteolytic cascades, which function as inflammatory mediators.[29] This response, in turn, results in a local inflammatory exudate: plasma proteins and leukocytes (mainly neutrophils) migrate from blood vessels to the extravascular tissues at the site of infection (or injury) through postcapillary venules. Once activated by local inflammatory mediators (ie, cytokines), the vascular endothelium becomes permeable, allowing selective extravasation of neutrophils first and other leukocytes later on in the process (**Fig. 4**). This event is mediated by several proinflammatory cytokines that induce the expression of several membrane glycoproteins (termed *selectins*) that act as adhesion molecules for circulating leukocytes.[30] Hence, circulating leukocytes flowing in the bloodstream first loosely adhere to the endothelium (*rolling*) through some constitutively expressed surface glycoproteins that serve to screen the local environment for signs of inflammation. The second step of leukocyte migration requires their firm adherence to endothelial cells. This step is ensured by other surface molecules constitutively expressed on circulating leukocytes called *integrins*.[31] Once rolling has occurred, a series of specific cytokines (*chemokines*) cause leukocytes to acquire integrin affinity. In the meanwhile, proinflammatory cytokines, such as IL-1 and TNF-α, regulate the induction of ligands that are specific for high-affinity integrins. In this way, a firm adhesion between leukocytes and endothelium is achieved. During ongoing inflammation, the very late antigen (VLA)-4 (or $\alpha_4\beta_1$) is selectively expressed on leukocytes and regulates their adhesion to its ligand, the vascular adhesion molecule (VCAM)-1, which is expressed on activated endothelial cells.[32] Similarly, the leukocyte function–associated antigen-1 (LFA-1 or CD11aCD18) binds to its specific ligand, the intracellular adhesion molecule (ICAM) (see **Fig. 4**).

Finally, the last step of leukocyte recruitment is the transmigration of cells across the endothelial lining to the site of inflammation. This process is promoted by the interaction between other integrins expressed on leukocytes and their specific ligands present at the level of the adherence junction between the endothelial cells.

During the process of acute inflammation, mast cells and platelets are induced to degranulate and massively release several vasoactive amines (histamine and serotonin) that act on vasculature and cause increased permeability and vasodilation in the targeted vessels. Furthermore, other vasoactive peptides (eg, Substance P) can be secreted by sensory neurons after their activation or they can be generated in the extracellular fluid by proteolysis of inactive precursors (eg, kinins, fibrinopeptide

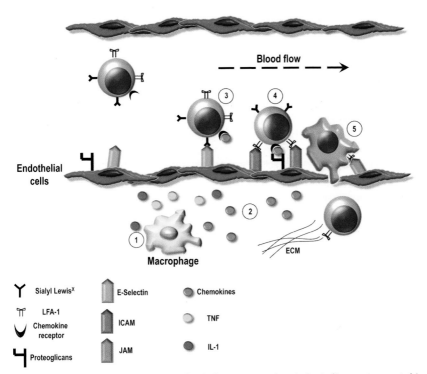

Fig. 4. Recruitment of leukocytes into the inflammatory site. 1. Proinflammatory cytokines produced by macrophages stimulate the expression of adhesion molecules (selectins and integrin ligands) on the endothelial cells. 2. Chemokines produced by stromal cells, inflammatory cells, and endothelial cells specifically attracts leukocytes bearing specific chemokine receptors. 3. Leukocytes bearing selectin ligands (ie, Sialyl Lewis^X weakly adheres to endothelium [rolling]). 4. Leukocytes display a process of integrin affinity maturation stimulated by chemokines. In this way, a firm adhesion between leukocytes and endothelium occurs (adhesion). 5. Transmigration of cells across the endothelial lining into the site of inflammation. The progression of cells through the endothelial cells is allowed by the interaction between other integrins expressed on leukocytes and their specific ligands present at the level of the adherence junction between the endothelial cells or in the subendothelial extracellular matrix.

A, fibrinopeptide B, and fibrin degradation products). Finally, the local environment also gets enriched with complement fragments C3a, C4a, and C5a (also termed *anaphylatoxins*), which are produced by several pathways of complement activation. Once released, C5a (and to a lesser extent C3a and C4a) contributes to granulocyte and monocyte recruitment and induces mast-cell degranulation.[29]

The neutrophils recruited in the site of inflammation attempt to kill the invading agents by releasing the toxic contents of their granules, which include reactive oxygen species (ROS) and reactive nitrogen species, and proteolytic enzymes (proteinase 3, cathepsin G, and elastase 5).

A successful acute inflammatory response results in the elimination of the infectious agents followed by a resolution and repair phase. However, if the acute inflammatory response fails to eliminate the pathogen, the inflammatory process persists and acquires new features. In such a circumstance, the neutrophil infiltration is gradually replaced by T cells and recently immigrated monocytes differentiating into macrophages. The aspects of this inflammatory state can display various characteristics depending on the effector class of the T cells (Th1, Th2, Th17) enrolled based on the pathogens involved (see later discussion).

If the combined actions of these cells are still insufficient to eliminate an invading pathogen, a chronic inflammatory state develops, eventually involving the formation of tertiary lymphoid tissues and granulomas.[33] Namely, failed attempts by macrophages to attack and destroy pathogens or foreign bodies can lead to the formation of granulomas, whereby intruders are walled off by layers of macrophages, in a final attempt to provide protection to the host.

However, a state of chronic inflammation can result not only from the persistence of pathogens but also during other types of tissue damage, such as autoimmune or auto-inflammatory responses, caused by the persistence of self-antigens or DAMPs.

ROLE OF THE ADAPTIVE IMMUNITY IN PERPETUATING THE INFLAMMATORY RESPONSE
B Cells and Immunoglobulins

Antibodies neutralize microbes and circulate microbial toxins by blocking their binding to host cellular receptors. Different immunoglobulin isotypes have distinct properties that enable them to promote the activation of different mechanisms. Namely,

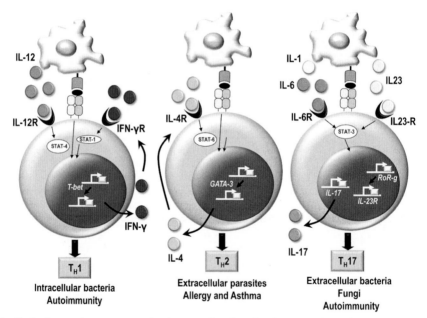

Fig. 5. During antigen presentation in secondary lymphoid organs, the regulatory cytokines IL-12 and IL-4 play a critical role in the orientation of the functional phenotype through the activation of signal transducer and activator of transcription 4 (STAT-4) or STAT-6 signaling pathways respectively. Differentiation signals regulate the expression of critical tissue-specific transcriptor factors that further specify the T_H1 or T_H2 orientation through regulation of chromatin structure and accessibility of cytokine genes. The T_H1 restricted transcription factor T-bet directly transactivates the *Ifng* promoter and induces remodeling of the *Ifng* locus. Conversely, the T_H2-restricted transcription factor GATA-3 is responsible for the induction of chromatin remodeling at the T_H2 cytokines locus acting on several control sequences, including *Il4*. RORγt was identified as the master regulator gene for T_H17 cells and activator of transcription 3 (STAT3) is required for signal transducer in T_H17 development.

antibodies can induce the activation of a variety of effector cells that bear a receptor for their respective fragment crystallizable region (Fc) portions. Only Fc portions of immunoglobulins that have interacted with their antigens can activate Fc receptors. This activation occurs because of the aggregation of immunoglobulin on the pathogen surface or because of conformational changes in the Fc portion occurring after antigen binding or both.

Antibodies can also coat (opsonize) the surface of microbes. The recognition of antibodies by Fc receptors on phagocytes triggers phagocytosis and killing of the opsonized microbes.

Furthermore, the Fc receptor can also induce the activation of other inflammatory cells, such as mast cells, basophils, and eosinophils. Fc receptors on NK cells and eosinophils may initiate *antibody-dependent cellular cytotoxicity* (ADCC) of antibody-coated infected cells and destroy them. The binding of antibodies to the C1 part of complement is an important modality of activation of the complement cascade (classical pathway).

T Cells

As stated previously, the functional development of Th cells is driven by several environmental factors at the moment of antigen presentation by APC, including cytokines

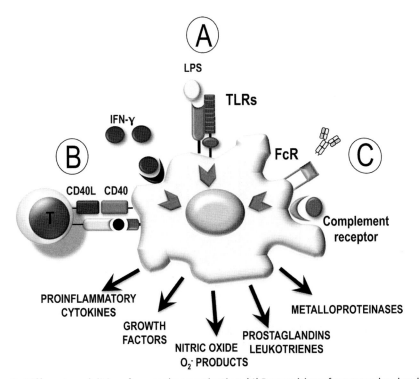

Fig. 6. Different modalities of macrophage activation. (*A*) Recognition of conserved molecular constituents of microbes (LPS, lipopolysaccharide) by specific receptors (ie, TLR, mannose-receptor, scavenger-receptor). (*B*) T-cell mediated activation via IFN-γ and CD40-CD40-ligand (L) interaction. (*C*) recognition of antibodies, immune complexes, and complement by the membrane receptors for the Fc fragment of immunoglobulins and complement receptors. The main effector soluble mediators produced after macrophage activation are also shown.

Table 2
Main cytokines of innate immunity

Cytokine	Size and Form	Receptors and Subunits	Main Cell Source	Principal Cellular Target and Biologic Effects
IL-1α IL-1β	17 kD, monomer 33 kD (precursors)	CD121a (IL-1R1), IL-1RAP CD121b (IL-1R2)	Macrophages, monocytes, DCs, fibroblasts, endothelial cells, keratinocytes, hepatocytes	Hypothalamus: fever; endothelial cells: activation (inflammation, coagulation); liver: synthesis of acute-phase reactants
TNF-α (TNFSF1)	17 kD, homotrimer	CD120a (TNFRSF1) or CD120b (TNFRSF2)	Macrophages, T cells, NK cells	Hypothalamus: fever; endothelial cells: activation (inflammation, coagulation); neutrophils: activation, apoptosis; liver: synthesis of acute-phase reactants; muscle, fat: cachexia
TNF-β (LT-α)	Homotrimer	CD120a (TNFRSF1) or CD120b (TNFRSF2)	T cells, B cells	Some as TNF
Type I IFNs	IFNα: 15–21 kD IFNβ: 20–25 kD monomers	IFNAR1 CD118 (IFNAR2)	Plasmacytoid dendritic cells, macrophages and fibroblasts	All cells: antiviral response; NK cells: activation
IL-6	19–26 kD, monomer	IL-6Rα, CD130 (gp130)	T cells, macrophages, endothelial cells	Liver: synthesis of acute phase reactants; B cell: proliferation of antibody-producing cells

IL-7	monomer	CD127 (IL-7R), CD132 (γc)	Fibroblasts, bone marrow stromal cells	Immature lymphoid progenitors: proliferation of pre-B cells and pre-T cells; T lymphocytes: survival of naïve and memory cells
IL-10	34–40 kD homodimer	CD210 (IL-10 R1), CD210B (IL-10R2)	Macrophages T cells (mainly Tregs)	Macrophages and DCs: inhibition of expression of IL-12, costimulators, and class II MHC
IL-12	Heterodimer of 35 and 40 kD[a]	IL-12 Rβ1, IL-12 Rβ2	Macrophages, DCs	T cells: differentiation of Th1 cells; NK cells: IFN-γ synthesis, increased cytotoxic activity
IL-15	3 kd, monomer	IL-15Rα, CD122 (IL-2Rb), CD132 (γc)	Macrophages and other non–T cells	NK cells: proliferation; T cells: survival and proliferation of memory CD8+ cells
IL-18	17 kD, monomer	CD218a (IL-18R1), CD218b (IL-18 RAP)	Monocytes, macrophages, DCs, keratinocytes, chondrocytes, synovial fibroblasts, osteoblasts	NK cells and T cells: IFN-γ synthesis; Monocytes: expression of GM-CSF, TNF, IL-1β; neutrophils: activation, cytokine release
IL-23	Heterodimer of 19 and 40 kD[a]	IL-23R IL-12 Rβ1, CD212 (IL-12 Rβ1)	Macrophages and DCs	T cells: maintenance of IL-17–producing T cells
IL-27	P28 and EBI3 heterodimer	IL-27Rα, CD130 (gp130)	Monocytes, macrophages, DCs	T cells: inhibition of Th1 cells; NK cells: IFN-γ synthesis

Abbreviation: Diacyl, lipopeptides; TNF, tumor necrosis factor; Tregs, regulatory T cells.
[a] IL-12 and IL-23 share the same p40 subunit.

Table 3
Main cytokines of adaptive immunity

Cytokine	Size and Form	Receptors and Subunits	Main Cell Source	Principal Cellular Target and Biologic Effects
IL-2	14–17 kD, monomer	CD25 (IL-2Rα) CD122 (IL-2Rβ) CD132 (γc)	T cells	T cells: proliferation and differentiation into effector and memory cells; promotes regulatory T-cell development, survival, and function; NK cells: proliferation, activation; B cells: proliferation, antibody synthesis (in vitro)
IL-4	18 kD, monomer	CD124 (IL-4Rα) CD132 (γc)	T cells (Th2), mast cells	B cells: Isotype switching to IgE; T cells: Th2 differentiation and proliferation; Macrophages: alternative activation and inhibition of IFN-γ- classical activation; Mast cells: proliferation (in vitro)
IL-5	45 kD, homodimer	CD125 (IL-5Rα) CD131 (βc)	T cells (Th2)	Eosinophils: activation and proliferation; B cells: proliferation and IgA production
IL-13	15 kD, monomer	CD213a1 (IL13Rα1) CD213a2 (IL13Rα2) CD132 (γc)	T cells (Th2), NKT cells, mast cells	B cell: isotype switching to IgE; Epithelial cells: increased mucus production; Fibroblasts: increased collagen synthesis; Macrophages: alternative activation
IL-17 A, F)	35 kD, 34 kD, monomer	CD217 (IL-17RA)	T cells	Endothelial cells: increased chemokine production; Macrophages: increased chemokine and cytokine production; Epithelial cells: GM-CSF and G-CSF production

IL-22	18,9 kD, homodimer	IL-22R1, CD210B (IL-10R2)	Th17 T cells, NK	Epithelial cells: production of defensins, increased barrier function; Hepatocytes: survival
IL-25	18 kD, monodimer	IL17BR	T cells, mast cells, eosinophils, macrophages, mucosal epithelial cells	T cells and various other cell types: expression of IL-4, IL-5, IL-13
IFN-γ	50 kD, homodimer	CD119 (IFNGR1), IFNGR2	T cells (Th1, CD8$^+$ T cells), NK cells	Macrophages: classical activation; B cells: isotype switching to opsonizing and complement-fixing IgG subclasses (established in mice); T cells: Th1 differentiation; Various cells: increased expression of class I and class II MHC molecules, increased antigen processing and presentation to T cells
LT-$\alpha\beta$	Heterotrimer	LTβR	T cells, NK cells, follicular B cells, lymphoid inducer cells	Lymphoid tissue stromal cells and follicular dendritic cells: chemokine expression and lymphoid organogenesis
TGF-β	25 kD, homodimer	TGF-βR	T cells (mainly T regs), macrophages	T cells: inhibition of proliferation and effector functions, differentiation of Th17 and Tregs; B cells: inhibition of proliferation, IgA production; Macrophages: inhibition of activation, stimulation of angiogenic factors; Fibroblasts: increased collagen synthesis

Abbreviations: LT, lymphotoxin; R, receptor; TGF, transforming growth factor; TNF, tumor necrosis factor; Tregs, regulatory T cells.

featuring the inflammatory milieu, the amount and sequence of the antigenic peptide, and possibly the nature of the APC (**Fig. 5**).[34–43]

The major Th1 effector cytokine is IFN-γ, which displays 2 main functions: (1) it causes macrophages to destroy microbes and (2) it induces the production of IgG antibody subclasses that bind to complement and high-affinity Fcγ receptors and, thus, are the principal antibodies involved in microbe opsonization and phagocytosis (**Fig. 6**). An additional mechanism driving macrophage activation is represented by the induction of the CD40 ligand on Th1 cells, which interacts with and activates the CD40 molecule on the macrophage surface (see **Fig. 6**). Th1 cells also play a key role in driving macrophage recruitment to the site of infection. This process occurs through the secretion by Th1 cells of several additional different cytokines, including (1) IL-3 and granulocyte/macrophage colony-stimulating factor (GM-CSF), which induce the production of new phagocytic cells in the bone marrow; (2) TNF-α, which stimulates the expression of adhesion molecules on endothelial cells; and (3) macrophage chemotactic factor (MCF) and other chemokines, which control macrophage migration from the endothelium toward the site of infection.

Th2 cells cause the production of immunoglobulin (Ig)M and non–complement-fixing IgG subclasses. IL-4 is the main inducer of the B-cell switch to IgE production, and IL-5 is the major cytokine that drives the activation of eosinophils. Th2 cells typically mediate the immune response to helminths, stimulating the production of specific IgE antibodies that opsonize the parasites. IL-5–activated eosinophils bind to IgE-coated helminths through Fc receptors specific for ε heavy chain and start to release their granule contents. The same mechanism of activation via IgE is also the trigger of mast cell degranulation in the immediate hypersensitivity immune response in allergic diseases.[44]

The role of Th17 cells in the pathogenesis of autoimmunity has been emphasized, primarily because the apparent limitations of the Th1/Th2 paradigm forced a reconsideration of the mechanisms of these disorders and, thereby led to the understanding of the role of this new subset. Th17 cells are characterized by the secretion of IL-17 and IL-22.[45] IL-17 and IL-22 can induce the expression of several proinflammatory cytokines and chemokines by a broad range of cellular targets, including epithelial cells, endothelial cells, and macrophages, but the most potent effect of both IL-17 and IL-22 is mobilization, recruitment, and activation of neutrophils.[46] The receptor for IL-17 is widely expressed on many cell types where it promotes the expression of chemokines, proinflammatory cytokines, and colony-stimulating factors. These factors, in turn, drive the recruitment of neutrophils and other myeloid cells, which is a critical feature of many infectious diseases.[47] Accordingly, it has been established that IL-17 is critical for the protection against gram-negative bacteria, including Klebsiella pneumoniae.[47] If fact, IL-17R, IL-12/IL-23, p40, IL-23, and p19 knockout mice are more susceptible to Klebsiella pneumoniae infection. Moreover, Th17 cells are also involved in antifungal defense both in mice and humans. Zymosan, a cell wall polysaccharide of yeast, and ω-1,3-glucan from *Candida albicans* preferentially induce IL-23 production.[48]

Although Th1 and Th2 cells protect against intracellular bacteria and helminths, a major function of Th17 cells is to protect against extracellular bacteria and fungi.

CD8+ cytolytic T lymphocyte's (CTL) main function is to eliminate intracellular microbes. Because such microbes cannot be eradicated through a T cell–mediated activation of phagocytes, the killing of infected cells is the only way to overcome the infection. After the recognition of a specific class I MHC-associated antigen and subsequent activation, CTLs deliver their cytoplasmic cytotoxic granule proteins (*perforin* and *granzymes*) to the target cell.[49] Perforin is a pore-forming protein present also in NK cells, which is able to polymerize in the lipid bilayer of the target cell membrane, thus, forming an aqueous channel. Granzymes are serine proteases that enter the target cell through the perforin-induced channels and activate intracellular enzymes, called caspases, that play a pivotal role in the induction of programmed cell death (apoptosis).

In conclusion, the inflammatory response is the consequence of a complex interaction among different cell types of the innate and adaptive immunity. The functional orientation of the inflammatory response is driven by the pathogens or by the type of cellular damage responsible for the activation of cells of the innate immunity. Several soluble factors, such as cytokines, chemokines, growth factors, proteolytic enzymes, and so forth, act as crucial mediators for the effector phase of the inflammatory response (**Tables 2** and **3**).

REFERENCES

1. Medzhitov R, Janeway C Jr. Innate immunity. N Engl J Med 2000;343(5):338–44.
2. Medzhitov R. Recognition of microorganisms and activation of the immune response. Nature 2007;449(7164):819–26.
3. Medzhitov R. Toll-like receptors and innate immunity. Nat Rev Immunol 2001;1(2): 135–45.
4. Takeda K, Akira S. Toll-like receptors in innate immunity. Int Immunol 2005;17(1): 1–14.
5. Mogensen TH. Pathogen recognition and inflammatory signaling in innate immune defenses. Clin Microbiol Rev 2009;22(2):240–73, Table.
6. Wilmanski JM, Petnicki-Ocwieja T, Kobayashi KS. NLR proteins: integral members of innate immunity and mediators of inflammatory diseases. J Leukoc Biol 2008;83(1):13–30.
7. Yoneyama M, Kikuchi M, Natsukawa T, et al. The RNA helicase RIG-I has an essential function in double-stranded RNA-induced innate antiviral responses. Nat Immunol 2004;5(7):730–7.
8. Kanneganti TD, Lamkanfi M, Nunez G. Intracellular NOD-like receptors in host defense and disease. Immunity 2007;27(4):549–59.
9. Chamaillard M, Hashimoto M, Horie Y, et al. An essential role for NOD1 in host recognition of bacterial peptidoglycan containing diaminopimelic acid. Nat Immunol 2003;4(7):702–7.
10. Girardin SE, Boneca IG, Viala J, et al. Nod2 is a general sensor of peptidoglycan through muramyl dipeptide (MDP) detection. J Biol Chem 2003;278(11):8869–72.
11. Agostini L, Martinon F, Burns K, et al. NALP3 forms an IL-1beta-processing inflammasome with increased activity in Muckle-Wells autoinflammatory disorder. Immunity 2004;20(3):319–25.
12. Bianchi ME. DAMPs, PAMPs and alarmins: all we need to know about danger. J Leukoc Biol 2007;81(1):1–5.
13. Banchereau J, Steinman RM. Dendritic cells and the control of immunity. Nature 1998;392(6673):245–52.
14. Sallusto F, Lanzavecchia A. Understanding dendritic cell and T-lymphocyte traffic through the analysis of chemokine receptor expression. Immunol Rev 2000;177: 134–40.
15. LeBien TW, Tedder TF. B lymphocytes: how they develop and function. Blood 2008;112(5):1570–80.
16. Fagarasan S, Honjo T. T-Independent immune response: new aspects of B cell biology. Science 2000;290(5489):89–92.

17. O'Neill LA, Bowie AG. The family of five: TIR-domain-containing adaptors in Toll-like receptor signaling. Nat Rev Immunol 2007;7(5):353–64.

18. Akira S, Uematsu S, Takeuchi O. Pathogen recognition and innate immunity. Cell 2006;124(4):783–801.

19. Kawai T, Takeuchi O, Fujita T, et al. Lipopolysaccharide stimulates the MyD88-independent pathway and results in activation of IFN-regulatory factor 3 and the expression of a subset of lipopolysaccharide-inducible genes. J Immunol 2001;167(10):5887–94.

20. Wang C, Deng L, Hong M, et al. TAK1 is a ubiquitin-dependent kinase of MKK and IKK. Nature 2001;412(6844):346–51.

21. Chang L, Karin M. Mammalian MAP kinase signaling cascades. Nature 2001; 410(6824):37–40.

22. Rubartelli A, Cozzolino F, Talio M, et al. A novel secretory pathway for interleukin-1 beta, a protein lacking a signal sequence. EMBO J 1990;9(5):1503–10.

23. Andrei C, Dazzi C, Lotti L, et al. The secretory route of the leaderless protein inter-leukin 1beta involves exocytosis of endolysosome-related vesicles. Mol Biol Cell 1999;10(5):1463–75.

24. Mariathasan S, Weiss DS, Newton K, et al. Cryopyrin activates the inflammasome in response to toxins and ATP. Nature 2006;440(7081):228–32.

25. Martinon F, Burns K, Tschopp J. The inflammasome: a molecular platform trig-gering activation of inflammatory caspases and processing of proIL-beta. Mol Cell 2002;10(2):417–26.

26. Martinon F, Petrilli V, Mayor A, et al. Gout-associated uric acid crystals activate the NALP3 inflammasome. Nature 2006;440(7081):237–41.

27. Kanneganti TD, Ozoren N, Body-Malapel M, et al. Bacterial RNA and small anti-viral compounds activate caspase-1 through cryopyrin/Nalp3. Nature 2006; 440(7081):233–6.

28. Muruve DA, Petrilli V, Zaiss AK, et al. The inflammasome recognizes cytosolic microbial and host DNA and triggers an innate immune response. Nature 2008; 452(7183):103–7.

29. Medzhitov R. Origin and physiological roles of inflammation. Nature 2008; 454(7203):428–35.

30. Patel KD, Cuvelier SL, Wiehler S. Selectins: critical mediators of leukocyte recruit-ment. Semin Immunol 2002;14(2):73–81.

31. Frenette PS, Wagner DD. Adhesion molecules–part II: blood vessels and blood cells. N Engl J Med 1996;335(1):43–5.

32. Pribila JT, Quale AC, Mueller KL, et al. Integrins and T cell-mediated immunity. Annu Rev Immunol 2004;22:157–80.

33. Drayton DL, Liao S, Mounzer RH, et al. Lymphoid organ development: from ontogeny to neogenesis. Nat Immunol 2006;7(4):344–53.

34. Bottomly K. T cells and dendritic cells get intimate. Science 1999;283(5405):1124–5.

35. Zhou L, Chong MM, Littman DR. Plasticity of CD4 + T cell lineage differentiation. Immunity 2009;30(5):646–55.

36. Bettelli E, Carrier Y, Gao W, et al. Reciprocal developmental pathways for the generation of pathogenic effector TH17 and regulatory T cells. Nature 2006; 441(7090):235–8.

37. Mangan PR, Harrington LE, O'Quinn DB, et al. Transforming growth factor-beta induces development of the T(H)17 lineage. Nature 2006;441(7090):231–4.

38. Acosta-Rodriguez EV, Napolitani G, Lanzavecchia A, et al. Interleukins 1beta and 6 but not transforming growth factor-beta are essential for the differentiation of interleukin 17-producing human T helper cells. Nat Immunol 2007;8(9):942–9.

39. Wilson NJ, Boniface K, Chan JR, et al. Development, cytokine profile and function of human interleukin 17-producing helper T cells. Nat Immunol 2007;8(9):950–7.
40. Annunziato F, Cosmi L, Santarlasci V, et al. Phenotypic and functional features of human Th17 cells. J Exp Med 2007;204(8):1849–61.
41. Murphy KM, Ouyang W, Farrar JD, et al. Signaling and transcription in T helper development. Annu Rev Immunol 2000;18:451–94.
42. Szabo SJ, Kim ST, Costa GL, et al. A novel transcription factor, T-bet, directs Th1 lineage commitment. Cell 2000;100(6):655–69.
43. Das J, Chen CH, Yang L, et al. A critical role for NF-kappa B in GATA3 expression and TH2 differentiation in allergic airway inflammation. Nat Immunol 2001;2(1): 45–50.
44. Abbas AK, Murphy KM, Sher A. Functional diversity of helper T lymphocytes. Nature 1996;383(6603):787–93.
45. Harrington LE, Hatton RD, Mangan PR, et al. Interleukin 17-producing CD4+ effector T cells develop via a lineage distinct from the T helper type 1 and 2 lineages. Nat Immunol 2005;6(11):1123–32.
46. Miossec P, Korn T, Kuchroo VK. Interleukin-17 and type 17 helper T cells. N Engl J Med 2009;361(9):888–98.
47. Matsuzaki G, Umemura M. Interleukin-17 as an effector molecule of innate and acquired immunity against infections. Microbiol Immunol 2007;51(12):1139–47.
48. Curtis MM, Way SS. Interleukin-17 in host defence against bacterial, mycobacterial and fungal pathogens. Immunology 2009;126(2):177–85.
49. Russell JH, Ley TJ. Lymphocyte-mediated cytotoxicity. Annu Rev Immunol 2002; 20:323–70.

Approach to the Child with Joint Inflammation

Roberta Berard, MD, MSc, FRCPC

KEYWORDS

- Pediatric • Approach • Monoarthritis • Polyarthritis

In pediatric practice, physicians are often faced with a child presenting with musculo-skeletal complaints. The differential diagnosis of musculoskeletal pain is broad and includes a variety of causes, including arthritis. Arthritis is manifested as a swollen joint or a joint having at least 2 of the following conditions: limited range of motion, pain on movement (stress pain), or warmth overlying the joint. The assessment of a child with arthritis must enable differentiation between acute and chronic causes of arthritis and, particularly, recognition of those who may require urgent medical or surgical intervention. Juvenile idiopathic arthritis (JIA) is only one of the many causes of arthritis. This review covers the evaluation of a child with arthritis of one (mono) or several (poly) joints.

MONOARTHRITIS

The differential diagnosis of monoarthritis includes entities in the broad categories of infection, postinfection, inflammation, malignancy, and trauma related to a systemic illness (**Table 1**). A carefully conducted history taking and physical examination are the initial and most important steps in narrowing the differential diagnosis and guiding the diagnostic evaluation.

History Taking

Important aspects to be considered in the history taking are as follows:

1. Characteristics of the pain and/or stiffness (site, number of joints, severity, frequency, duration, pattern, and association of warmth or discoloration). Morning stiffness is a characteristic feature of inflammatory arthritis. Night pain should alert the clinician to a malignancy or an osteoid osteoma
2. Review of systems focused on the presence of fever or other constitutional symptoms (eg, weight loss, anorexia, night sweats, or nocturnal pain)
3. Precipitating factors: traumas, infections (streptococcal, enteric, viral), immunizations, medication exposures, and history of sexual activity

Pediatrics Western University, Pediatric Rheumatology, Children's Hospital, London Health Sciences Centre, 800 Commissioners Road East, London, Ontario N6A 5W9, Canada
E-mail address: roberta.berard@lhsc.on.ca

Pediatr Clin N Am 59 (2012) 245–262
doi:10.1016/j.pcl.2012.03.003
0031-3955/12/$ – see front matter Crown Copyright © 2012 Published by Elsevier Inc. All rights reserved.

Table 1
Differential diagnosis of monoarthritis

Infection-related	Septic arthritis
	Osteomyelitis
	Transient synovitis
	Reactive arthritis
	Lyme disease
	Tuberculosis
Trauma	Fracture: accidental and nonaccidental
	Internal derangement: ligament rupture
	Foreign body: synovitis
Malignancy	Leukemia
	Neuroblastoma
Inflammation	JIA
	Inflammatory bowel disease
	Familial Mediterranean fever
Hemarthrosis	Hemophilia
	Pigmented villonodular synovitis
	Synovial hemangioma

4. Travel to Lyme disease–endemic or tuberculosis (TB)-endemic areas or other risk factors for TB (born in Africa, Asia, Latin America, or Eastern Europe; exposure to a person with TB; close contact with a person with a positive TB skin test result)
5. Presence of extra-articular features (diarrhea, urethral discharge, ocular symptoms, rash)
6. Personal or family history of a bleeding diathesis or HLA-B27–associated diseases (inflammatory bowel disease [IBD], acute anterior uveitis, psoriasis, ankylosing spondylitis).

Physical Examination

Abnormalities detected on physical examination are important clues to the diagnosis of monoarthritis. A detailed general physical examination should include growth parameters and vital signs. The presence of fever should alert the clinician to the potential for more severe conditions requiring urgent treatment (eg, septic arthritis). On general examination, clues to underlying diagnosis include rash (psoriasis, viral exanthema), iritis (IBD or enthesitis-related arthritis), and hepatosplenomegaly/lymphadenopathy suggestive of malignancy. The musculoskeletal examination should include a review of all joints and examination of the gait but with a focus on the affected joints. A recently developed and validated tool is the pGALS (pediatric Gait, Arms, Legs, Spine), which is a simple screening examination that can be performed in a few minutes (**Fig. 1**).[1,2]

The focused examination of the affected joint should include inspection of the skin for warmth, redness, swelling, and soft tissue involvement, using the contralateral side for comparison. Importantly, the distinction whether the swelling is of articular or extra-articular (eg, bursitis) origin must be made. Palpation of the surrounding bone is important because the presence of pinpoint bony tenderness is suggestive of fracture, osteomyelitis, or malignancy. Passive and active range of motion should be observed. An exquisite pain in the joint on range of motion or a joint that is severely restricted in its range of motion suggests an etiology other than inflammatory arthritis (eg, septic joint). In the presence of a significant trauma history, stress maneuvers for ligamentous instability should also be performed.

A

FIGURE	SCREENING MANOEUVRES (Note the manoeuvres in bold are additional to those in adult GALS²)	WHAT IS BEING ASSESSED?
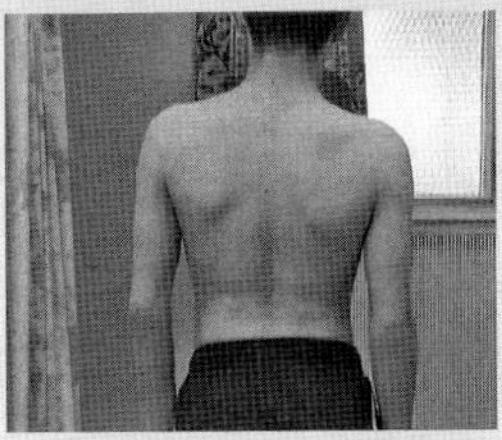	Observe the child standing (from front, back and sides)	• Posture and habitus • Skin rashes – e.g. psoriasis • Deformity – e.g. leg length inequality, leg alignment (valgus, varus at the knee or ankle), scoliosis, joint swelling, muscle wasting, flat feet
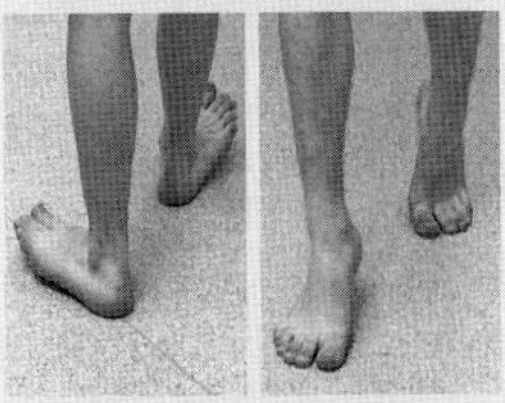	Observe the child walking and **'Walk on your heels' and 'Walk on your tiptoes'**	• Ankles, subtalar, midtarsal and small joints of feet and toes • Foot posture (note if presence of normal longitudinal arches of feet when on tiptoes)
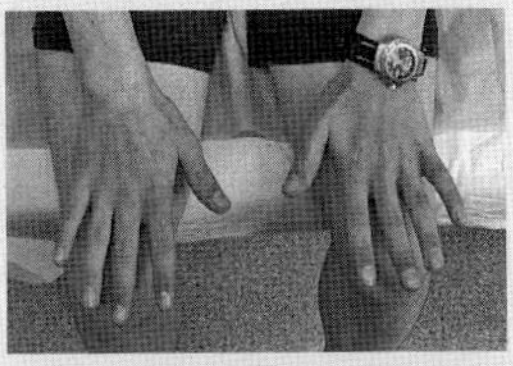	'Hold your hands out straight in front of you'	• Forward flexion of shoulders • Elbow extension • Wrist extension • Extension of small joints of fingers
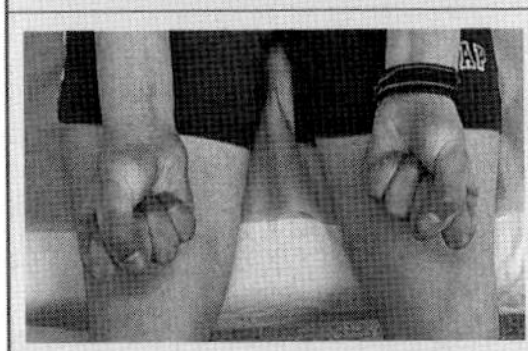	'Turn your hands over and make a fist'	• Wrist supination • Elbow supination • Flexion of small joints of fingers
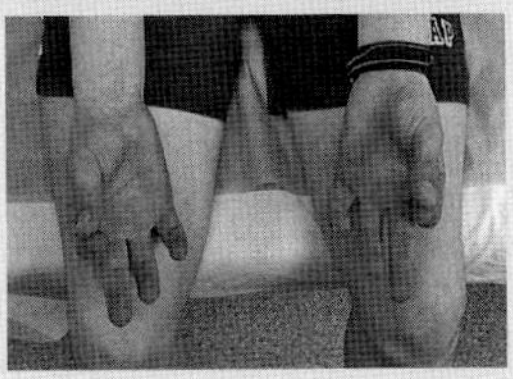	'Pinch your index finger and thumb together'	• Manual dexterity • Coordination of small joints of index finger and thumb and functional key grip

The screening table is titled **The pGALS musculoskeletal screen**

Screening questions
- Do you (or does your child) have any pain or stiffness in your (their) joints, muscles or back?
- Do you (or does your child) have any difficulty getting yourself (him/herself) dressed without any help?
- Do you (or does your child) have any problem going up and down stairs?

Fig. 1. (*A–C*) The pGALS musculoskeletal screen. (*From* Foster HE, Jandial S. pGALS— a screening examination of the musculoskeletal system in school-aged children. Reports on the Rheumatic Diseases (Series 5), Hands On 15: Arthritis Research Campaign; 2008. p. 4–6. Copyright © 2008 Arthritis Research Campaign; with permission.)

B

FIGURE	SCREENING MANOEUVRES	WHAT IS BEING ASSESSED?
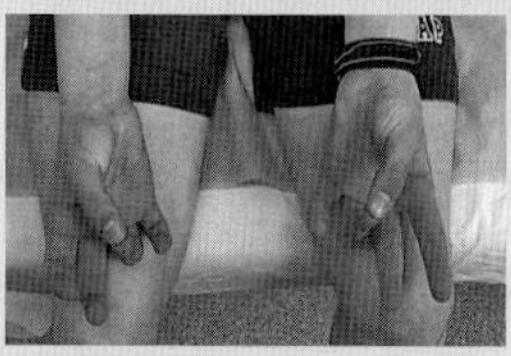	'Touch the tips of your fingers'	• Manual dexterity • Coordination of small joints of fingers and thumbs
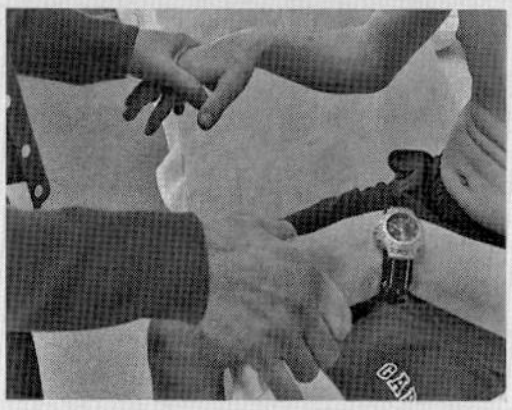	Squeeze the metacarpo-phalangeal joints for tenderness	• Metacarpophalangeal joints
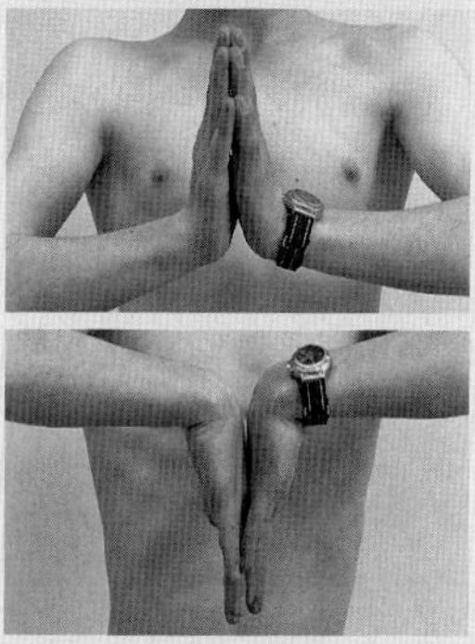	**'Put your hands together palm to palm'** and **'Put your hands together back to back'**	• Extension of small joints of fingers • Wrist extension • Elbow flexion
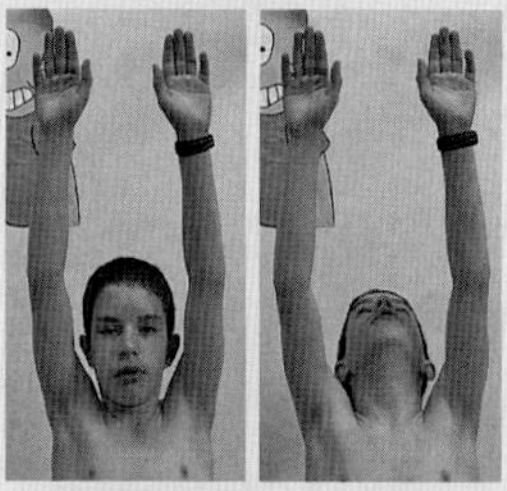	**'Reach up, "touch the sky"'** and **'Look at the ceiling'**	• Elbow extension • Wrist extension • Shoulder abduction • Neck extension
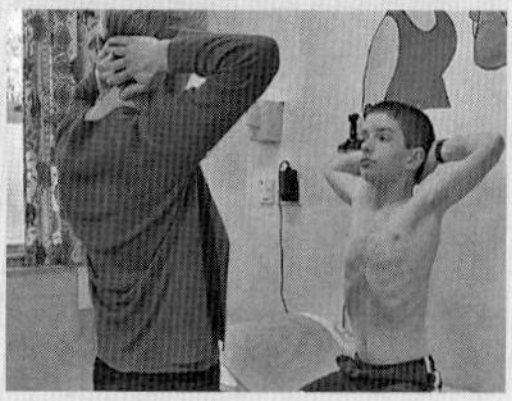	'Put your hands behind your neck'	• Shoulder abduction • External rotation of shoulders • Elbow flexion

Fig. 1. (*continued*)

C

FIGURE	SCREENING MANOEUVRES	WHAT IS BEING ASSESSED?
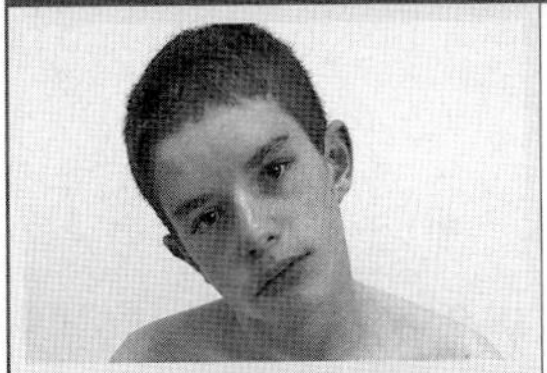	'Try and touch your shoulder with your ear'	• Cervical spine lateral flexion
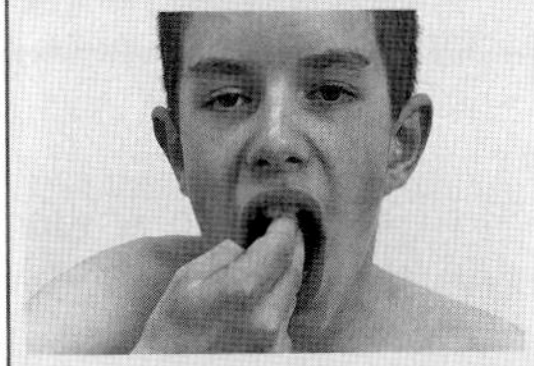	**'Open wide and put three (*child's own*) fingers in your mouth'**	• Temporomandibular joints (and check for deviation of jaw movement)
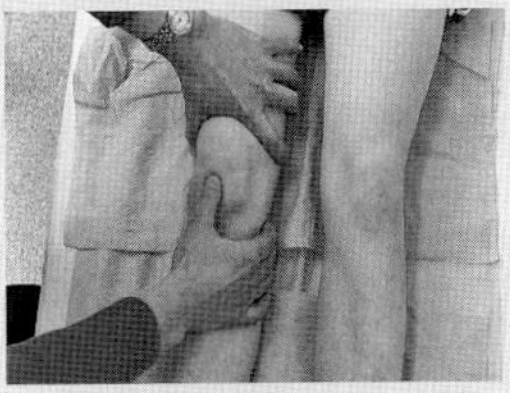	Feel for effusion at the knee (patella tap, or cross-fluctuation)	• Knee effusion (small effusion may be missed by patella tap alone)
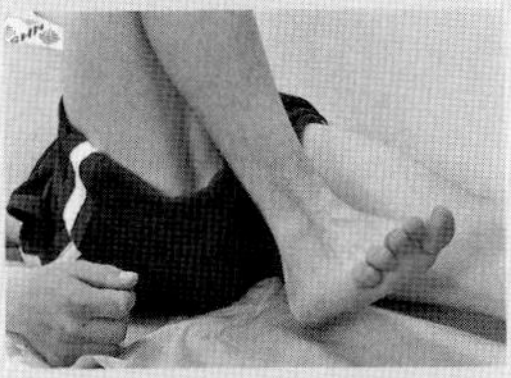	Active movement of knees (flexion and extension) and feel for crepitus	• Knee flexion • Knee extension
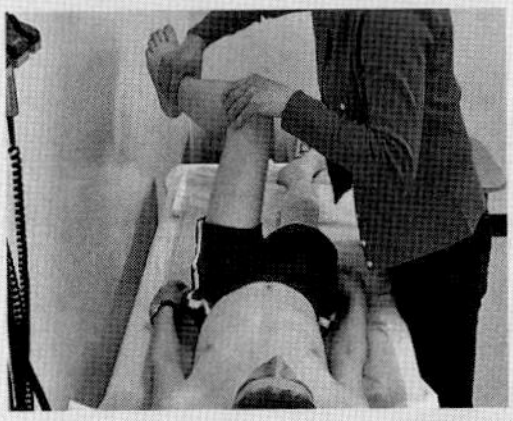	Passive movement of hip (knee flexed to 90°, and internal rotation of hip)	• Hip flexion and internal rotation
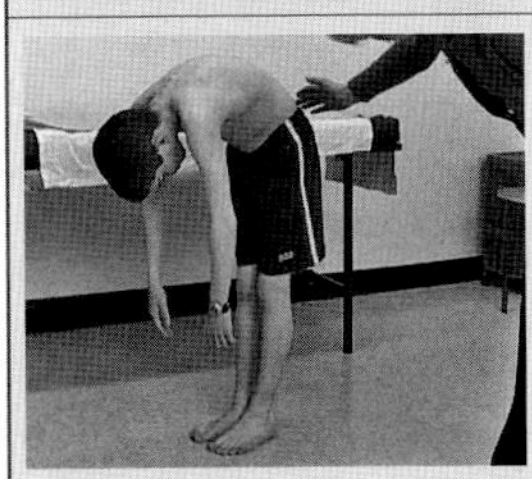	'Bend forwards and touch your toes?'	• Forward flexion of thoraco-lumbar spine (and check for scoliosis)

Fig. 1. (*continued*)

Preliminary investigations that are to be considered for the evaluation of monoarthritis are presented in **Box 1**. Laboratory investigations of acute or chronic monoarthritis are performed to confirm the clinician's impression regarding the suspected diagnosis or to exclude conditions. A diagnosis of JIA is made based on history taking and physical examination and after exclusion of other causes.

Laboratory Investigations

Complete blood cell count (CBC) and differential white blood cell (WBC) count, inflammatory markers, and liver and renal functions should be considered in any child with monoarthritis. If the presentation is acute (<72 hours), a joint aspiration must be performed if the clinician is concerned about a septic joint, with the fluid sent for blood cell count, Gram stain, and culture. In addition, culture of the throat, blood, stool, and/or urine should be considered to identify a potential organism in the case of reactive arthritis. An acute presentation is also observed with hematologic and malignant diseases (eg, hemophilia and leukemia), highlighting the importance of CBC and coagulation studies. Antistreptolysin-O (ASO) and anti–deoxyribonuclease B (anti–DNase B) titers are useful to identify a recent streptococcal infection.

In chronic monoarthritis, Lyme serology (when history is suggestive of an exposure) and antinuclear antibody (ANA) and rheumatoid factor (RF) titers should be considered. HLA-B27 testing is most relevant in chronic arthritis when the child is suspected of having a specific category of JIA (enthesitis-related arthritis), which is generally seen

---

Box 1
Preliminary investigations to be considered for the evaluation of monoarthritis

Basic screening

- Complete blood cell count and differential white blood cell count
- Erythrocyte sedimentation rate
- C-reactive protein
- Renal function and liver enzyme
- Serum lactate dehydrogenase
- Radiographs

Further investigations

- Cultures of throat, blood, joint fluid, stool, and/or urine
- Partial thromboplastin time
- Antinuclear antibody titer
- Serologic testing for Lyme disease
- Antistreptolysin-O titer
- Urinalysis
- Tuberculin skin test
- Further imaging (ultrasonography, magnetic resonance imaging)
- Bone marrow aspiration
- Slit lamp examination of the eyes

Data from Tse SM, Laxer RM. Approach to acute limb pain in childhood. Pediatr Rev 2006;27(5):170–9 [quiz: 180].

in boys older than 8 years and often associated with enthesitis, lumbosacral back pain, and a family history of HLA-B27–associated diseases (eg, IBD, ankylosing spondylitis). The presence of ANA or RF is neither necessary nor sufficient to make a diagnosis of JIA.[3] ANA should not be used as a screening test for rheumatic illness in a primary care setting, because it may be positive in up to 15% of healthy children. ANA is used as a diagnostic test for children with probable systemic lupus erythematosus (SLE) or mixed connective tissue disease (MCTD) and other overlap-like illnesses. In the context of JIA, a positive ANA titer is associated with a significantly increased risk of developing chronic anterior uveitis.[4,5]

RF has been associated with aging (>60 years), infections (bacterial endocarditis, hepatitis B or C, parasitic disease, viral infection), pulmonary disease (sarcoidosis, interstitial pulmonary fibrosis), malignancy, and primary biliary cirrhosis[6] and thus is not a specific test for the diagnosis of rheumatic disease. Only 5% to 10% of patients with JIA have a positive RF, highlighting the lack of sensitivity for the diagnosis of JIA.[7]

A joint aspiration must be performed when a septic joint (bacterial) is suspected but is also recommended for the diagnosis of TB arthritis. The presence of hemarthrosis suggests coagulation disorder, trauma, or rare causes, including synovial hemangioma or pigmented villonodular synovitis.

The more common and/or serious causes of monoarthritis are addressed in the following sections.

Monoarthritis Related to Infection

Septic arthritis

Septic arthritis is a medical emergency that requires prompt antibiotic therapy and orthopedic intervention (drainage and irrigation). This condition is estimated to account for 6.5% of all childhood arthritides.[8] Septic arthritis results from direct puncture injury to a joint, hematogenous spread, or spread from a contiguous infection (eg, osteomyelitis or cellulitis). In children and adolescents, the most common causative agents are *Staphylococcus aureus*, group A streptococci (GAS), and *Streptococcus pneumoniae*.[9,10] In children younger than 2 years, *Haemophilus influenzae* type B had been the most common pathogen identified, but vaccination of infants for *H influenzae* has significantly decreased the frequency of infection with this organism.[11] Other important agents are *Salmonella* in patients with sickle cell disease and *Neisseria gonorrhoeae* in sexually active adolescents. *Kingella kingae* has emerged as an important pathogen, particularly in children younger than 4 years.[12,13] This organism grows better in aerobic conditions; hence synovial fluid and bone aspirates from patients should be inoculated in an aerobic blood culture system in addition to the traditional solid culture media.[13,14] *K kingae* is difficult to isolate on routinely used solid culture media, which is why it is proposed that this organism may account for a significant portion of culture-negative cases of septic arthritis. *Mycobacterium tuberculosis* is an unusual causative agent of septic monoarthritis but must be considered in an at-risk individual.

As outlined earlier, the presence of fever, localized erythema, warmth, and significant pain on passive range of motion are highly suggestive of a septic joint. Children (particularly neonates) can present with pseudoparalysis of the affected limb. Investigations usually demonstrate an elevated WBC count (predominance of neutrophils) and inflammatory marker levels (erythrocyte sedimentation rate [ESR], C-reactive protein [CRP]). However, an urgent joint aspiration and a synovial fluid analysis with blood cell count and Gram stain is essential for the diagnosis. The causative agent is recovered in 50% to 70% of cases (blood or synovial fluid).

Initial radiologic examination is not diagnostic and may demonstrate only soft tissue and capsular swelling. The characteristic findings of osteopenia and joint space loss may not be present until 10 days into the illness. Despite prompt recognition with appropriate surgical and antibiotic management, permanent damage is common. A septic hip joint is particularly vulnerable to early damage, with chronic debilitating changes seen within 24 to 48 hours if aspiration and treatment are delayed. Such a delay may result in avascular necrosis related to increased intra-articular pressure that compromises the blood vessels that supply the cartilage and femoral head.

Reactive arthritis

The term reactive arthritis refers to arthritis that develops during or after an infection elsewhere in the body but in which the microorganisms cannot be recovered from the joint. The classic organisms causing reactive arthritis are enteric (*Campylobacter*, *Yersinia*, *Salmonella*, *Shigella*) and genitourinary organisms (*Chlamydia trachomatis*). The triad of conjunctivitis, urethritis, and arthritis, formerly known as Reiter syndrome, may be seen after one of these infections. More recently, reactive arthritis has also been reported after infection with *Mycoplasma pneumoniae*[15] and *Chlamydia pneumoniae*.[16] Although the precise role of HLA-B27 in the development of arthritis is not fully elucidated, there is a higher frequency of HLA-B27 positivity in patients who develop reactive arthritis after infection with one of these organisms.[11] The generally short-lived arthritis may be monoarticular or polyarticular, involving the larger joints of the lower extremities; can be quite painful; and usually responds well to nonsteroidal antiinflammatory drugs (NSAIDs). In addition, acute rheumatic fever (ARF) and poststreptococcal reactive arthritis (PSRA) are postinfectious arthritides and are discussed in the differential diagnosis of polyarthritis.

Hip monoarthritis

Transient synovitis of the hip Transient (toxic) synovitis (TS) of the hip presents as a painless limp or a painful hip or knee (referred pain) typically affecting boys younger than 4 years (occasionally up to 8 years). The cause of TS is unknown but it has been postulated to be related to previous infection, most commonly involving the upper respiratory tract. In a large incidence study of family practice visits for nontraumatic hip pain in children, which determined an incidence rate of 148.1 per 100,000 person-years, TS had the highest incidence rate of all diagnoses considered (76.2 per 100,000 person-years).[17] On inspection, the child is generally well appearing (afebrile or only mildly elevated temperature) and can ambulate but may do so with a limp. The affected leg is often held in a position of external rotation and flexion. A few attempts have been made to develop predictors to differentiate septic arthritis from TS. A non–weight bearing status, a history of fever, an ESR greater than 40 mm/h, and a WBC count greater than 12,000 cells/mm is highly predictive of septic arthritis.[18,19] A radiograph of the affected area should be sought to rule out other pathologic conditions (eg, osteoid osteoma, fracture). Because the diagnosis of TS is one of exclusion, in the case of a child who looks well, with no fever and normal WBC count and ESR, conservative management with close follow-up (1–2 days) is sensible. If there is any concern for an infection being the cause of hip pain and limp (fever, abnormal ESR or WBC count, localized tenderness), an ultrasonography is recommended to document evidence of an effusion followed by a diagnostic aspiration (if an effusion is present).[20]

With conservative use of NSAIDs and bed rest, this self-limited process tends to resolve in 3 to 10 days. It has been suggested that patients with TS should have a repeat radiography within 6 months to exclude Legg-Calvé-Perthes (LCP) disease, which is estimated to be a complication of TS in 1% to 3% of cases. The recurrence rate is 4% to 17%, occurring mostly within 6 months. There has been no identified increased risk of developing JIA after a diagnosis of TS.

When the presentation is one of monoarticular pain involving the hip, additional important considerations are slipped capital femoral epiphysis (SCFE) and LCP disease. Both these conditions are noninflammatory and not typically associated with arthritis.

SCFE SCFE classically occurs in overweight boys aged 10 to 14 years or in children with endocrine disorders, such as hypothyroidism or pituitary deficiencies (eg, growth hormone deficiency). SCFE is diagnosed radiographically. Both hips should be imaged because SCFE is bilateral in 30% of cases in which the presenting symptoms are unilateral. On diagnosis, an urgent referral should be made to orthopedics; in the meantime, the child should be non–weight bearing and on bed rest and prescribed crutches.

LCP syndrome LCP syndrome, an idiopathic avascular necrosis of the capital femoral epiphysis, typically affects boys aged between 4 and 10 years. A high index of suspicion is needed to make the diagnosis because initial radiographs are often normal. At this early stage, magnetic resonance imaging (MRI) is most sensitive for the diagnosis, showing changes in the bone marrow related to hypoperfusion. Subsequently, radiographs show fragmentation and then healing of the femoral head, often with residual deformity. Patients with LCP should be made non–weight bearing, with an urgent referral to orthopedics. Treatment focuses on maintaining containment of the femoral head within the acetabulum with the use of abduction splints or, occasionally, surgically with an osteotomy of the proximal femur.

Lyme disease

Lyme arthritis is most commonly recognized in the Northeastern, Mid-Atlantic, and North-Central United States and less commonly in the West Coast and Southern Canada, attributable to the distribution of the white-tailed deer.[21] This tick-borne illness is primarily caused by 3 species of the spirochete *Borrelia burgdorferi*. The clinical manifestations of Lyme disease vary but early disease manifestations include a flu-like illness, rash (erythema migrans), lymphocytic meningitis, cranial nerve VII palsy, arthralgia, and rarely carditis. Arthritis is a late manifestation occurring months to years after the original infection. Often, the child is asymptomatic and may not recall having been bitten by a tick. This underscores the importance of eliciting a history of travel or residence in a Lyme-endemic area. The most frequently involved joint is the knee (in two-thirds of cases), but any large joint may be affected,[22] and more than one joint may be involved at presentation. The arthritis may be painless and episodic; however, chronic arthritis has been described in up to 18% of patients.[23]

The diagnosis is based on suggestive clinical characteristics in addition to confirmatory laboratory tests. Indirect methods to detect infection are preferred over direct detection methods (cultures, stains, or polymerase chain reactions) because the latter have higher rates of false-negative results and it often takes a prolonged period before the results are known. Of the indirect methods, the enzyme immunoassay (enzyme-linked immunosorbent assay) has high sensitivity and low specificity and thus is used as a targeted screening test. In the case of a positive result, Western blot is the confirmatory test with high specificity.[11]

Malignancy

A malignancy must always be considered at the top of the differential diagnosis, even if it can be immediately discounted. Clues that suggest a malignancy as the cause for arthritis include the following: pain out of keeping with the degree of arthritis, the child being irritable and difficult to examine, fever, lymphadenopathy or hepatosplenome-galy, leukocyte or platelet count that are lower than expected, bone pain, and meta-physeal lucencies seen on the radiograph (**Fig. 2**).[24] Joint involvement in malignancy tends to be oligoarticular ($\leq$4 joints) rather than polyarticular.[25]

One study looking at the factors differentiating acute leukemia from chronic arthritis found that the presence of a low WBC count (<4 $\times$ 10^9/L), low-normal platelet count (150–250 $\times$ 10^9/L), and history of nighttime pain was 100% specific and 85% sensitive for the diagnosis of acute lymphoblastic leukemia (ALL).[26] Moreover, when pain is the chief complaint of the patient, this may have a strong negative predictive value for the diagnosis of JIA. Isolated musculoskeletal pain, in the absence of other signs or symp-toms, is almost never a presenting complaint in children with JIA, and, instead, chil-dren (with JIA) more commonly complain of joint swelling and/or gait disturbance.[27]

JIA

Chronic arthritis is the most common rheumatic disease in children, affecting about 1 in 1000 children worldwide.[28] JIA is an umbrella term describing a group of arthritides of unknown etiology lasting more than 6 weeks in children younger than 16 years.[29] JIA is an important consideration in chronic monoarthritis because it is a significant cause of short-term and long-term disability. In addition, there is mounting evidence that early disease identification and treatment may lead to improved quality of life. The most frequently affected joints are the knee, ankle, wrist, and elbow. Chronic monoarthritis can be the presenting manifestation of oligoarthritis, enthesitis-related arthritis, and psoriatic arthritis. JIA rarely presents as monoarthritis involving the hip or shoulder. Consequently, there is a low threshold for further imaging (MRI) once an infectious cause has been ruled out. Up to 20% of children with JIA (oligoarthritis) may develop chronic anterior uveitis. Therefore, a slit lamp examination should be considered for a child with suspected JIA because detection of uveitis would support this diagnosis. JIA is reviewed in detail in this issue of *The Clinics*.

Other Important Diagnostic Considerations

Hemophilia may cause recurrent monoarthritis. Chronic joint pain and damage is one of the most important causes of morbidity in this X-linked recessive coagulopathy. Hemorrhage into the soft tissues, particularly intramuscularly, may mimic hemarthrosis.

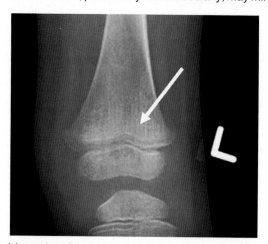

Fig. 2. Metaphyseal lucencies observed in leukemia. Arrow, metaphysis of femur; arrow-head, metaphyseal lucency.

The most commonly affected joints are the knees, elbows, and ankles. The classic presentation of hemarthrosis is one of acute onset of increasing fullness in a joint, with loss of range of motion. On examination, the joint is warm and distended. Recurrent hemarthrosis can lead to bone and joint damage and early osteoarthritis, causing a significant effect on the patients' quality of life. A rarer cause of hemarthrosis is pigmented villonodular synovitis, which may represent a benign neoplasm of the synovium.

An acute or a chronic monoarthritis may easily be confused with extra-articular joint swelling, particularly around the knee joint. Bursitis is another important consideration in the approach to monoarthritis. A bursa is a synovial-lined sac designed to reduce friction between moving structures (eg, tendons rubbing against bones, ligaments, or other tendons). A bursa may communicate with the joint (eg, suprapatellar and popliteal); however, other bursae around the knee do not necessarily do so (eg, infrapatellar and medial collateral ligament). Bursitis typically presents with maximal tenderness at the site of the bursa and localized swelling. In the case of communication with the knee joint, a small joint effusion may also be observed. Although the prevalence of bursitis in childhood is low, it may be higher in athletes[30] and patients with JIA.[31] When bursitis is suspected, an MRI is the preferred imaging modality to confirm the diagnosis. It is important to distinguish between monoarthritis and bursitis because the treatment differs; bursitis may not respond to an intra-articular corticosteroid injection and may require a direct injection into the affected bursa.

POLYARTHRITIS

The differential diagnosis of polyarthritis essentially includes infectious, inflammatory, and malignant causes (**Table 2**). Although mechanical causes (eg, hypermobility and skeletal dysplasia) and diffuse idiopathic pain syndromes are considered in the

Table 2
Differential diagnosis of polyarthritis

Infection-related	N gonorrhea infection
	Viral infections (eg, parvovirus B19, rubella virus/vaccine)
	Infective endocarditis
	ARF
	PSRA
	Reactive arthritis
Inflammatory	JIA
	SLE
	Juvenile dermatomyositis
	Systemic vasculitides
	• Henoch-Schönlein purpura
	• Kawasaki disease
	Hereditary autoinflammatory syndromes
	Sarcoidosis
	IBD related
Malignancy	Leukemia
	Neuroblastoma
Mechanical	Hypermobility
	Skeletal dysplasia
Other systemic illness	Immunodeficiency-associated arthritis
	Serum sickness

Data from Cassidy J, Petty RE, Laxer RM, et al. Textbook of pediatric rheumatology. 6th edition. Philadelphia: Saunders; 2011.

differential diagnosis of polyarthralgia, they do not routinely cause polyarthritis. The review of systems and physical examination is critical to establishing a diagnosis because there are clues in the characteristics of the arthritis, fever, rash, and other system involvements that often provide the correct diagnosis (**Table 3**). When polyarthritis is the presenting complaint, in addition to the investigations outlined in **Box 1**, additional investigations may include serum C3 and C4 complement levels, serum levels of quantitative immunoglobulins, urinalysis, serologic testing for viral

Table 3
Review of systems in the differential diagnosis of polyarthritis

System Involved	Review of System or Physical Finding	Diagnoses
Ophthalmologic	• Uveitis • Conjunctival injection without exudate	• JIA • KD
Dermatologic	• Malar rash, alopecia • Heliotrope rash, Gottron papules • Polymorphous rash, perineal desquamation, edema, and erythema of hands • Evanescent salmon-colored rash • Palpable purpura • Nail pitting or onycholysis • Oral ulcers	• SLE • JDM • KD • SJIA • HSP, SLE • JIA (psoriatic) • SLE
Cardiovascular	• New heart murmur • Pericarditis • Raynaud phenomenon	• ARF, IE • SJIA, SLE, ARF • SLE, MCTD, scleroderma
Respiratory tract	• Pleuritis • Acute or chronic sinusitis, pulmonary nodules, or hemorrhage • Interstitial lung disease	• SJIA, SLE • GPA • SLE or scleroderma
Gastrointestinal/ Genitourinary tract	• Weight loss or poor growth • Diarrhea/hematochezia, colicky abdominal pain • History of gastroenteritis • History of urethritis or cervicitis	• IBD, malignancy, SLE • IBD, HSP • Reactive arthritis • Reactive arthritis, gonococcal arthritis
Neurologic	• Seizures, psychosis, mood disorder, decline in school performance • Stroke • Proximal muscle weakness	• SLE • SLE, vasculitis • JDM, MCTD

Abbreviations: GPA, granulomatosis with polyangiitis (Wegener); HSP, Henoch-Schönlein purpura; IE, infective endocarditis; JDM, juvenile dermatomyositis; KD, Kawasaki disease; SJIA, systemic JIA.
Data from Singh S, Mehra S. Approach to polyarthritis. Indian J Pediatr 2010;77(9):1005–10.

pathogens, swabs for gonococcal infection as indicated, ASO and anti–DNase B titers, cardiac evaluation (electrocardiography and echocardiography), chest radiography, ANA titer, other autoantibodies (anti-Ro, anti-La, anti-Sm, anti-RNP, anti–Scl 70), and antineutrophil cytoplasmic antibody.

Important and serious causes of polyarthritis are discussed.

Rheumatic Diseases

Polyarthritis is a presenting feature of many rheumatic diseases including JIA, autoimmune connective tissue diseases, and systemic vasculitides. The most common cause of rheumatic diseases is polyarticular JIA (both RF negative and RF positive).

Systemic JIA (SJIA) classically presents with a quotidian fever of at least 2 weeks' duration. The typical pattern is once or twice daily spikes, with return to normal or even subnormal temperatures between spikes. In SJIA, the rash is evanescent, often occurring with the fever, which helps to distinguish this diagnosis from the rashes of erythema marginatum in ARF, palpable purpura in vasculitis, or Gottron papules in juvenile dermatomyositis. SLE commonly presents in adolescence with low-grade fevers, constitutional symptoms of anorexia, weight loss, malar rashes, and painful polyarthritis affecting both the large and small joints.[32]

Generally, the ANA titer is strongly positive in SLE but may also be positive in polyarticular JIA. Both SLE and SJIA can present with serositis and hepatosplenomegaly; however, the presence of nephritis, cytopenias, hypocomplementemia, anti-dsDNA, and other autoantibodies differentiates SLE from SJIA (see articles by Levy and Kamphuis; Gowdie and Tse elsewhere in this issue).

Patients with systemic sclerosis and idiopathic inflammatory myositis frequently have mild nonpainful arthritis, but there are other clues to these diagnoses (weakness, heliotrope rashes, and Gottron papules seen in juvenile dermatomyositis and sclerotic skin changes; Raynaud phenomenon; skin and gum telangiectasias; respiratory symptoms; or gastrointestinal [GI] tract dysmotility seen in systemic sclerosis). MCTD is characterized by Raynaud phenomenon, myositis, polyarthritis and sclerodactyly with positive ANA titer and high titers of anti-RNP autoantibodies.

The painful oligoarthritis or polyarthritis associated with Kawasaki disease can occur in up to one-third of patients and is typically observed in the subacute phase of the illness; however, it may also be seen in the acute phase.[33] Arthritis is also seen in 75% of patients[34] with Henoch-Schönlein purpura, but other features, such as lower extremity palpable purpura, abdominal pain, and nephritis, help to clarify this diagnosis.

Pediatric sarcoidosis is a rare chronic noncaseating granulomatous disease characterized by arthritis, eczematous-like rash, anterior or posterior uveitis, and polyarthritis often associated with marked tenosynovitis.[35] Fever, constitutional symptoms, hepatosplenomegaly, bone marrow involvement, and pulmonary manifestations are seen more with the adult-onset form of sarcoidosis.

Polyarthritis may also be a presenting feature of several of the autoinflammatory syndromes (familial Mediterranean fever, cryopyrin-associated periodic syndrome, hyperimmunoglobulinemia D syndrome).

Polyarthritis Related to Infection

Bacterial pathogens

Bacterial pathogens are generally associated with monoarthritis (septic joint). However, N gonorrhoeae is associated with fever, chills, vesiculopustular rashes, and migratory arthritis often accompanied by painful tenosynovitis. Purulent synovitis of several joints may be observed. Gonococcal arthritis usually develops in association with primary asymptomatic genitourinary tract infection or gonococcal infection of the throat or rectum. Thus, if suspected, cultures from the genital tract, throat, rectum, and any vesicle in addition to the joint fluid should be obtained.

The arthritis of infective endocarditis can precede other immune-mediated manifestations (Osler nodes, Janeway lesions, Roth spots) by weeks. This symmetric polyarthritis is thought to be an immune complex–mediated process as demonstrated by the presence of hypocomplementemia, circulating immune complexes, and sometimes RFs.[11]

Reactive arthritis related to streptococcal infection: ARF and PSRA

The diagnosis of ARF is established mainly on clinical grounds. The initial description of the clinical manifestations, now known as the Jones criteria, was revised most recently in 1992. The major criteria include (1) carditis, (2) polyarthritis, (3) chorea, (4) erythema marginatum, and (5) subcutaneous nodules. The minor criteria include (1) arthralgia (counted only when arthritis is not present), (2) fever, (3) elevated acute phase reactants, and (4) an electrocardiogram showing prolonged PR interval (first-degree heart block). Evidence of a preceding GAS infection is necessary for the diagnosis and indicates a high probability of ARF when present with 2 major manifestations or 1 major and 2 minor manifestations.[36]

Evidence of prior GAS infection is necessary for the diagnosis of both ARF and PSRA. Microbiological confirmation can be obtained by throat culture or rapid antigen detection tests. However, both throat culture and rapid antigen detection tests cannot differentiate a true GAS infection from a carrier state, which can be found in as many as 15% of school-aged children.[37] Confirmation of a recent GAS infection may also be achieved by serologic testing. A preceding GAS infection can be identified in the presence of elevated or increasing antistreptococcal antibody titers. The most commonly used tests are ASO and anti–DNase B.

After the initial GAS infection, ASO titers begin to increase in 1 week and peak 3 to 6 weeks later. Anti–DNase B titers begin to increase in 1 to 2 weeks and peak 6 to 8 weeks after the infection. Elevated titers for both tests may persist for months after GAS infection.[11]

Differentiating between ARF and PSRA can be a challenge. PSRA tends to occur sooner after a streptococcal infection than the arthritis of ARF (7–10 vs 10–28 days). The arthritis of ARF is typically migratory in nature, involving the large joints; is often associated with erythema over the joints and significant elevation in the acute phase reactants; and is dramatically responsive to NSAIDs. This is in contrast to the additive arthritis seen in PSRA, which tends to be more persistent, involves large and small joints and axial involvement, is associated with only moderate elevation in acute phase reactants, and is more resistant to NSAIDs.[38]

Viral pathogens

Arthralgia and arthritis are well recognized and relatively common occurrences with viral infections. The most widely recognized viral-induced arthritis (in adults) is caused by parvovirus B19. This virus causes fifth disease/erythema infectiosum, a self-limited exanthem of childhood. Joint symptoms occur in about 10% of children and 60% of adults. In pediatrics, arthritis may be asymmetric and oligoarticular (<4 joints) in contrast to the acute-onset symmetric arthritis more commonly seen in adults.[39] The diagnosis is made if circulating IgM antibodies to parvovirus are present. Treatment is supportive with NSAIDs.

Although a primary rubella virus infection is associated with arthritis, a general pediatrician is more likely to observe arthritis associated with the rubella vaccine. Joint symptoms usually develop approximately 2 weeks (10–28 days) after vaccination. Symmetric, migratory, and additive arthritis typically resolve within 2 to 4 weeks.[11]

Several herpesviruses, including varicella-zoster virus, Epstein-Barr virus, herpes simplex virus, and cytomegalovirus, have been associated with arthritis, in addition to hepatitis B and C. There are many immune phenomena related to human immunodeficiency virus infection, one of which is reactive arthritis.[40]

Other Important Diagnostic Considerations

IBD can be associated with arthritis in 7% to 21% of children affected by this disease.[11] There are 2 patterns of joint disease that can occur in association with IBD. The first pattern is involvement of the lower extremity joints, especially the ankles and knees. The activity of this peripheral arthritis tends to parallel the activity of the GI tract inflammation. Medical management is aimed at optimizing control of the GI tract inflammation, resulting in improvement in arthritis. The second pattern is of axial involvement and is often associated with HLA-B27. The involvement bears little relation to the GI disease. Clues to this would include a positive history of cramping abdominal pain, anorexia, diarrhea/hematochezia, weight loss, anemia, fever, or poor growth.

As outlined earlier, malignancy should always be considered in the differential diagnosis of arthritis. Infiltration of the bone or synovium can mimic polyarthritis, although in most instances this is periarticular. ALL can cause polyarthritis as a result of leukemic infiltration into the synovium. In addition to constitutional symptoms, laboratory evaluation may show moderate to severe anemia or an elevation of the ESR, with a normal or low platelet count; a low WBC count; or high lactate dehydrogenase or uric acid levels.

Serum sickness is an important consideration in the differential diagnosis of transient polyarthritis. Serum sickness is an immune complex–mediated disease that is most commonly seen after a drug exposure (eg, cefaclor, penicillin, NSAIDs, thiazide diuretics, phenytoin). This disease is characterized by onset 7 to 14 days after exposure to an antigen, with the presenting symptoms of fever, arthralgia (two-thirds of patients), true arthritis (minority), myalgia, lymphadenopathy, and pruritic rash. The affected joints are characteristically quite tender to palpation and movement, with predominance of periarticular swelling, making it challenging to differentiate from true arthritis. The findings on CBC are nonspecific and may include neutropenia, reactive lymphocytes, mild thrombocytopenia, and eosinophilia. The ESR and CRP levels are frequently elevated, and hypoalbuminemia may be present in patients with edema. There may be mild proteinuria. C3, C4, and total hemolytic complement levels are often low, reflecting the consumptive process.

SUMMARY

The differential diagnosis for monoarthritis and polyarthritis is broad. An organized approach within the framework presented, including carefully attending to clues in the history taking and physical examination allows for correct diagnosis in most cases. Laboratory evaluation is performed to support the clinician's impression. Serious and/or potentially life-threatening infectious, malignant, or orthopedic causes need to be identified, and the patient is referred for surgical or medical management. Given that monoarthritis and polyarthritis can be the presenting features of serious chronic rheumatic illness, persistent symptoms or concerning results arising from the diagnostic evaluation should be referred to a rheumatologist for assessment.

REFERENCES

1. Goff I, Bateman B, Myers A, et al. Acceptability and practicality of musculoskeletal examination in acute general pediatric assessment. J Pediatr 2010;156(4): 657–62.
2. Foster HE, Kay LJ, Friswell M, et al. Musculoskeletal screening examination (pGALS) for school-age children based on the adult GALS screen. Arthritis Rheum 2006;55(5):709–16.
3. Malleson PN, Mackinnon MJ, Sailer-Hoeck M, et al. Review for the generalist: the antinuclear antibody test in children—when to use it and what to do with a positive titer. Pediatr Rheumatol Online J 2010;8:27.
4. American Academy of Pediatrics Section on Rheumatology and Section on Ophthalmology: guidelines for ophthalmologic examinations in children with juvenile rheumatoid arthritis. Pediatrics 1993;92(2):295–6.
5. Saurenmann RK, Levin AV, Feldman BM, et al. Risk factors for development of uveitis differ between girls and boys with juvenile idiopathic arthritis. Arthritis Rheum 2010;62(6):1824–8.
6. Shmerling RH, Delbanco TL. The rheumatoid factor: an analysis of clinical utility. Am J Med 1991;91(5):528–34.
7. Oen K, Tucker L, Huber AM, et al. Predictors of early inactive disease in a juvenile idiopathic arthritis cohort: results of a Canadian multicenter, prospective inception cohort study. Arthritis Rheum 2009;61(8):1077–86.
8. Kunnamo I, Kallio P, Pelkonen P, et al. Clinical signs and laboratory tests in the differential diagnosis of arthritis in children. Am J Dis Child 1987;141(1):34–40.
9. Wang CL, Wang SM, Yang YJ, et al. Septic arthritis in children: relationship of causative pathogens, complications, and outcome. J Microbiol Immunol Infect 2003;36(1):41–6.
10. Kocher MS, Mandiga R, Murphy JM, et al. A clinical practice guideline for treatment of septic arthritis in children: efficacy in improving process of care and effect on outcome of septic arthritis of the hip. J Bone Joint Surg Am 2003;85(6):994–9.
11. Cassidy J, Petty RE, Laxer RM, et al. Textbook of pediatric rheumatology. 6th edition. Philadelphia: Saunders; 2011.
12. Dubnov-Raz G, Ephros M, Garty BZ, et al. Invasive pediatric Kingella kingae infections: a nationwide collaborative study. Pediatr Infect Dis J 2010;29(7):639–43.
13. Yagupsky P, Porsch E, St Geme JW 3rd. Kingella kingae: an emerging pathogen in young children. Pediatrics 2011;127(3):557–65.
14. American Academy of Pediatrics. Summary of Major Changes in the 2009 Red Book. In: Pickering LK, editors. Red Book: 2009 Report of the Committee on Infectious Diseases. 28th edition. Elk Grove Village, IL: American Academy of Pediatrics; 2009. p. XXIX.
15. Cimolai N, Malleson P, Thomas E, et al. Mycoplasma pneumoniae associated arthropathy: confirmation of the association by determination of the antipolypeptide IgM response. J Rheumatol 1989;16(8):1150–2.
16. Hannu T, Puolakkainen M, Leirisalo-Repo M. Chlamydia pneumoniae as a triggering infection in reactive arthritis. Rheumatology 1999;38(5):411–4.
17. Krul M, van der Wouden JC, Schellevis FG, et al. Acute non-traumatic hip pathology in children: incidence and presentation in family practice. Fam Pract 2010;27(2):166–70.
18. Kocher MS, Mandiga R, Zurakowski D, et al. Validation of a clinical prediction rule for the differentiation between septic arthritis and transient synovitis of the hip in children. J Bone Joint Surg Am 2004;86(8):1629–35.

19. Luhmann SJ, Jones A, Schootman M, et al. Differentiation between septic arthritis and transient synovitis of the hip in children with clinical prediction algorithms. J Bone Joint Surg Am 2004;86(5):956–62.

20. Do TT. Transient synovitis as a cause of painful limps in children. Curr Opin Pediatr 2000;12(1):48–51.

21. Bacon RM, Kugeler KJ, Mead PS. Surveillance for Lyme disease—United States, 1992-2006. MMWR Surveill Summ 2008;57(10):1–9.

22. Gerber MA, Zemel LS, Shapiro ED. Lyme arthritis in children: clinical epidemiology and long-term outcomes. Pediatrics 1998;102(4 Pt 1):905–8.

23. Huppertz HI, Karch H, Suschke HJ, et al. Lyme arthritis in European children and adolescents. The Pediatric Rheumatology Collaborative Group. Arthritis Rheum 1995;38(3):361–8.

24. Cabral DA, Tucker LB. Malignancies in children who initially present with rheumatic complaints. J Pediatr 1999;134(1):53–7.

25. Spasova MI, Stoyanova AA, Moumdjiev IN, et al. Childhood acute lymphoblastic leukemia presenting with osteoarticular syndrome—characteristics and prognosis. Folia Med (Plovdiv) 2009;51(1):50–5.

26. Jones OY, Spencer CH, Bowyer SL, et al. A multicenter case-control study on predictive factors distinguishing childhood leukemia from juvenile rheumatoid arthritis. Pediatrics 2006;117(5):e840–4.

27. McGhee JL, Burks FN, Sheckels JL, et al. Identifying children with chronic arthritis based on chief complaints: absence of predictive value for musculoskeletal pain as an indicator of rheumatic disease in children. Pediatrics 2002;110(2 Pt 1):354–9.

28. Hayward K, Wallace CA. Recent developments in anti-rheumatic drugs in pediatrics: treatment of juvenile idiopathic arthritis. Arthritis Res Ther 2009;11(1):216.

29. Petty RE, Southwood TR, Manners P, et al. International League of Associations for Rheumatology classification of juvenile idiopathic arthritis: second revision, Edmonton, 2001. J Rheumatol 2004;31(2):390–2.

30. Barclay C, Springgay G, van Beek EJ, et al. Medial collateral ligament bursitis in a 12-year-old girl. Arthroscopy 2005;21(6):759.

31. Alqanatish JT, Petty RE, Houghton KM, et al. Infrapatellar bursitis in children with juvenile idiopathic arthritis: a case series. Clin Rheumatol 2011;30(2):263–7.

32. Hiraki LT, Benseler SM, Tyrrell PN, et al. Clinical and laboratory characteristics and long-term outcome of pediatric systemic lupus erythematosus: a longitudinal study. J Pediatr 2008;152(4):550–6.

33. Gong GW, McCrindle BW, Ching JC, et al. Arthritis presenting during the acute phase of Kawasaki disease. J Pediatr 2006;148(6):800–5.

34. Saulsbury FT. Clinical update: Henoch-Schönlein purpura. Lancet 2007; 369(9566):976–8.

35. Rose CD, Wouters CH, Meiorin S, et al. Pediatric granulomatous arthritis: an international registry. Arthritis Rheum 2006;54(10):3337–44.

36. Guidelines for the diagnosis of rheumatic fever. Jones Criteria, 1992 update. Special Writing Group of the Committee on Rheumatic Fever, Endocarditis, and Kawasaki Disease of the Council on Cardiovascular Disease in the Young of the American Heart Association. JAMA 1992;268(15):2069–73.

37. Gerber MA, Baltimore RS, Eaton CB, et al. Prevention of rheumatic fever and diagnosis and treatment of acute streptococcal pharyngitis. A scientific statement from the American Heart Association Rheumatic Fever, Endocarditis, and Kawasaki Disease Committee of the Council on Cardiovascular Disease in the Young, the Interdisciplinary Council on Functional Genomics and Translational

Biology, and the Interdisciplinary Council on Quality of Care and Outcomes Research: endorsed by the American Academy of Pediatrics. Circulation 2009; 119(11):1541–51.

38. Uziel Y, Perl L, Barash J, et al. Post-streptococcal reactive arthritis in children: a distinct entity from acute rheumatic fever. Pediatr Rheumatol Online J 2011; 9(1):32.

39. Moore TL. Parvovirus-associated arthritis. Curr Opin Rheumatol 2000;12(4): 289–94.

40. Nguyen BY, Reveille JD. Rheumatic manifestations associated with HIV in the highly active antiretroviral therapy era. Curr Opin Rheumatol 2009;21(4):404–10.

Laboratory Testing in Pediatric Rheumatology

Jay Mehta, MD, MS

KEYWORDS

- Pediatric rheumatology • Diagnosis • Laboratory testing
- Biologic markers • Autoantibodies • Prognosis

Although pediatric rheumatic disorders are primarily diagnosed through history and physical examination, laboratory studies are valuable adjuncts to the care of patients with such disorders. Laboratory evaluations can assist in the screening of patients for inflammatory disorders, confirm diagnoses, allow for monitoring of disease activity and response to therapy, and suggest prognoses and risk of morbidities associated with rheumatic diseases.

Which laboratory tests are ordered should be dictated by a thorough history and physical examination, rather than by the indiscriminate use of a rheumatology screen. Although commonly ordered tests such as the complete blood count (CBC), antinuclear antigen (ANA), erythrocyte sedimentation rate (ESR), and C-reactive protein (CRP) are useful in the appropriate clinical setting, they lack specificity and abnormal values may be found in the well child. This review provides an overview of the usefulness and interpretation of both the commonly ordered tests ordered by the general pediatrician as well as those frequently used in the pediatric rheumatology clinic for diagnosis and disease monitoring.

CBC

The CBC provides information about the 3 major cellular components of whole blood. Rheumatic diseases may be associated with alterations in each of them.

Red Blood Cell Count

Anemia is seen in many of the rheumatic diseases and can be multifactorial. An anemia of chronic disease is usually normocytic, but may be microcytic, and can be associated with any inflammatory disease. The cause likely relates to cytokine-mediated shortened red blood cell (RBC) survival and impaired bone marrow response to erythropoietin.[1] Another major contribution to the anemia of chronic

---

Division of Pediatric Rheumatology, Albert Einstein College of Medicine, Children's Hospital at Montefiore, 3415 Bainbridge Avenue, Bronx, NY 10467, USA
E-mail address: jmehta@montefiore.org

Pediatr Clin N Am 59 (2012) 263–284
doi:10.1016/j.pcl.2012.03.008
0031-3955/12/$ – see front matter © 2012 Elsevier Inc. All rights reserved.

disease is the inflammation-induced activation of the interleukin 6 (IL-6)-hepcidin axis, which leads to decreased intestinal iron absorption and decreased iron release from stores.[2] This condition must be distinguished from iron-deficiency anemia, which can also be seen in any of the rheumatic diseases. **Table 1** contrasts these 2 conditions based on commonly used serum parameters. Complicating factors include the frequent coexistence of these 2 conditions and the fact that ferritin is an acute phase reactant so it may be normal, or even increased, in iron deficiency. Measurement of the soluble transferrin receptor, which is gaining acceptance, may help to more reliably distinguish anemia of chronic disease from iron-deficiency anemia.[3]

Autoimmune hemolytic anemia may be seen in systemic lupus erythematosus (SLE) and related conditions (ie, Sjögren syndrome and mixed connective tissue disease [MCTD]). This diagnosis is made through a positive direct Coombs test and evidence of hemolysis (decreased hemoglobin or hematocrit, increased reticulocyte count, increased serum lactate dehydrogenase (LDH), increased unconjugated bilirubin, decreased haptoglobin, and hemoglobinuria). Nonimmune-mediated hemolysis is seen in the macrophage activation syndrome (MAS) (see later discussion) and thrombotic thrombocytopenic purpura.

White Blood Cell Count

SLE and related conditions frequently cause leukopenia, specifically lymphopenia and neutropenia. These abnormalities may confer an increased risk of infection in patients with SLE.[4–6] Increased white blood cell (WBC) counts can be seen in other inflammatory diseases, and particularly increased counts may be seen in systemic juvenile idiopathic arthritis (sJIA; often >30,000 cells/mm^3). Malignancies can cause either increased or depressed WBC counts, and they must be considered in any patient who presents with WBC abnormalities.

Platelet Count

Because of their role as an acute phase reactant, platelets are frequently modestly increased in the rheumatic diseases. Significant increases (occasionally more than 1,000,000 cells/mm^3) may be seen in sJIA, Kawasaki disease, or Takayasu arteritis. SLE and related conditions often cause thrombocytopenia, and a depressed platelet count in the face of signs of systemic inflammation or arthritis should raise suspicion for these diseases or for malignancy. Thrombocytopenia may also be seen in the antiphospholipid antibody syndrome (APS) and in thrombotic thrombocytopenic purpura.

Table 1
Distinguishing features of anemia of chronic disease and iron-deficiency anemia

Parameter	ACD	IDA
MCV	Normal (can be ↓ in prolonged disease)	↓
Serum iron	↓	↓
Transferrin	↓	↑
Ferritin	Normal or ↑	↓ (can be normal if ACD+IDA)
STfR-ferritin index	<1.0	>2.0 (can also indicate ACD+IDA)
Transferrin saturation %	Normal (can be ↓)	↓

Abbreviations: ACD, anemia of chronic disease; IDA, iron-deficiency anemia; MCV, mean corpuscular volume; STfR, soluble transferrin receptor.

Special Considerations

MAS is a potentially life-threatening complication of any of the rheumatic diseases, and is particularly associated with sJIA. An overwhelming inflammatory reaction is seen and phagocytosis of all hematopoietic components ensues. Thus, any of WBC, RBC, and platelets may decrease. Therefore, normalization of previously increased WBC or platelets (and significantly increased ferritin level) in the face of a clinically worsening patient should alert the provider to the possibility of MAS.

ACUTE PHASE REACTANTS

The acute phase reactants are nonspecific markers of inflammation. Although they are frequently increased in inflammatory conditions, normal acute phase reactants should not be reassuring in a patient who presents with other signs of systemic inflammation (eg, fever, arthritis, failure to thrive). Conversely, in a child who is otherwise growing and developing normally, is afebrile, and has no persistent musculoskeletal complaints, checking acute phase reactants is of low yield and could lead to unnecessary further investigations.

ESR

The ESR evaluates the distance RBCs sediment in 1 hour. Its increase in inflammatory conditions primarily reflects increased fibrinogen production because fibrinogen is an acute phase reactant and causes RBCs to form rouleaux, which decrease at a faster rate than free RBCs. As an indirect measure of inflammation, the ESR can be influenced by several nonpathologic conditions. One of the most commonly encountered of these conditions in the pediatric outpatient setting is obesity, which can cause the ESR to be increased outside the normal age-specific range.[7] Other increasing factors include anemia, increasing age, and pregnancy.[8] For these reasons, mild increases in the ESR (ie, ESR <50 mm/h) in the absence of signs and symptoms of localized or systemic inflammation should not prompt further investigation or subspecialty referral. Conversely, an ESR of more than 100 mm/h is frequently associated with infection, malignancy, or inflammatory disease[9] and warrants further workup.

Although it is not specific for inflammatory diseases, the ESR is valuable as a tool to monitor disease activity and determine prognosis in patients with these conditions. Persistently increased ESR is predictive of a more aggressive course or worse outcome in sJIA,[10] enthesitis-related arthritis (ERA),[11] and oligoarticular JIA.[12,13] Increased ESR is associated with active synovitis in JIA[14] and a normal ESR is one of the provisional criteria for inactive disease in JIA.[15] The ESR is frequently normal in oligoarticular, and occasionally polyarticular, JIA, in contrast to malignancy (eg, leukemia or neuroblastoma), which may present with pain in 1 or a few joints but often has an extremely increased ESR. In SLE, an increased ESR has been shown to be associated with disease activity and damage accrual.[16] However, ESR increases are not always associated with disease activity. Likewise, a normal ESR does not invariably suggest inactive disease.

As previously mentioned, MAS is a severe complication of pediatric rheumatic diseases, most frequently seen with sJIA. Consequent to the intense systemic inflammation seen in MAS, hypofibrinogemia occurs, likely because of both liver dysfunction and fibrinogen consumption from coagulopathy.[17–19] This situation leads to a paradoxic decrease in the ESR. Therefore, a decreasing ESR in a patient who otherwise has active rheumatologic disease by clinical and other laboratory parameters should raise suspicion of MAS and indicate the need for emergent rheumatology consultation.

CRP

In contrast to the indirect association of ESR increase with inflammation, the CRP is produced by the liver as an acute phase reactant and plays a role in the innate host defense system.[20] It is a sensitive, but not specific, marker of inflammation. Plasma CRP more rapidly increases, in response to inflammation, and decreases, with its resolution, than does the ESR.

Similarly to the ESR, the CRP is predictive of disease course in JIA, although it may more closely reflect severe disease in polyarthritis.[21] Its normalization is a criterion for disease inactivity in JIA. One particular usefulness of the CRP in rheumatology is in the differentiation of flare from active infection in a patient with SLE. Given that either flare or infection can present with constitutional symptoms and that the immunosuppressive therapy used in SLE increases patients' risk for serious infection, this is often a difficult distinction to make clinically. Whereas the ESR can be increased in both disease flare and infection, the CRP tends not to increase with disease flare (with the exception of serositis) but does increase with active infection.[22] In a recent study of adult patients with SLE, a CRP greater than 5 mg/dL was 80% specific for infection.[23]

Ferritin

Ferritin is central to iron homeostasis and its synthesis and expression are regulated at multiple steps by iron, cytokines (IL-1, IL-6, and tumor necrosis factor α), hormones (thyroid hormones, insulin, and insulinlike growth factor 1), and oxidative stress.[24] During inflammation, serum ferritin level frequently increases in response to a decrease in serum iron. In sJIA, ferritin levels correlate with disease activity, with mild to moderate increases with active disease and normalization with quiescence.[25] Ferritin levels also correlate with disease activity in SLE,[26,27] but this is not a widely used method of monitoring patients, unlike in sJIA, in which it is part of routine surveillance and helps to guide treatment. In MAS, the ferritin level is often increased, and in hemophagocytic lymphohistiocytosis, which shares many similarities to MAS, the ferritin level is frequently more than 10,000 ng/mL.[28] Very low glycosylated ferritin percentage (<20%) has been seen in both adult-onset Still disease[29] and other hemophagocytic syndromes.[30] It remains to be established whether glycosylated ferritin measurement has a role in diagnosis of MAS associated with pediatric rheumatic diseases.

TESTS SPECIFIC TO RHEUMATOLOGIC DISEASES
ANA

Since the first description more than 50 years ago by Friou[31] of the binding to nuclear antigens by serum of patients with SLE, the ANA has been used as a serologic marker to aid in the diagnosis of SLE as well as other rheumatic diseases. The ANA also has special significance in pediatric rheumatology because of the well-recognized association of a positive ANA with an increased risk of chronic uveitis in patients with JIA.[32,33] However, up to 20% of children who are either healthy or have benign musculoskeletal complaints have a positive ANA,[34–36] and, therefore, results of ANA testing must be interpreted in combination with clinical findings. Although this positivity may persist,[35] most patients who present to a rheumatology clinic with a positive ANA but no autoimmune condition do not go on to develop any autoimmune disease.[36] For these reasons, the ANA should not be used as a screening tool without concerning joint symptoms (morning stiffness, persistent swelling) or signs of SLE (**Box 1**). Conversely, a negative ANA has a strong (0.96–1) negative predictive value for SLE, MCTD, and overlap syndromes.[37]

Box 1
Common signs of lupus

1. Persistent malar rash

2. Discoid rash

3. Photosensitivity: rash in reaction to sunlight

4. Oral or nasopharyngeal ulcers: usually painless

5. Arthritis: tenderness, swelling or effusion

6. Serositis: by history, examination, electrocardiography, or imaging

7. Proteinuria: >0.5 g/d or 3+ protein on dipstick

8. Urinary cellular casts

9. Seizures or psychosis in absence of other causes

10. Cytopenia

11. Alopecia: rapid loss of large amount of scalp hair

12. Raynaud phenomenon (RP)

The method used to perform the ANA testing influences interpretation of the results. The gold standard method[38] is immunofluorescence (IF) against human epithelial (HEp-2) cells, which have large nuclei and express a large number (>100) of nuclear antigens. From the IF, information about the pattern and intensity of staining is provided. The pattern of ANA staining on IF reflects the specific nuclear antigens to which the ANA is binding (**Fig. 1**). However, using the ANA pattern to diagnose specific autoimmune disorders has low sensitivity and specificity, and is being replaced by specific antinuclear antibody tests (see later discussion).

Some laboratories have moved to more automated commercial enzyme-linked immunosorbent assays (ELISAs), which allow for higher throughput of samples. The ELISA tests for serum absorbance to specified nuclear antigens. A disadvantage of this method arises when a patient has an ANA that binds to a nuclear antigen not present among the ones tested, which may lead to a false-negative test. This finding is of particular concern in patients with JIA, because the antigen specificity in ANA-positive patients is not known and is likely heterogenous.[39] Exclusive use of the ELISA in these patients could lead to misclassification of chronic uveitis risk.[40] The practice at our institution is to order both IF and ELISA on all patients with JIA.

In addition to SLE and JIA, other rheumatologic conditions are associated with a positive ANA (**Box 2**). In children with RP, the ANA predicts the risk of an underlying connective tissue disease, such as lupus or systemic sclerosis. In a retrospective study, 85% of children with secondary RP (RP associated with an underlying connective tissue disease) had a positive ANA, whereas only 25% of those with RP alone (primary RP) were ANA positive.[41]

As mentioned earlier, a positive ANA correlates with an increased risk of chronic, insidious uveitis in patients with JIA. ANA positivity more than triples the risk of uveitis in JIA,[42] and more than 80% of patients with JIA who develop uveitis are ANA positive.[42,43] Therefore, patients with JIA and a positive ANA are screened more frequently for chronic uveitis,[44] which is generally asymptomatic and detected only through slit-lamp examination by an ophthalmologist.

Indications for ordering an ANA are listed in **Box 3**.

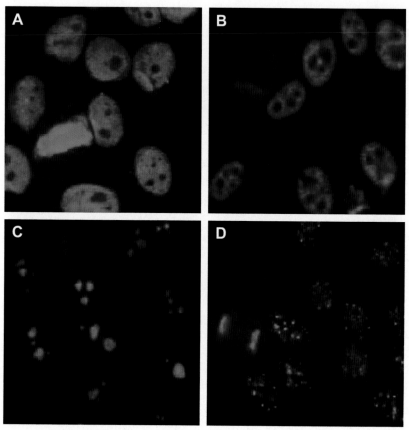

Fig. 1. ANA patterns on Immunofluorescence. (*A*) Homogenous; (*B*) Speckled; (*C*) Nucleolar; (*D*) Centromere. (*From* Damoiseaux JG, Tervaert JW. From ANA to ENA: how to proceed? Autoimmun Rev 2006;5:10–7; with permission.)

Specific Antinuclear Antibodies

Antibodies to specific nuclear antigens can be associated with specific diseases (**Table 2**). In addition, testing for anti-dsDNA antibodies has special value in the management of SLE, because increasing levels are predictive of flares of glomerulonephritis in patients with a history of renal disease.[45] For nonrenal manifestations of SLE, the relationship between persistently high or increasing anti-dsDNA levels and flare is less certain.[46–48]

Other than antihistone antibodies, tests for specific antinuclear antibodies are not usually positive in JIA. Therefore, the presence of specific antinuclear antibodies in a patient with chronic arthritis should suggest an alternative diagnosis than JIA.

Rheumatoid Factor

Rheumatoid factor (RF) is an antibody (typically IgM) directed against the F_c portion of IgG. The primary usefulness of RF measurement in the pediatric rheumatology clinic is differentiating between the 2 subtypes of polyarticular JIA: RF positive and RF negative. Unlike adult rheumatoid arthritis, most children with JIA do not have RF. Of patients with polyarthritis, approximately 85% are RF negative.[49,50] Testing for RF is generally not helpful in establishing or ruling out a diagnosis of JIA,[51] and it is indicated

---

Box 2
Conditions associated with a positive ANA

1. SLE
2. Drug-induced lupus
3. JIA
4. MCTD
5. Sjögren syndrome
6. Systemic sclerosis
7. RP
8. Juvenile dermatomyositis (JDM)
9. Malignancy
10. Autoimmune thyroiditis
11. Graves disease
12. Autoimmune hepatitis
13. Primary biliary cirrhosis
14. Autoimmune cholangitis
15. Chronic infections
16. Idiopathic pulmonary hypertension

---

only in patients who have objective signs of polyarthritis ($\geq$4 affected joints). In those patients with polyarthritis who are RF positive, the course tends to be more aggressive, with more long-term disability[52] and the lowest remission rates among juvenile arthritis subtypes.[53] Other rheumatologic conditions are associated with a positive RF (**Box 4**). The clinical significance of RF in these conditions is unknown.

Anticyclic Citrullinated Peptide Antibodies

In rheumatoid arthritis, inflamed synovium contains citrullinated peptides, and patients with RA produce antibodies that bind specifically to substrates that contain citrulline.[54] In adults, anticyclic citrullinated peptide (anti-CCP) antibodies are highly specific for RA and may be present before the onset of symptoms.[55] These antibodies are found primarily in children with polyarticular, and rarely other subsets of, JIA.[56–58] Anti-CCP antibodies have been associated with more aggressive disease,[58] even in RF-negative polyarticular patients, and may indicate the need for more aggressive therapy. The precise role of anti-CCP testing in JIA has not been established.

Antineutrophil Cytoplasmic Antibodies

Antineutrophil cytoplasmic antibodies (ANCA) were discovered to have an association with granulomatosis with polyangiitis (GPA; formerly known as Wegener granulomatosis)

Box 3
Indications for ordering an ANA

1. A patient with signs or symptoms suggestive of SLE (see **Box 1**)
2. Assessment of the risk of uveitis in a patient with JIA
3. Assessment of the risk of an underlying connective tissue disease in a patient with RP

Table 2
Specific antinuclear antibody disease associations

Antibody Specificity	Disease Association
SS-A (Ro)	Sjögren syndrome. SLE. NLE
SS-B (La)	Sjögren syndrome. SLE. NLE
Smith	SLE
Double-stranded DNA	SLE
Centromere	Limited cutaneous systemic sclerosis
Topoisomerase 1 (Scl-70)	Diffuse cutaneous systemic sclerosis
Pm-Scl	Myositis-scleroderma overlap
Ribonucleoprotein	MCTD
Histone	SLE. Drug-induced SLE

Abbreviation: NLE, neonatal lupus erythematosus.

in 1985.[59,60] Since then, it has been found to be closely associated with 2 other systemic vasculitides: microscopic polyangiitis (MPA) and Churg-Strauss syndrome. In these conditions, the target of ANCA-binding is usually either myeloperoxidase (MPO) or serine protease 3 (PR3), which are found in granules of neutrophils and macrophages. The binding of ANCA to its target likely plays a pathogenic role in the pathophysiology of ANCA-associated vasculitis (AAV).[61] This topic is discussed in more detail in the article on vasculitis by Weiss elsewhere in this issue.

Two methods are used to measure the ANCA: indirect IF and ELISA. Each method has clinical usefulness and both are usually ordered in patients in whom systemic vasculitis is suspected. IF is more sensitive, whereas ELISA is more specific. On IF, one of 2 staining patterns (**Fig. 2**) may be seen: cytoplasmic (c-ANCA) or perinuclear (p-ANCA). ELISA measures antibodies against MPO and PR3. c-ANCA staining on IF usually correlates with a positive ELISA for PR3, and this pattern is primarily seen in GPA. p-ANCA staining usually correlates with a positive MPO ELISA, and this pattern is primarily seen in MPA. However, the associations among IF staining, ELISA, and disease are not rigid and some crossover may be seen (**Table 3**). There are other conditions in which a positive ANCA by IF is found (**Box 5**). Other than drug exposure, these conditions are generally not associated with positive ELISA for anti-PR3 or anti-MPO antibodies.

Box 4
Rheumatologic conditions associated with a positive RF

1. Polyarticular JIA
2. Rheumatoid arthritis
3. SLE
4. Systemic sclerosis
5. MCTD
6. Sjögren syndrome
7. Sarcoidosis

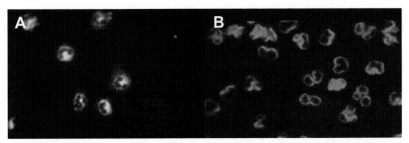

Fig. 2. ANCA patterns on immunofluorescence. (*A*) Cytoplasmic (c-ANCA); (*B*) Perinuclear (p-ANCA). (*From* Calabrese LH, Molloy ES, Duna G. Antineutrophil cytoplasmic antibody–associated vasculitis. In: Firestein GS, Budd RC, Harris ED, et al, editors. Kelley's Textbook of Rheumatology, 8th edition. Philadelphia: WB Saunders, 2008; with permission.)

Given the protean presentation of systemic vasculitis, the question of when to order ANCA testing arises. Situations in which systemic vasculitis should be suspected are listed in **Box 6**.

Antiphospholipid Antibodies

Antiphospholipid antibodies (APLs) are a group of antibodies that, through effects on platelets, endothelial cells, neutrophils, and monocytes, lead to an increased risk of arterial and venous thromboembolic events. These antibodies may be transiently found in healthy children, and, therefore, diagnosis of the APS requires at least 2 positive measurements (for the same positive antibody) 12 weeks apart along with clinical criteria (**Table 4**). Persistently positive APLs or the APS may be found in patients with no other findings or in patients with an underlying rheumatologic disorder (most commonly SLE).

There are 3 commonly used tests to assay for APLs: (1) lupus anticoagulant (LA) tests; (2) ELISA for anticardiolipin (ACL) IgG and IgM; (3) ELISA for anti-β_2-glycoprotein-I (anti-β_2GPI) IgG and IgM. LA is tested for through either the activated partial thromboplastin time (aPTT) or the dilute Russell viper venom time (DRVVT). In patients with APLs, the aPTT is paradoxically prolonged, despite the prothrombotic state that APLs confer. However, only half of patients with LA have a prolonged aPTT and the DRVVT is a more sensitive test for LA. The DRVVT test uses the ability of the venom of the Russell viper to activate factor X and set off the intrinsic clotting cascade. However, as with the aPTT test, APLs interfere with the ability of phospholipids to promote in vitro thrombosis and thus prolong the DRVVT. The prolongation of both

Table 3		
ANCA by IF, ELISA, and disease association in AAV		
Disease	**IF (%)**	**ELISA (%)**
Granulomatosis with	66 c-ANCA	68 PR3
polyangiitis (Wegener)[a]	21 p-AWCA	14 MPO
Microscopic polyangiitis[b]	23 c-ANCA	25 PR3
	58 p-ANCA	58 MPO

[a] *Data from* Cabral DA, Uribe AG, Benseler SM, et al. Classification, presentation and initial treatment of Wegener's granulomatosis in childhood. Arthritis Rheum 2009;60:3413–24.
[b] *Data from* Hagen EC, Daha MR, Hermans J, et al. Diagnostic value of standardized assays for antineutrophil cytoplasmic antibodies in idiopathic systemic vasculitis. EC/BCR Project for ANCA Assay Standardization. Kidney Int 1998;53:743–53.

Box 5
Conditions associated with a positive ANCA

1. Inflammatory bowel disease (IBD)

2. Rheumatoid arthritis

3. SLE

4. Myositis

5. Cystic fibrosis

6. Sclerosing cholangitis

7. Autoimmune hepatitis

8. Infections

   a. Endocarditis

   b. Human immunodeficiency virus

9. Drugs

   a. Hydralazine

   b. Propylthiouracil

   c. D-penicillamine

   d. Minocycline

---

the aPTT and DRVVT is not reversed when patient's plasma is mixed with normal plasma. In children, a persistently positive LA test is only somewhat sensitive (72%)[62] for the APS, but confers a strong risk for thrombotic events,[63] especially in patients with underlying SLE.[64–66]

ELISA for ACL is the most sensitive test for APS in children,[62] and its specificity increases with increasing titer.[67] Many APLs are directed against β_2-glycoprotein-I and the anti-β_2GPI ELISA tests for these antibodies. Anti-β_2GPI ELISA is the least sensitive of the APLs in children[62] but is more specific than the ACL for thrombosis, especially in patients with SLE.[68] It is unknown whether other frequently tested APLs, such as ACL IgA and anti-β_2GPI IgA antibodies, and antibodies to prothrombin, phosphatidylserine, and phosphatidylethanolamine confer an increased thrombosis risk.[69]

Recent work by Wahezi and colleagues[70] has suggested that the annexin A5 resistance assay, a newly developed test of annexin A5 anticoagulant activity, is strongly associated with persistent APLs. In addition, decreased annexin A5 resistance was seen in children with rheumatic diseases who had thrombotic events. At our institution, we obtain annexin A5 resistance testing on all lupus patients and on those with suspected APS.

Box 6
When to consider ANCA testing

1. Fever of unclear cause >2 weeks

2. Multiple organ disease (especially lung, kidney, or neurologic disease)

3. Petechial or purpuric rash

4. Unexplained signs of systemic inflammation (increased ESR of CRP, anemia of chronic disease, thrombocytosis

Table 4 Classification criteria for APS	
Clinical Criteria	
1 Vascular thrombosis	≥ 1 clinical episode of arterial, venous, or small vessel thrombosis in any tissue or organ
2 Pregnancy morbidity	a. ≥ 1 unexplained deaths of a morphologically normal fetus at or beyond the 10th week of gestation
	OR
	b. ≥ 1 premature births of a morphologically normal neonate before the 34th week of gestation because of: (1) eclampsia or severe preeclampsia or (2) placental insufficiency
	OR
	c. ≥ 3 unexplained consecutive spontaneous abortions before the 10th week of gestation
Laboratory Criteria (require 2 or more positive tests at least 12 weeks apart):	
1 Lupus anticoagulant present in plasma	
2 Anticardiolipin antibody of IgG or IgM isotype in serum or plasma, present in medium or high titer (ie, >40 GPL or MPL, or >99th percentile)	
3 Anti-β2 glycoprotein-I antibody of IgG or IgM isotype in serum or plasma (in titer >99th percentile)	

APS criteria met if ≥ 1 clinical criteria and ≥ 1 laboratory criteria.
Abbreviations: GPL, IgG phospholipid standardized units; MPL, IgM phospholipid standardized units.

Adapted from Miyakis S, Lockshin MD, Atsumi T, et al. International consensus statement on an update of the classification criteria for definite antiphospholipid syndrome. J Thromb Haemost 2006;4:295–306; with permission.

APS should be suspected and APLs testing obtained in patients with a history of any of the clinical criteria in **Table 4** or with the suggestive findings described in **Box 7**.

LABORATORY TESTS FREQUENTLY USED IN RHEUMATOLOGY
Muscle Enzymes

Serum levels of muscle enzymes are most commonly used in pediatric rheumatology for the diagnosis and management of JDM. Individual patients may have increases in any of the commonly tested enzymes throughout their disease course, and, therefore, serial measurement of creatine kinase (CK), alanine aminotransferase (ALT), aspartate aminotransferase (AST), LDH, and aldolase is recommended. However, normal values for these enzymes do not rule out a diagnosis of JDM; up to 26% of children with JDM, in a retrospective study, had a normal value for at least 1 enzyme at presentation.[71] In a retrospective study in adults with dermatomyositis or polymyositis, increases in CK heralded a flare of disease up to a month before relapse and normalization of CK was present weeks before muscle strength improvement.[72] However, in children with JDM, it was reported that LDH and AST predicted flares, and neither CK nor ALT was associated with disease flare.[73] It has been suggested that LDH is the most useful muscle enzyme because it best predicts global disease activity in patients with long-standing disease.[74]

Each of these enzymes has sources other than muscle, and, therefore, other conditions may lead to their increase (**Table 5**).

Box 7
Nonthrombotic clinical findings suggestive of APS

1. Dermatologic
   a. Livedo reticularis
   b. RP
   c. Digital necrosis
   d. Splinter hemorrhages
   e. Skin ulcers
2. Hematologic
   a. Thrombocytopenia
   b. Autoimmune hemolytic anemia
3. Neurologic
   a. Migraine headaches
   b. Seizures
   c. Chorea
4. Cardiac
   a. Sterile endocarditis
   b. Cardiomyopathy

Serum Complement Levels

Complement C3 and C4 levels are frequently measured as an adjunct to the clinical diagnosis and monitoring of patients with SLE. The rationale for this situation is activation of the classic and alternative pathways with antibody-antigen binding in SLE. Multiple studies have shown that decreased C3 or C4 levels correlate with increased renal and extrarenal activity or disease flare.[75–79] In addition, normalization of complement levels has been associated with disease improvement.[75] However, flares are not always accompanied by decreases in C3 and C4,[80] and some patients have persistently low complement levels despite disease inactivity.[48,81] Therefore, complement levels need to be considered in the context of clinical findings and other markers of disease activity when making decisions about therapy.

Inherited and acquired deficiencies of certain complement components (C1, C2, C3, C4, mannose-binding lectin, and C1-inhibitor) are associated with SLE or SLE-like diseases.[82] The CH_{50} is a reliable screen for homozygous deficiencies in the classic pathway components, which have the strongest association with lupus and

---

Table 5
Nonmuscle sources of muscle enzymes

Enzyme	Sources
CK	Heart, brain
ALT	Liver
AST	Liver, heart, kidney, brain, erythrocytes
LDH	Liver, erythrocytes, heart, kidney, brain, lung
Aldolase	Liver, heart, erythrocytes, brain, kidney

lupuslike illnesses. This test quantifies complement activity by assaying the ability of patient's serum to lyse sheep erythrocytes coated with rabbit antisheep IgM. A homozygous deficiency in any of the classic pathway components gives an undetectable CH_{50} (except homozygous C9 deficiency, which may give a low CH_{50}). Indications for screening for complement deficiencies are listed in **Box 8**.

Urinalysis

The kidney can be affected as a primary manifestation of SLE (and related disorders) and the AAV, as well as a complication of amyloidosis in sJIA and the periodic fever syndromes. The American College of Rheumatology criteria for renal involvement in SLE require either persistent proteinuria of greater than 0.5 g/d (or 3+ albumin on dipstick) or cellular casts of any type.[83] For proteinuria measurements, urine spot protein/creatinine ratios have been increasingly accepted as a more convenient method for determining protein excretion. The rule of thumb that the ratio of spot urine protein to creatinine approximates the grams of urine protein excretion per day has been shown to hold true in lupus nephritis[84] and other glomerular diseases.[85] Thus, a ratio of greater than 0.2 is of concern and may warrant further monitoring and testing. Conversely, the urine dipstick for albumin lacks precision and correlation with the 24-hour total protein measurement and should not be used for diagnosis or monitoring of glomerular disease.[86]

Detection of cellular casts, which may be seen in SLE and AAV, requires prompt examination of urine as casts deteriorate over time. Community-based clinical laboratories often are not able to reliably detect pathologic casts,[87] and, therefore, urine from those patients for whom the clinician has a high suspicion of renal disease should be examined microscopically by an experienced hospital-based clinical pathology laboratory or by a nephrologist. Whereas proteinuria may be seen with any of the classes of lupus nephritis, the presence of RBC casts reflects a nephritic syndrome that is typically seen only with diffuse proliferative (class IV), advanced sclerotic (class VI), or a thrombotic microangiopathy.[88]

Angiotensin-converting Enzyme and Lysozyme

The angiotensin-converting enzyme (ACE) level is frequently increased in sarcoidosis, and the level of increase corresponds to clinical disease activity.[89] The source of increased ACE in sarcoidosis is alveolar macrophages[90] and granulomatous epithelioid cells.[91] A large, multicenter study of patients with sarcoidosis revealed the sensitivity of ACE for sarcoidosis to be 57%, specificity of 90%, positive predictive value of 90%, and negative predictive value of 60%.[92] Increases in the ACE level in an individual patient may reflect progressive, rather than stable, disease.[93] ACE gene polymorphisms contribute to interindividual variability in ACE levels between both

---

Box 8
Indications for suspecting a complement deficiency

1. Recurrent, unexplained pyogenic or *Neisseria* infections

2. Patients with SLE with a family history of SLE

3. Subacute cutaneous lupus

4. Very young (<7 years old) patient with SLE or SLE-like disease

5. Recurrent angioedema

patients with sarcoidosis[82] and normal controls,[54] and it has been suggested that ACE genotyping be used in the interpretation of ACE levels.[66]

Stimulated mononuclear phagocytes in sarcoidosis secrete lysozyme, and increased lysozyme levels are seen in patients with sarcoidosis.[94] The serum lysozyme level, like the ACE, can be followed as an indicator of disease activity.[95] Lysozyme is more sensitive than ACE for sarcoidosis (79% vs 59% in 1 study[96]). However, the specificity is only 60% and abnormal values can be seen in many other diseases, including tuberculosis. In patients for whom sarcoidosis is suspected, assaying both ACE and lysozyme is recommended.

Streptococcal Antibody Tests

Streptococcal antibody tests provide evidence for previous infection with group A streptococcus (GAS) and are used in pediatric rheumatology to aid in the diagnosis of acute rheumatic fever (ARF) and poststreptococcal reactive arthritis (PSRA). The most commonly used ones are the antistreptolysin O (ASO), anti-DNase B (ADB), and streptozyme. The streptozyme provides no useful information beyond that provided by the ASO and ADB and, furthermore, lacks reproducibility. It should, therefore, not be used as a test of GAS exposure.

Antibodies to GAS peak approximately 3 weeks after an acute infection.[70] Both ASO and ADB should be obtained in patients for whom either of these diseases are suspected because almost 20% of patients with ARF, in 1 study, had a negative result for at least 1 of the tests[29] but 92% were positive for at least 1 of these 2 tests. In contrast, a study of 25 patients with PSRA showed an increase in at least 1 antibody for all patients.[30] After treatment of ARF, ASO levels may begin to normalize after 2 months but can stay increased for 6 to 12 months[97] (longer if reinfection occurs). There is no correlation between level of ASO and clinical manifestations of ARF.[98] The height of ASO increase does not help in differentiating between ARF (mean 1011 IU) and PSRA (mean 889 IU).[99]

GENETIC TESTS USED IN RHEUMATOLOGY
HLA-B27

There is a well-established relationship between the HLA class I allele HLA-B27 and ankylosing spondylitis (AS) in both children (in whom it is known as ERA)[100] and adults.[101] ERA is one of a group of diseases known as the juvenile spondyloarthropathies (JSpA), which have as their defining characteristic inflammation of the axial skeleton and entheses (the sites of tendon, ligament, fascia, and capsule attachment to bone). JSpA is an umbrella term encompassing ERA, juvenile AS, reactive arthritis (ReA), arthritis associated with IBD, and juvenile psoriatic arthritis (PsA). Detailing the nuances in classification of JSpA is beyond the scope of this review, but each of these diseases is associated with HLA-B27. Testing for HLA-B27 is most useful in a male older than 8 years who presents with any of the symptoms listed in **Box 9**. The presence of a first-degree relative with similar symptoms increases the usefulness of testing.

Although the diagnosis of JSpA is made on clinical grounds, testing for HLA-B27 helps for classification purposes, because patients with JAS are more likely to be positive than those with other types of JSpA and the presence of HLA-B27 in patients with undefined JSpA predicts evolution to an identifiable disease. However, 5% to 10% of the normal population is positive for HLA-B27,[102,103] and only about 1% of all HLA-B27–positive individuals in the general population go on to develop AS.[103]

Box 9
Indications for testing HLA-B27

1. Arthritis in a male >8 years old

2. ReA

3. Inflammatory back pain[a]

4. Sacroiliac joint tenderness

5. Enthesitis

6. Arthritis in a patient with a family history of AS, ERA, PsA, ReA, acute uveitis, or IBD

7. Acute uveitis

[a] Inflammatory back pain is pain that is present in the morning (or the second half of the night), improves with exercise, has an insidious onset, and does not improve with rest.

Genetic Testing for Hereditary Periodic Fever Syndromes

Periodic fever syndromes (PFS) are defined as 3 or more episodes of fever, with no other defined medical illness to explain the fevers, in a 6-month period, with at least 7 days between episodes.[104] The hereditary PFS, which can be distinguished by their clinical characteristics and gene abnormalities, are listed in **Table 6**. Further details on the clinical presentation, genetics, and ethnic predilection for each of these PFS are found in the article on autoinflammatory diseases by Hashkes and Toker elsewhere in this issue. Commercial testing (GeneDx; Gaithersburg, MD) for mutations underlying familial Mediterranean fever (FMF); tumor necrosis factor receptor-associated periodic syndrome (TRAPS); hyper-IgD syndrome (HIDS); Muckle-Wells syndrome; familial cold autoinflammatory syndrome; neonatal-onset multisystem inflammatory disorder; cyclic hematopoiesis; pyogenic arthritis, pyoderma gangrenosum, and acne syndrome; and Majeed syndrome is available as a single panel. The sensitivity

---

Table 6
Gene abnormalities and clinical features of hereditary PFS

Syndrome	Gene	Distinctive Clinical Features
FMF	MEFV	Arthritis, peritonitis, erysipeloidlike rash
TRAPS	TNFRS1A	Macular migratory erythema, myalgia
HIDS	MVK	Erythematous macules, oral and vaginal ulcers
FCAS	CIAS1	Cold-induced symptoms, urticarial rash
MWS	CIAS1	Urticarial rash, sensorineural hearing loss
NOMID	CIAS1	Urticarial rash, meningitis, bone abnormalities
CH	ELA2	ANC <200/μL, recurrent oral infections
PAPA	PSTPIP1/CD2BP1	Recurrent arthritis, pyoderma gangrenosum, acne

Abbreviations: CH, cyclic hematopoiesis; FCAS, familial cold autoinflammatory syndrome; FMF, familial Mediterranean fever; HIDS, hyper-IgD syndrome; MWS, Muckle-Wells syndrome; NOMID, neonatal-onset multisystem inflammatory disorder; PAPA, pyogenic arthritis, pyoderma gangrenosum, and acne syndrome; TRAPS, tumor necrosis factor receptor-associated periodic syndrome.

and specificity of the individual tests varies widely, because only the most common mutations are tested and some mutations may be polymorphisms in certain ethnicities. Given this situation, only patients whose clinical symptoms, ethnicity, or family history lead to a strong clinical suspicion of a hereditary PFS should be tested. Gottorno and colleagues[105] used a set of clinical criteria including age, abdominal pain, aphthosis, thoracic pain, diarrhea, and family history to develop a decision tree for which patients should receive genetic testing for FMF, HIDS, and TRAPS. This algorithm had good sensitivity (82%) and moderate specificity (72%).

SUMMARY

Laboratory tests can suggest or confirm diagnoses, offer prognosis, and guide therapy in children with rheumatic diseases. They may also be a source of unnecessary consternation and cost for patients, families, and health care providers, especially given the varied sensitivity and specificity of many of these tests. Therefore, primary care and rheumatology providers are encouraged to let the patient's signs and symptoms guide the laboratory workup. The otherwise well child with occasional musculoskeletal complaints likely does not need an extensive laboratory evaluation; conversely, the child who presents with persistent complaints or signs of systemic illness is well served by a focused and sequential workup. When used in this way, these tests play an invaluable role in the care of our patients.

REFERENCES

1. Greer J, Foerster J, Rodgers GM, et al, editors. Wintrobe's Clinical Hematology. 11th edition. Philadelphia: Lippincott Williams & Wilkins; 2008.
2. Nemeth E, Rivera S, Gabayan V, et al. IL-6 mediates hypoferremia of inflammation by inducing the synthesis of the iron regulatory hormone hepcidin. J Clin Invest 2004;113:1271–6.
3. Koulaouzidis A, Said E, Cottier R, et al. Soluble transferrin receptors and iron deficiency, a step beyond ferritin. A systematic review. J Gastrointestin Liver Dis 2009;18:345–52.
4. Dias AM, do Couto MC, Duarte CC, et al. White blood cell count abnormalities and infections in one-year follow-up of 124 patients with SLE. Ann N Y Acad Sci 2009;1173:103–7.
5. Kinder BW, Freemer MM, King TE Jr, et al. Clinical and genetic risk factors for pneumonia in systemic lupus erythematosus. Arthritis Rheum 2007;56:2679–86.
6. Ng WL, Chu CM, Wu AK, et al. Lymphopenia at presentation is associated with increased risk of infections in patients with systemic lupus erythematosus. QJM 2006;99:37–47.
7. Leff RD, Akre SP. Obesity and the erythrocyte sedimentation rate. Ann Intern Med 1986;105:143.
8. Sox HC Jr, Liang MH. The erythrocyte sedimentation rate. Guidelines for rational use. Ann Intern Med 1986;104:515–23.
9. Fincher RM, Page MI. Clinical significance of extreme elevation of the erythrocyte sedimentation rate. Arch Intern Med 1986;146:1581–3.
10. Singh-Grewal D, Schneider R, Bayer N, et al. Predictors of disease course and remission in systemic juvenile idiopathic arthritis: significance of early clinical and laboratory features. Arthritis Rheum 2006;54:1595–601.
11. Flato B, Hoffmann-Vold AM, Reiff A, et al. Long-term outcome and prognostic factors in enthesitis-related arthritis: a case-control study. Arthritis Rheum 2006;54:3573–82.

12. Guillaume S, Prieur AM, Coste J, et al. Long-term outcome and prognosis in oligoarticular-onset juvenile idiopathic arthritis. Arthritis Rheum 2000;43: 1858–65.
13. Al-Matar MJ, Petty RE, Tucker LB, et al. The early pattern of joint involvement predicts disease progression in children with oligoarticular (pauciarticular) juvenile rheumatoid arthritis. Arthritis Rheum 2002;46:2708–15.
14. Gilliam BE, Chauhan AK, Low JM, et al. Measurement of biomarkers in juvenile idiopathic arthritis patients and their significant association with disease severity: a comparative study. Clin Exp Rheumatol 2008;26:492–7.
15. Wallace CA, Giannini EH, Huang B, et al. American College of Rheumatology provisional criteria for defining clinical inactive disease in select categories of juvenile idiopathic arthritis. Arthritis Care Res (Hoboken) 2011;63:929–36.
16. Vila LM, Alarcon GS, McGwin G Jr, et al. Systemic lupus erythematosus in a multiethnic cohort (LUMINA): XXIX. Elevation of erythrocyte sedimentation rate is associated with disease activity and damage accrual. J Rheumatol 2005;32:2150–5.
17. Hadchouel M, Prieur AM, Griscelli C. Acute hemorrhagic, hepatic, and neurologic manifestations in juvenile rheumatoid arthritis: possible relationship to drugs or infection. J Pediatr 1985;106:561–6.
18. Stephan JL, Zeller J, Hubert P, et al. Macrophage activation syndrome and rheumatic disease in childhood: a report of four new cases. Clin Exp Rheumatol 1993;11:451–6.
19. Sawhney S, Woo P, Murray KJ. Macrophage activation syndrome: a potentially fatal complication of rheumatic disorders. Arch Dis Child 2001;85:421–6.
20. Volanakis JE. Human C-reactive protein: expression, structure, and function. Mol Immunol 2001;38:189–97.
21. Gwyther M, Schwarz H, Howard A, et al. C-reactive protein in juvenile chronic arthritis: an indicator of disease activity and possibly amyloidosis. Ann Rheum Dis 1982;41:259–62.
22. Pepys MB, Lanham JG, De Beer FC. C-reactive protein in SLE. Clin Rheum Dis 1982;8:91–103.
23. Firooz N, Albert DA, Wallace DJ, et al. High-sensitivity C-reactive protein and erythrocyte sedimentation rate in systemic lupus erythematosus. Lupus 2011; 20:588–97.
24. Zandman-Goddard G, Shoenfeld Y. Ferritin in autoimmune diseases. Autoimmun Rev 2007;6:457–63.
25. Pelkonen P, Swanljung K, Siimes MA. Ferritinemia as an indicator of systemic disease activity in children with systemic juvenile rheumatoid arthritis. Acta Paediatr Scand 1986;75:64–8.
26. Lim MK, Lee CK, Ju YS, et al. Serum ferritin as a serologic marker of activity in systemic lupus erythematosus. Rheumatol Int 2001;20:89–93.
27. Beyan E, Beyan C, Demirezer A, et al. The relationship between serum ferritin levels and disease activity in systemic lupus erythematosus. Scand J Rheumatol 2003;32:225–8.
28. Allen CE, Yu X, Kozinetz CA, et al. Highly elevated ferritin levels and the diagnosis of hemophagocytic lymphohistiocytosis. Pediatr Blood Cancer 2008;50: 1227–35.
29. Van Reeth C, Le Moel G, Lasne Y, et al. Serum ferritin and isoferritins are tools for diagnosis of active adult Still's disease. J Rheumatol 1994;21:890–5.
30. Fardet L, Coppo P, Kettaneh A, et al. Low glycosylated ferritin, a good marker for the diagnosis of hemophagocytic syndrome. Arthritis Rheum 2008;58:1521–7.

31. Friou GJ, Finch SC, Detre KD. Interaction of nuclei and globulin from lupus erythematosis serum demonstrated with fluorescent antibody. J Immunol 1958; 80:324–9.

32. Schaller JG, Johnson GD, Holborow EJ, et al. The association of antinuclear antibodies with the chronic iridocyclitis of juvenile rheumatoid arthritis (Still's disease). Arthritis Rheum 1974;17:409–16.

33. Egeskjold EM, Johansen A, Permin H, et al. The significance of antinuclear antibodies in juvenile rheumatoid arthritis associated with chronic bilateral iridocyclitis. Acta Paediatr Scand 1982;71:615–20.

34. Allen RC, Dewez P, Stuart L, et al. Antinuclear antibodies using HEp-2 cells in normal children and in children with common infections. J Paediatr Child Health 1991;27:39–42.

35. Cabral DA, Petty RE, Fung M, et al. Persistent antinuclear antibodies in children without identifiable inflammatory rheumatic or autoimmune disease. Pediatrics 1992;89:441–4.

36. Deane PM, Liard G, Siegel DM, et al. The outcome of children referred to a pediatric rheumatology clinic with a positive antinuclear antibody test but without an autoimmune disease. Pediatrics 1995;95:892–5.

37. Malleson PN, Sailer M, Mackinnon MJ. Usefulness of antinuclear antibody testing to screen for rheumatic diseases. Arch Dis Child 1997;77:299–304.

38. American College of Rheumatology Position Statement: Methodology of testing for antinuclear antibodies. Available at: www.rheumatology.org/practice/clinical/position/ana_position_stmt.pdf. Accessed March 20, 2012.

39. Reiff A, Haubruck H, Amos MD. Evaluation of a recombinant antigen enzyme-linked immunosorbent assay (ELISA) in the diagnostics of antinuclear antibodies (ANA) in children with rheumatic disorders. Clin Rheumatol 2002;21:103–7.

40. Nordal EB, Songstad NT, Berntson L, et al. Biomarkers of chronic uveitis in juvenile idiopathic arthritis: predictive value of antihistone antibodies and antinuclear antibodies. J Rheumatol 2009;36:1737–43.

41. Nigrovic PA, Fuhlbrigge RC, Sundel RP. Raynaud's phenomenon in children: a retrospective review of 123 patients. Pediatrics 2003;111:715–21.

42. Saurenmann RK, Levin AV, Feldman BM, et al. Prevalence, risk factors, and outcome of uveitis in juvenile idiopathic arthritis: a long-term followup study. Arthritis Rheum 2007;56:647–57.

43. Heiligenhaus A, Niewerth M, Ganser G, et al. Prevalence and complications of uveitis in juvenile idiopathic arthritis in a population-based nation-wide study in Germany: suggested modification of the current screening guidelines. Rheumatology (Oxford) 2007;46:1015–9.

44. American Academy of Pediatrics Section on Rheumatology and Section on Ophthalmology: Guidelines for ophthalmologic examinations in children with juvenile rheumatoid arthritis. Pediatrics 1993;92:295–6.

45. Linnik MD, Hu JZ, Heilbrunn KR, et al. Relationship between anti-double-stranded DNA antibodies and exacerbation of renal disease in patients with systemic lupus erythematosus. Arthritis Rheum 2005;52:1129–37.

46. ter Borg EJ, Horst G, Hummel EJ, et al. Measurement of increases in anti-double-stranded DNA antibody levels as a predictor of disease exacerbation in systemic lupus erythematosus. A long-term, prospective study. Arthritis Rheum 1990;33:634–43.

47. Esdaile JM, Abrahamowicz M, Joseph L, et al. Laboratory tests as predictors of disease exacerbations in systemic lupus erythematosus. Why some tests fail. Arthritis Rheum 1996;39:370–8.

48. Gladman DD, Urowitz MB, Keystone EC. Serologically active clinically quiescent systemic lupus erythematosus: a discordance between clinical and serologic features. Am J Med 1979;66:210–5.
49. Saurenmann RK, Rose JB, Tyrrell P, et al. Epidemiology of juvenile idiopathic arthritis in a multiethnic cohort: ethnicity as a risk factor. Arthritis Rheum 2007; 56:1974–84.
50. Adib N, Hyrich K, Thornton J, et al. Association between duration of symptoms and severity of disease at first presentation to paediatric rheumatology: results from the Childhood Arthritis Prospective Study. Rheumatology (Oxford) 2008;47: 991–5.
51. Eichenfield AH, Athreya BH, Doughty RA, et al. Utility of rheumatoid factor in the diagnosis of juvenile rheumatoid arthritis. Pediatrics 1986;78:480–4.
52. Packham JC, Hall MA. Long-term follow-up of 246 adults with juvenile idiopathic arthritis: functional outcome. Rheumatology (Oxford) 2002;41:1428–35.
53. Wallace CA, Huang B, Bandeira M, et al. Patterns of clinical remission in select categories of juvenile idiopathic arthritis. Arthritis Rheum 2005;52:3554–62.
54. Schellekens GA, de Jong BA, van den Hoogen FH, et al. Citrulline is an essential constituent of antigenic determinants recognized by rheumatoid arthritis-specific autoantibodies. J Clin Invest 1998;101:273–81.
55. Rantapaa-Dahlqvist S, de Jong BA, Berglin E, et al. Antibodies against cyclic citrullinated peptide and IgA rheumatoid factor predict the development of rheumatoid arthritis. Arthritis Rheum 2003;48:2741–9.
56. Brunner J, Sitzmann FC. The diagnostic value of anti-cyclic citrullinated peptide (CCP) antibodies in children with Juvenile Idiopathic Arthritis. Clin Exp Rheumatol 2006;24:449–51.
57. Ferucci ED, Majka DS, Parrish LA, et al. Antibodies against cyclic citrullinated peptide are associated with HLA-DR4 in simplex and multiplex polyarticular-onset juvenile rheumatoid arthritis. Arthritis Rheum 2005;52:239–46.
58. Syed RH, Gilliam BE, Moore TL. Prevalence and significance of isotypes of anti-cyclic citrullinated peptide antibodies in juvenile idiopathic arthritis. Ann Rheum Dis 2008;67:1049–51.
59. Hall JB, Wadham BM, Wood CJ, et al. Vasculitis and glomerulonephritis: a subgroup with an antineutrophil cytoplasmic antibody. Aust N Z J Med 1984;14:277–8.
60. van der Woude FJ, Rasmussen N, Lobatto S, et al. Autoantibodies against neutrophils and monocytes: tool for diagnosis and marker of disease activity in Wegener's granulomatosis. Lancet 1985;1:425–9.
61. Kallenberg CG. Pathophysiology of ANCA-associated small vessel vasculitis. Curr Rheumatol Rep 2010;12:399–405.
62. Avcin T, Cimaz R, Silverman ED, et al. Pediatric antiphospholipid syndrome: clinical and immunologic features of 121 patients in an international registry. Pediatrics 2008;122:e1100–7.
63. Galli M, Luciani D, Bertolini G, et al. Lupus anticoagulants are stronger risk factors for thrombosis than anticardiolipin antibodies in the antiphospholipid syndrome: a systematic review of the literature. Blood 2003;101:1827–32.
64. Levy DM, Massicotte MP, Harvey E, et al. Thromboembolism in paediatric lupus patients. Lupus 2003;12:741–6.
65. Male C, Foulon D, Hoogendoorn H, et al. Predictive value of persistent versus transient antiphospholipid antibody subtypes for the risk of thrombotic events in pediatric patients with systemic lupus erythematosus. Blood 2005;106: 4152–8.

66. Berube C, Mitchell L, Silverman E, et al. The relationship of antiphospholipid antibodies to thromboembolic events in pediatric patients with systemic lupus erythematosus: a cross-sectional study. Pediatr Res 1998;44:351–6.

67. Neville C, Rauch J, Kassis J, et al. Thromboembolic risk in patients with high titre anticardiolipin and multiple antiphospholipid antibodies. Thromb Haemost 2003;90:108–15.

68. Galli M, Luciani D, Bertolini G, et al. Anti-beta 2-glycoprotein I, antiprothrombin antibodies, and the risk of thrombosis in the antiphospholipid syndrome. Blood 2003;102:2717–23.

69. Miyakis S, Lockshin MD, Atsumi T, et al. International consensus statement on an update of the classification criteria for definite antiphospholipid syndrome (APS). J Thromb Haemost 2006;4:295–306.

70. Wahezi DM, Ilowite NT, Rajpathak S, et al. Prevalence of annexin A5 resistance in children and adolescents with rheumatic diseases. J Rheumatol 2012;39(2):382–8.

71. Pachman LM, Abbott K, Sinacore JM, et al. Duration of illness is an important variable for untreated children with juvenile dermatomyositis. J Pediatr 2006; 148:247–53.

72. Oddis CV, Medsger TA Jr. Relationship between serum creatine kinase level and corticosteroid therapy in polymyositis-dermatomyositis. J Rheumatol 1988;15: 807–11.

73. Guzman J, Petty RE, Malleson PN. Monitoring disease activity in juvenile dermatomyositis: the role of von Willebrand factor and muscle enzymes. J Rheumatol 1994;21:739–43.

74. Rider LG. Outcome assessment in the adult and juvenile idiopathic inflammatory myopathies. Rheum Dis Clin North Am 2002;28:935–77.

75. Lloyd W, Schur PH. Immune complexes, complement, and anti-DNA in exacerbations of systemic lupus erythematosus (SLE). Medicine (Baltimore) 1981;60: 208–17.

76. Valentijn RM, van Overhagen H, Hazevoet HM, et al. The value of complement and immune complex determinations in monitoring disease activity in patients with systemic lupus erythematosus. Arthritis Rheum 1985;28:904–13.

77. Ricker DM, Hebert LA, Rohde R, et al. Serum C3 levels are diagnostically more sensitive and specific for systemic lupus erythematosus activity than are serum C4 levels. The Lupus Nephritis Collaborative Study Group. Am J Kidney Dis 1991;18:678–85.

78. Ting CK, Hsieh KH. A long-term immunological study of childhood onset systemic lupus erythematosus. Ann Rheum Dis 1992;51:45–51.

79. Singsen BH, Bernstein BH, King KK, et al. Systemic lupus erythematosus in childhood correlations between changes in disease activity and serum complement levels. J Pediatr 1976;89:358–69.

80. Gawryl MS, Chudwin DS, Langlois PF, et al. The terminal complement complex, C5b-9, a marker of disease activity in patients with systemic lupus erythematosus. Arthritis Rheum 1988;31:188–95.

81. Abrass CK, Nies KM, Louie JS, et al. Correlation and predictive accuracy of circulating immune complexes with disease activity in patients with systemic lupus erythematosus. Arthritis Rheum 1980;23:273–82.

82. Pickering MC, Botto M, Taylor PR, et al. Systemic lupus erythematosus, complement deficiency, and apoptosis. Adv Immunol 2000;76:227–324.

83. Hochberg MC. Updating the American College of Rheumatology revised criteria for the classification of systemic lupus erythematosus. Arthritis Rheum 1997;40: 1725.

84. Christopher-Stine L, Petri M, Astor BC, et al. Urine protein-to-creatinine ratio is a reliable measure of proteinuria in lupus nephritis. J Rheumatol 2004;31: 1557–9.

85. Chitalia VC, Kothari J, Wells EJ, et al. Cost-benefit analysis and prediction of 24-hour proteinuria from the spot urine protein-creatinine ratio. Clin Nephrol 2001; 55:436–47.

86. Siedner MJ, Gelber AC, Rovin BH, et al. Diagnostic accuracy study of urine dipstick in relation to 24-hour measurement as a screening tool for proteinuria in lupus nephritis. J Rheumatol 2008;35:84–90.

87. Rasoulpour M, Banco L, Laut JM, et al. Inability of community-based laboratories to identify pathological casts in urine samples. Arch Pediatr Adolesc Med 1996;150:1201–4.

88. Cassidy JTPR, Laxer RM, Lindsley CB. Textbook of pediatric rheumatology. 6th edition. Philadelphia: Saunders Elsevier; 2010.

89. Lieberman J. Elevation of serum angiotensin-converting-enzyme (ACE) level in sarcoidosis. Am J Med 1975;59:365–72.

90. Hinman LM, Stevens C, Matthay RA, et al. Angiotensin convertase activities in human alveolar macrophages: effects of cigarette smoking and sarcoidosis. Science 1979;205:202–3.

91. Silverstein E, Pertschuk LP, Friedland J. Immunofluorescent localization of angiotensin converting enzyme in epithelioid and giant cells of sarcoidosis granulomas. Proc Natl Acad Sci U S A 1979;76:6646–8.

92. Studdy RP, James DG. The specificity and sensitivity of serum angiotensin converting enzyme in sarcoidosis and other disease: experience in twelve centers in six different countries. In: Chretien J, editor. Sarcoidosis and other granulomatous disorders. Paris: Pergamon; 1983. p. 332–44.

93. Turton CW, Grundy E, Firth G, et al. Value of measuring serum angiotensin I converting enzyme and serum lysozyme in the management of sarcoidosis. Thorax 1979;34:57–62.

94. Pascual RS, Gee JB, Finch SC. Usefulness of serum lysozyme measurement in diagnosis and evaluation of sarcoidosis. N Engl J Med 1973;289:1074–6.

95. Selroos O, Klockars M. Serum lysozyme in sarcoidosis. Evaluation of its usefulness in determination of disease activity. Scand J Respir Dis 1977;58:110–6.

96. Tomita H, Sato S, Matsuda R, et al. Serum lysozyme levels and clinical features of sarcoidosis. Lung 1999;177:161–7.

97. Stollerman GH, Lewis AJ, Schultz I, et al. Relationship of immune response to group A streptococci to the course of acute, chronic and recurrent rheumatic fever. Am J Med 1956;20:163–9.

98. Roodpeyma S, Kamali Z, Zare R. Rheumatic fever: the relationship between clinical manifestations and laboratory tests. J Paediatr Child Health 2005;41: 97–100.

99. Barash J, Mashiach E, Navon-Elkan P, et al. Differentiation of post-streptococcal reactive arthritis from acute rheumatic fever. J Pediatr 2008;153:696–9.

100. Hafner R. [Juvenile spondarthritis. Retrospective study of 71 patients]. Monatsschr Kinderheilkd 1987;135:41–6.

101. Brewerton DA, Hart FD, Nicholls A, et al. Ankylosing spondylitis and HL-A 27. Lancet 1973;1:904–7.

102. Hofer M. Spondylarthropathies in children–are they different from those in adults? Best Pract Res Clin Rheumatol 2006;20:315–28.

103. van der Linden SM, Valkenburg HA, de Jongh BM, et al. The risk of developing ankylosing spondylitis in HLA-B27 positive individuals. A comparison of relatives

of spondylitis patients with the general population. Arthritis Rheum 1984;27:
241–9.

104. John CC, Gilsdorf JR. Recurrent fever in children. Pediatr Infect Dis J 2002;21:
1071–7.

105. Gattorno M, Sormani MP, D'Osualdo A, et al. A diagnostic score for molecular
analysis of hereditary autoinflammatory syndromes with periodic fever in children. Arthritis Rheum 2008;58:1823–32.

Rheumatologic Emergencies in Newborns, Children, and Adolescents

Jonathan D. Akikusa, MBBS[a,b,*]

KEYWORDS

- Neonatal heart block • Macrophage activation syndrome
- Pulmonary renal syndrome
- Catastrophic antiphospholipid syndrome • Cardiac tamponade

Pediatric rheumatic diseases can present with a wide spectrum of clinical illness, affecting virtually any organ in the body. Although they have the potential to cause significant morbidity and even mortality if not recognized and managed appropriately, in most situations the institution of treatment is not time critical. There are a few situations, however, in which prompt recognition and treatment is essential to preserve organ function and even life. This article provides a problem-oriented review of five such rheumatologic emergencies. Although each may occur in the context of known preexisting rheumatic disease, they may also be the initial presentation of the diseases concerned and may, therefore, be encountered by general pediatricians, intensivists, or emergency room physicians. This article does not deal with the extensive list of disease- and treatment-related complications that may occur in patients with known rheumatic illness, because although they require timely recognition and management, the patient's prior history is likely to prompt consideration of rheumatologic differentials and involvement of a pediatric rheumatologist. It also does not deal with other conditions, such as septic arthritis and osteomyelitis, which although occasionally a diagnostic challenge – particularly in the neonate – and important to recognize and treat promptly, are rarely life threatening. The reader is referred to another article in this issue for more information on these conditions.

Disclosures: None.
[a] Rheumatology Service, Department of General Medicine, Royal Children's Hospital, 3 West Clinical Offices, 50 Flemington Road, Parkville, 3052, Victoria, Australia; [b] Murdoch Childrens Research Institute, Royal Children's Hospital, 50 Flemington Road, Parkville, 3052, Victoria, Australia
* Corresponding author. Rheumatology Service, Department of General Medicine, Royal Children's Hospital, 3 West Clinical Offices, 50 Flemington Road, Parkville, 3052, Victoria, Australia.
E-mail address: Jonathan.akikusa@rch.org.au

Pediatr Clin N Am 59 (2012) 285–299
doi:10.1016/j.pcl.2012.03.001
0031-3955/12/$ – see front matter © 2012 Elsevier Inc. All rights reserved.

pediatric.theclinics.com

The objective of this article is to assist pediatricians, intensivists, and emergency room physicians in the recognition of clinical scenarios involving critically unwell children in which rheumatic diseases are an important, and in some cases the main, differential. Included is a guide to the key clinical and laboratory features that may be used to identify the relevant illness and an overview of initial treatment approaches. It is not the intention of this review to present detailed diagnostic criteria for the conditions considered, many of which are dealt with elsewhere in this issue. Similarly, although broad treatment principles are presented, the assumption is that after a diagnosis is confirmed the assistance of a physician experienced in the management of pediatric rheumatologic disease will be sought or the reader will consult a more detailed text.

THE FETUS OR NEONATE WITH COMPLETE HEART BLOCK

Rheumatologic Differential
Neonatal lupus erythematosus with complete heart block

The diagnosis of complete atrioventricular heart block (CAVB) in the perinatal period is uncommon, with an estimated incidence of approximately 1 in 15,000 live births. As an isolated finding it is associated with the presence of transplacentally acquired maternal antibodies to Ro/SSA or La/SSB in more than 85% of cases, in a condition termed "neonatal lupus erythematosus" (NLE).[1,2] Without treatment the prognosis of affected infants is guarded, with reported rates of in utero and 1-year mortality of 23% and 54%, respectively.[3] It is important that pediatricians recognize the implications of this finding and the need for urgent assessment to confirm its cause and institution of appropriate monitoring and referrals for ongoing management.

Clinical Presentation

The development of CAVB in utero in fetuses with NLE may be preceded by second-degree heart block or may occur rapidly in the apparent absence of preceding lesser degrees of block.[4] Onset may be at any time after 16 weeks gestation. Although most cases occur before the 30th week, fetuses remain at risk to term.[5] Affected fetuses with lesser degrees of heart block at the time of delivery remain at risk of developing CAVB in the neonatal period and beyond.[6]

The clinical presentation of CAVB in the fetus and neonate is with bradycardia.[5] Complications of significant bradycardia, such as hydrops and pericardial effusion in the fetus and congestive cardiac failure in the neonate, may also be seen.[5] Second-degree heart block also presents with bradycardia (heart rate <120 beats per minute), although of a lesser degree than CAVB. The detection of bradycardia in the fetus or neonate mandates immediate referral for assessment as to cause. The confirmation of heart block is by estimation of the PR interval using specialized echocardiographic techniques antenatally or by electrocardiogram after birth. Neonates with heart block in the setting of NLE may manifest other findings typical of the condition, which might serve as a clue to the underlying diagnosis. These include an annular skin rash, typically of the face and scalp; elevation of hepatic enzymes; and thrombocytopenia.

Approach to Investigation

The detection of isolated CAVB or lesser degrees of heart block in the fetus or neonate should prompt testing for the presence of antinuclear antibodies, specifically those against Ro/SSA and La/SSB, in maternal and neonatal serum. Found in approximately

0.5% of asymptomatic pregnant women, these antibodies are associated with a 1% to 2% risk of CAVB in the fetus in the absence of a prior affected pregnancy. This risk is increased to 15% to 20% if there is a history of a prior pregnancy complicated by fetal CAVB.[4] In association with fetal heart block, these antibodies confirm the presence of neonatal lupus syndrome and appropriate monitoring and treatment should be instigated.

Treatment Overview

The management of fetuses with heart block has not been the subject of randomized trials and some aspects remain controversial. Fetal conduction block in NLE is thought to be the result of immune-mediated damage to the atrioventricular (AV) node.[7] This damage results in scarring with CAVB as the end result. The suspected role of the immune system in this process raises the possibility that immunosuppression administered to the at-risk fetus might reduce AV node damage and prevent CAVB.

Based on data from observational studies it is generally accepted that treatment of the fetus using fluoridated corticosteroids, such as dexamethasone, administered to the mother has a role in the treatment of second-degree heart block. Such treatment may prevent progression to CAVB and in some cases may result in regression of the degree of block.[4,8] More controversial is their use, with their potential side effects on the mother and fetus, in the management of first-degree heart block and established CAVB. This controversy has arisen because it is unclear if the former is a risk factor for the development of CAVB or if the latter is reversible.[4,8]

Irrespective of whether corticosteroids are used, an essential component of the management of fetal heart block is frequent monitoring for complications of bradycardia, or for other cardiac abnormalities associated with neonatal lupus syndrome, such as endocardial fibroelastosis. Fetal heart rates greater than 55 to 60 beats per minute are usually tolerated and early delivery of the fetus is not required in the absence of other complications. Early delivery should be considered if the fetal heart rate is less than 55 to 60 beats per minute. β-Sympathomimetic agents may be used as a temporizing measure. A significant proportion of babies with CAVB require cardiac pacing after birth and delivery should be effected at a center with ready access to this capability.[5]

Neonates who present with CAVB should be managed according to their degree of circulatory decompensation. The rate of pacemaker placement in the neonatal period is lower in this group than in those diagnosed in utero, although over the longer term the rate of both groups is similar.[5] Neonates followed in utero with first- and second-degree heart block require ongoing follow-up because they remain at risk for the development of higher degrees of heart block over time.

THE FEBRILE CHILD WITH PANCYTOPENIA

Rheumatologic Differential
Macrophage activation syndrome secondary to:
Systemic lupus erythematosus
Systemic juvenile idiopathic arthritis
Kawasaki disease

The differential diagnosis of fever in association with pancytopenia includes such entities as sepsis, myelodysplastic syndromes, and malignancy, all of which pediatricians are familiar with and routinely work-up, treat, and refer when appropriate. Less commonly appreciated is the rheumatologic differential of macrophage activation syndrome (MAS). This potentially fatal disorder, a secondary form of hemophagoctyic lymphohistiocytosis (HLH), may complicate the initial presentation and subsequent course of a number of pediatric rheumatic diseases.[9–12] Although it may also be seen in the context of infection, malignancy, and immunodeficiency, this discussion is limited to rheumatic disease–triggered MAS. Without appropriate treatment MAS has the potential to cause rapid clinical deterioration and death. Because many of the routine laboratory findings associated with this condition are protean and overlap with those of other disorders, particularly sepsis, misdiagnosis through lack of awareness is a significant risk.[13] The reader is referred elsewhere in this issue for more comprehensive information. This section provides an overview of the key features helpful in the recognition of MAS triggered by rheumatic disease and provides a guide to making the diagnosis and its initial management.

Clinical Presentation

Cytopenias in association with fever and splenomegaly are important clues to the possibility of MAS. In the absence of formal diagnostic criteria, those used for the diagnosis of familial HLH have become the default in this condition (See article by Gowdie and Tse elsewhere in this issue for further exploration of this topic). Caution needs to be exercised, however, in the rigid application of these criteria to rheumatic disease-triggered MAS, where significant cell count changes associated with the underlying disease may mask the presence of evolving cytopenias (eg, in Kawasaki disease [KD] and systemic juvenile idiopathic arthritis [sJIA]) or result in misattribution with respect to cause (eg, in systemic lupus erythematosus [SLE]). Under these circumstances falling cell counts, particularly platelets and/or neutrophils, even if still within the normal range, may be an important clue to the presence of MAS. Other suggestive abnormalities of common laboratory parameters are extreme hyperferritinemia, fasting hypertriglyceridemia, or hypofibrinogenemia with coagulopathy and elevation of hepatic enzymes. In rheumatic disease–triggered MAS, clinical or laboratory findings of the underlying rheumatic disorder are also present. These must be carefully sought in all cases of suspected MAS. The most common rheumatologic disorders associated with MAS are SLE, sJIA, and KD. The important clinical and laboratory features that must be looked for when evaluating a patient for the presence of these disorders are outlined in **Table 1**. Formal diagnostic criteria for these conditions are dealt with elsewhere in this issue. It should be noted that SLE itself may cause fever and cytopenias; however, the profound neutropenia typically seen in MAS is uncommon and its presence should alert the clinician to the possibility of the latter.

Approach to Investigation

The investigations that should be ordered when MAS is suspected and the values that suggest its presence, based on the current criteria for HLH,[14] are outlined in **Box 1**. The current criteria also include testing natural killer cell activity and levels of soluble CD25; however, these may not be available in all laboratories. Although demonstrating excessive hemophagocytosis in bone marrow or lymph node biopsies provides good evidence of the presence of MAS, its absence does not exclude MAS. Even in fatal cases of HLH the sensitivity of autopsy samples from these tissues for the detection of hemophagocytosis has been reported to be just 39% and 74%, respectively.[15]

Investigations that may be useful in the diagnosis of an underlying rheumatologic disorder are outlined in **Table 1**. Because MAS may be triggered by conditions

Table 1
Important clinical and laboratory features of rheumatic diseases that may present with macrophage activation syndrome

	Kawasaki Disease	Systemic Juvenile Idiopathic Arthritis	Systemic Lupus Erythematosus
M:F	M = F	M = F	M<F
Typical age	Less than 5 yr	No age peak, may occur at any age, uncommon <1 yr	Older children, adolescents
Rash	Polymorphous	Evanescent, salmon pink, macules	Photosensitive, esp. malar distribution. Discoid
Oromucosal changes	Strawberry tongue Cracked lips	—	Oral ulceration, esp hard palate
Conjunctivitis	Nonpurulent		
Lymphadenopathy	Cervical >1.5 cm	Generalized, may be associated hepatosplenomegaly	Generalized, may be associated hepatosplenomegaly
Arthritis	Present in ~25% Mostly large joint	Required for diagnosis, may not be present initially	Present in ~60% Both large and small joint
Peripheral changes	Palmar erythema, edema, peeling subacutely	—	Edema if nephrotic, vasculitic skin changes
Serositis	Pericarditis	Pericarditis, pleural effusions	Pericarditis, pleural effusions
Neurologic	Irritability, aseptic meningitis	—	Chorea, psychosis, headache, seizures
Urinalysis	Sterile pyuria	—	Active sediment, Hematuria and/or proteinuria
Changes in common laboratory parameters without MAS	Elevation of ESR, CRP, WCC, Thrombocytosis subacutely	Elevation of ESR, CRP, WCC, PLT Ferritin markedly raised Anemia common	Elevation of ESR. CRP usually normal. Hemolytic Anemia, low PLT and WCC may occur
Autoantibodies	—	—	Positive ANA, aPL, anti-dsDNA, anti-Sm antibodies

Italicized features are diagnostic criteria for the indicated condition. The reader is referred to the relevant article in this issue for more detailed information on each of these conditions.

Abbreviations: ANA, antinuclear antibody; aPL, antiphospholipid; CRP, C-reactive protein; dsDNA, double-stranded DNA; ESR, erythrocyte sedimentation rate; PLT, platelets; Sm, Smith; WCC, white cell count.

Box 1
Useful investigations in suspected MAS

Full blood examination ($\geq$2 of three cell lines affected)

  Hemoglobin <90 g/L

  Neutrophils <1 $\times$ 10^9/L

  Platelets <100 $\times$ 10^9/L

Fasting triglycerides

  $\geq$3 mmol/L

Fibrinogen

  $\leq$1.5 g/L

Ferritin

  $\geq$500 μg/L

Bone marrow or lymph node biopsy:

  Excessive hemophagocytosis

---

other than rheumatic diseases, in particular infection and malignancy, appropriate investigations to exclude these possibilities should also be undertaken. In the absence of an identifiable trigger, genetic testing for primary HLH should be performed irrespective of the age of the child. Although primary HLH typically manifests in infancy, presentations in older children and adults are being increasingly recognized.[16,17]

Treatment Overview

After the diagnosis of MAS is confirmed or, in a critically ill child in whom a complete evaluation is not possible, considered highly likely, treatment should be commenced without delay. In situations where infection cannot be excluded, concurrent treatment with appropriate antimicrobial therapy should be given. In general, the initial treatment of MAS is the same irrespective of the underlying trigger. High-dose intravenous steroid pulsed methylprednisolone (30 mg/kg/dose over 30–60 minutes, maximum 1 g) administered daily is considered first-line therapy. This is typically continued for 3 days or until clinical and laboratory parameters begin to improve. Therapy is usually then switched to daily divided-dose steroids, starting at 2 mg/kg/d. Other treatments that may be used in the acute management of MAS complicating rheumatic diseases include cyclosporin, intravenous immunoglobulin, and anakinra.[18–20] These agents are most often considered in critically unwell children or those who fail to respond to corticosteroids. On rare occasions, in children whose disease is resistant to the previously mentioned measures, the chemotherapy protocol designed for the treatment of primary HLH involving the administration of dexamethasone and etoposide is required. In general, the therapy needed to control rheumatic disease-triggered MAS will also treat the underlying rheumatic disorder. Additional disease-specific therapy is required only in patients with KD for whom intravenous immunoglobulin remains the only therapy proved to reduce the risk of coronary artery aneurysms. After the episode of MAS is controlled, the long-term management of these patients is determined by their underlying rheumatic disorder.

THE CHILD WITH RESPIRATORY DISTRESS AND RENAL FAILURE

Rheumatologic Differentials
Pulmonary renal syndrome secondary to:
Antineutrophil cytoplasmic antibody (ANCA)–associated vasculitis
Systemic lupus erythematosus
Goodpasture syndrome

An important differential diagnosis for the child presenting with respiratory distress and renal failure is pulmonary renal syndrome (PRS), a term describing the clinical presentation of diffuse alveolar hemorrhage in combination with rapidly progressive glomerulonephritis. It has been reported as a manifestation of several multisystem illnesses; however, three main causes predominate: (1) antineutrophil cytoplasmic antibody (ANCA)–associated vasculitis (primarily granulomatosis with polyangiitis and microscopic polyangiitis); (2) SLE; and (3) less commonly in children, Goodpasture syndrome.[21–24] It may be the presenting feature of each of these conditions and, if unrecognized, can be rapidly fatal as a result of devastating pulmonary hemorrhage.[24]

Clinical Presentation

Patients typically present with dyspnea and cough in association with hypoxemia in air.[25] Hemoptysis in this context is a strong clue to the presence of pulmonary hemorrhage but may not be present in all cases. Chest radiography demonstrates a diffuse alveolar filling process (**Fig. 1**) and a full blood count reveals anemia or falling hemoglobin. Renal involvement is evident as elevation of serum creatinine and urea, the finding of which should prompt analysis of urinary sediment for evidence of glomerulonephritis. In

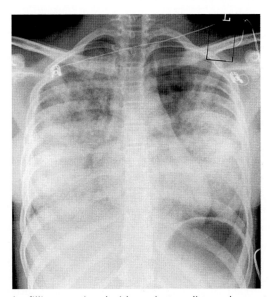

Fig. 1. Diffuse alveolar filling associated with respiratory distress, hemoptysis, and anemia in a 13-year-old girl subsequently diagnosed with an ANCA-associated vasculitis.

addition to these generic features of PRS, patients may have clinical findings related to the specific underlying disorder. Clinical features suggestive of ANCA-associated vasculitis include prominent constitutional symptoms, such as fever and arthralgias; concurrent upper airway disease including oral or nasal ulceration, sinusitis, saddle nose, and subglottic stenosis; the presence of conjunctivitis, scleritis, or episcleritis; and the presence of peripheral palpable purpura or petechiae-like skin lesions suggestive of leukocytoclastic vasculitis.[21,26] The specific type of ANCA-vasculitis diagnosed is determined by the particular combination of clinical and serologic features found. Clinical features suggestive of SLE are outlined in **Table 1**. The clinical features of Goodpasture syndrome are typically those arising from its effect on the kidneys and lungs.[24]

Approach to Investigation

Respiratory distress in combination with renal failure may be the result of PRS or may occur as the result of coincidental pathologies in the respiratory and renal systems.[23] Because clinical deterioration in the former can be very rapid, the priority in the investigation of patients with this combination of clinical features is to determine whether pulmonary hemorrhage and glomerulonephritis are present. If they are then the presence of

---

Box 2
Investigation of suspected PRS

A. Tests to confirm the presence of PRS

  First-line testing

    Chest radiograph: diffuse alveolar filling

    Full blood count: anemia, falling hemoglobin

    Creatinine and urea: abnormal elevation

    Urinalysis: proteinuria, hematuria, cellular casts

  Second-line testing (if first-line testing inconclusive for pulmonary hemorrhage)

    D_{LCO}: increased in the presence of intra-alveolar bleeding

    Bronchoalveolar lavage: presence of red cells, hemosiderin-laden macrophages

B. Tests to confirm the cause of PRS

  Autoantibody screening for

    ANCA-associated vasculitis: ANCA, if positive then test for anti-PR3 or anti-MPO specificity

    SLE: ANA, anti-ENA, anti-dsDNA, anti-Sm, anticardiolipn, lupus anticoagulant

    Goodpasture syndrome: anti-GBM antibodies

  Tissue diagnostics

    Renal biopsy: ANCA vasculitides: pauci-immune, necrotizing, crescentic glomerulonephritis

    SLE: glomerular immune deposits with histologic changes of lupus nephritis

    Goodpasture syndrome: typical pattern of IgG deposition in glomeruli with crescentic changes

Abbreviations: ANCA, antineutrophil cytoplasmic antibody; ANA, antinuclear antibodies; D_{LCO}, diffusing capacity of lung for carbon monoxide; ENA, extractible nuclear antigens; GBM, glomerular basement membrane; MPO, myeloperoxidase; PR3, proteinase 3.

PRS is confirmed and subsequent investigations should be directed toward determining the underlying cause. **Box 2** outlines investigations and expected findings useful in establishing the presence and cause of PRS. In most cases the patient's history, examination, and simple first-line investigations are sufficient to confirm the presence of PRS and allow commencement of presumptive treatment.

Treatment Overview

Patients with PRS are frequently critically ill at presentation or have a high risk of becoming so if treatment is delayed. Once the presence of PRS is confirmed, presumptive treatment should be commenced. Investigations to determine the underlying cause are rarely available acutely and do not significantly alter immediate therapy requirements. If the presence of concurrent infection cannot be excluded, appropriate antimicrobial cover should be administered. Patients should be managed in a setting in which renal and respiratory support can be provided if needed because they continue to be at risk of significant deterioration until treatment measures are well underway.

Initial therapy for PRS consists of high-dose intravenous pulsed methylprednisolone (30 mg/kg/dose over 30–60 minutes, maximum 1 g) daily for at least 3 days followed by high-dose prednisolone (1–2 mg/kg/d). Plasmapheresis is standard therapy in Goodpasture syndrome and has been shown to be of benefit for renal survival in patients with severe ANCA-associated vasculitis.[27] Although not proved to increase survival, in the context of significant alveolar hemorrhage, particularly in patients requiring respiratory support, it has become standard adjunctive therapy in PRS irrespective of the underlying cause. The third component of therapy for PRS is cyclophosphamide, administered either orally or intravenously.

THE CHILD WITH MULTIPLE ORGAN DYSFUNCTION WITH OR WITHOUT OBVIOUS THROMBOSIS

Rheumatologic Differential
Catastrophic antiphospholipid syndrome

One of the most difficult differentials in pediatric rheumatology is catastrophic antiphospholipid syndrome (CAPS), which as its name implies may be rapidly fatal if not recognized promptly. The difficulty in recognizing this syndrome arises as a result of its rarity and the nonspecific manner in which it may present. Patients with CAPS have an underlying predisposition to thrombosis as a result of persistent antiphospholipid antibodies (lupus anticoagulant and anticardiolipin). These may occur as a primary phenomenon or in the context of an underlying connective tissue disease, the commonest of which is SLE. Whether primary or secondary, their presence may not be suspected until an index event, of which CAPS may be one.[28,29] In approximately two-thirds of patients with CAPS an underlying triggering event can be identified.[28,30] The commonest trigger is infection. Others include surgery; trauma; malignancy; and in cases associated with SLE, flares of the underlying disease. The primary pathology in CAPS is multisystem microvascular thrombosis with a secondary systemic inflammatory response as a result of tissue damage.[29] Patients present with progressive multiorgan dysfunction in the context of an apparently primary inflammatory disease. They may not have obvious features to suggest a thrombotic process, in which case more subtle features must be carefully sought. There are other rheumatologic differentials for multiorgan dysfunction in the context of acute inflammatory disease including

SLE and the primary systemic vasculitides, particularly those affecting medium and small vessels. The reader is referred to the relevant articles of this issue to familiarize themselves with the key features of those conditions.

Clinical Presentation

No one symptom or clinical finding is diagnostic of CAPS. Diagnostic criteria for the syndrome have been proposed and subsequently validated (**Box 3**).[31,32] They provide a conceptual framework for the evaluation of patients presenting with complex multi-system disease in whom the diagnosis of CAPS is being considered.

Data regarding the common clinical features of CAPS are derived from a registry of predominantly adult patients.[28–30] Manifestations resulting from thrombosis are a key feature, although because of the size of the vessels involved may not initially be appreciated as such. Large-vessel thrombosis, as seen in antiphospholipid syndrome, does occur in CAPS; however, small-vessel and microvascular thrombosis is more common. Cardiopulmonary manifestations are the most frequent at presentation. These typically include acute dyspnea and respiratory failure in the context of acute respiratory distress syndrome. Pulmonary embolus and alveolar hemorrhage may also occur. The next commonest organ involvement is the central nervous system, typically as cerebral infarction, seizures, and encephalopathy. Cerebral venous sinus thrombosis may also be seen and be a more obvious clue to an underlying thrombotic tendency. Renal and abdominal involvement are the third and fourth most frequently involved systems at presentation, with renal failure, proteinuria, and significant abdominal pain common presenting features. Over the course of an episode of CAPS more than 80% of patients experience an intra-abdominal thrombotic event; therefore, any new abdominal symptom should be carefully evaluated. Less common organ involvement includes the skin, with livedo reticularis, purpura, and ulcers all being described.

In addition to clinical manifestations related to thrombosis, patients may also exhibit systemic inflammation and have laboratory features suggestive of disseminated intra-vascular coagulation or thrombotic microangiopathy, including thrombocytopenia,

---

Box 3
Criteria for the diagnosis of CAPS

Definite CAPS requires all of the following

1. Evidence of vessel occlusion, or effect of vessel occlusion, in ≥3 organs, systems, or tissues

2. Occurrence of diagnostic features simultaneously or in <1 week

3. Histopathology demonstrating small-vessel occlusion in at least one affected organ or tissue

4. Presence of antiphospholipid antibodies (LAC/aCL) persistent over at least 6 weeks

Probable CAPS if

• Only two organ systems affected, or

• Occurrence of two diagnostic features in <1 week and the third within 4 weeks, or

• Histopathologic demonstration of small-vessel occlusion not possible, or

• Persistence of APL unable to be demonstrated because of death of patient

Abbreviations: aCL, anticardiolipin antibodies; APL, antiphospholipid antibodies; LAC, lupus anticoagulant.

anemia, and features of hemolysis on blood film.[29,33] For patients with CAPS in the context of associated diseases, such as SLE or malignancy, clinical features of the associated condition may be apparent. The reader is referred to **Table 1** and elsewhere in this issue for a description of the key features of SLE. Patients may have features of underlying infection, the single most common trigger for CAPS. If the possibility of CAPS is not considered, the clinical and laboratory picture may be mistaken for overwhelming sepsis.

Approach to Investigation

Bearing in mind the specific requirements of the criteria reviewed previously, the investigation of a patient with suspected CAPS has three main objectives: (1) to confirm the presence of a thrombotic disorder; (2) to confirm the presence of antiphospholipid antibodies (ie, lupus anticoagulant and anticardiolipin antibodies); and (3) to detect underlying triggers for the episode.

Identifying the presence of a thrombotic disorder is relatively straightforward when large vessels are involved. However, in CAPS thrombosis more commonly affects smaller vessels, which may be more difficult to detect.[28,30] Clues to such involvement include evidence of organ infarction (eg, kidney, spleen, or bowel) on imaging, or organ failure (eg, cardiac or renal) in association with markers of abnormal activation of coagulation and peripheral destruction of blood elements, such as elevated fibrin degradation products, thrombocytopenia, hemolytic anemia (with or without features of microangiopathy, such as schistocytes), or fully manifested disseminated intravascular coagulation. Tissue samples (eg, skin or kidney) may provide further evidence of small-vessel thrombosis and occlusion.

Assays for antiphospholipid antibodies should be performed as soon as the diagnosis of CAPS is suspected. In patients with no prior history of antiphospholipid antibodies, their persistence must be demonstrated to meet criteria for CAPS.

Approximately two-thirds of patients have an identifiable trigger for the episode of CAPS.[28] The commonest is infection, particularly of the respiratory system, skin, and urinary tract, for which patients should be carefully screened. Other common triggers that should be excluded in the absence of another obvious cause are malignancy and flare of an underlying connective tissue disease, most commonly SLE.

Therapy Overview

Patients with CAPS are often critically ill. The need for management in an intensive care setting should be anticipated; general supportive measures including ventilation and dialysis are frequently required acutely. It is often not possible to exclude infection as an underlying trigger for CAPS acutely and empiric antimicrobial therapy should be strongly considered. Specific therapy for CAPS is directed toward the two underlying pathologic processes in this disorder: thrombosis and the secondary systemic inflammatory response. Although there have been no randomized trials of therapy, early institution of currently suggested treatments has reduced mortality in CAPS from 50% to 30%.[29] Thrombosis is managed using parenteral and subsequently oral anticoagulation. Systemic corticosteroids, typically in high dose, are administered to mitigate systemic inflammation. Plasmapheresis is also frequently used, particularly in those with evidence of microangiopathy, and intravenous immunoglobulin may be of benefit. Other measures including vasodilators, fibrinolyics, and embolectomy may have a role in individual patients.

THE CHILD WITH PERICARDIAL TAMPONADE

Rheumatologic Differentials

Serositis secondary to:
    Systemic lupus erythematosus
    Systemic juvenile idiopathic arthritis

Pericardial tamponade is an uncommon life-threatening complication of pericarditis with effusion. Autoimmune disorders account for between 5% and 12% of pericardial effusions in adults and 13% and 30% in children.[34–36] The most common rheumatic diseases associated with pericardial effusions in children are SLE and sJIA, which are the most commonly reported in association with pericardial tamponade.[34,35,37–41] In both conditions pericardial tamponade may occur in the course of established disease or as an initial manifestation.[37–40,42] Although the immediate management of pericardial tamponade is similar irrespective of cause, it is important to identify the presence of an associated rheumatic condition because disease involvement of other organ systems may require management distinct from that of the pericardial issues and tamponade may recur if the underlying disease is not treated.[38,39] It is also important to be aware of, and investigate appropriately for, other causes of pericardial effusion including infection and malignancy.[34,35] In up to 48% of children no cause is identified.[34]

Clinical Presentation

Pericardial tamponade typically presents with dyspnea, tachypnea, and chest pain. Clinical signs include distended neck veins, facial suffusion, tachycardia, pulsus paradoxus, muffled heart sounds, and in advanced stages hypotension. Fever is common.[34] In addition to signs of tamponade, there may be clinical features of the underlying rheumatic disease. **Table 1** provides an overview of clinical features suggestive of SLE and sJIA. These entities are discussed in more detail elsewhere in this issue.

Approach to Investigation

Urgent echocardiography is required in all cases of suspected pericardial tamponade. This confirms the presence of pericardial fluid, provides an assessment of its effect on cardiac mechanics, and allows planning of therapeutic intervention. In patients with subacute presentations, common in those with rheumatic disease–associated pericardial tamponade, the clinical features of tamponade may be more subtle than those described previously and a chest radiograph demonstrating gross enlargement of the cardiac silhouette may be the first clue to the diagnosis (**Fig. 2**). After the diagnosis has been established and treatment instituted, identification of an underlying cause is the next priority. This should begin with sending pericardial fluid obtained during therapeutic pericardiocentesis for appropriate microbial studies and other serologic investigations relevant for identifying possible infective causes of pericardial effusion. Investigations relevant in the work-up for SLE and sJIA are outlined in **Table 1**.

Therapy Overview

The first priority in management of pericardial tamponade is to restore adequate cardiac output by removal of the pericardial fluid. Temporizing measures to maintain cardiac output, such as giving intravenous volume and sympathomimetics, may be

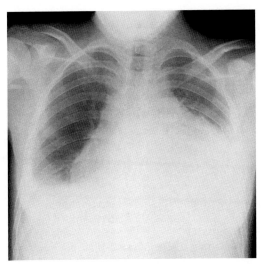

Fig. 2. Bilateral pleural effusions and gross enlargement of the cardiac silhouette in a 13-year-old girl presenting with a 1-week history of increasing chest pain and dyspnea. Echocardiogram confirmed pericardial effusion with tamponade, relieved by drainage of 1000 mL of fluid from the pericardial sac. Subsequent testing revealed the presence of antinuclear antibody, anti–double stranded DNA, and anticardiolipin antibodies and nephritis, confirming a diagnosis of SLE.

considered until this is achieved based on clinical circumstances. Once the adequate cardiac output has been restored and the cause identified, specific treatments can begin. For SLE and sJIA this involves a period of immunosuppression with corticosteroids with or without other agents based on clinical response and other organ involvement.

REFERENCES

1. Buyon JP, Clancy RM, Friedman DM. Cardiac manifestations of neonatal lupus erythematosus: guidelines to management, integrating clues from the bench and bedside. Nat Clin Pract Rheumatol 2009;5(3):139–48.
2. Taylor PV, Taylor KF, Norman A, et al. Prevalence of maternal Ro (SS-A) and La (SS-B) autoantibodies in relation to congenital heart block. Br J Rheumatol 1988;27(2): 128–32.
3. Jaeggi ET, Fouron JC, Silverman ED, et al. Transplacental fetal treatment improves the outcome of prenatally diagnosed complete atrioventricular block without structural heart disease. Circulation 2004;110(12):1542–8.
4. Friedman DM, Kim MY, Copel JA, et al. Utility of cardiac monitoring in fetuses at risk for congenital heart block: the PR Interval and Dexamethasone Evaluation (PRIDE) prospective study. Circulation 2008;117(4):485–93.
5. Jaeggi ET, Hamilton RM, Silverman ED, et al. Outcome of children with fetal, neonatal or childhood diagnosis of isolated congenital atrioventricular block. A single institution's experience of 30 years. J Am Coll Cardiol 2002;39(1):130–7.
6. Askanase AD, Friedman DM, Copel J, et al. Spectrum and progression of conduction abnormalities in infants born to mothers with anti-SSA/Ro-SSB/La antibodies. Lupus 2002;11(3):145–51.

7. Clancy RM, Kapur RP, Molad Y, et al. Immunohistologic evidence supports apoptosis, IgG deposition, and novel macrophage/fibroblast crosstalk in the pathologic cascade leading to congenital heart block. Arthritis Rheum 2004; 50(1):173–82.

8. Friedman DM, Kim MY, Copel JA, et al. Prospective evaluation of fetuses with autoimmune-associated congenital heart block followed in the PR Interval and Dexamethasone Evaluation (PRIDE) Study. Am J Cardiol 2009;103(8):1102–6.

9. Avcin T, Tse SM, Schneider R, et al. Macrophage activation syndrome as the presenting manifestation of rheumatic diseases in childhood. J Pediatr 2006;148(5): 683–6.

10. Kounami S, Yoshiyama M, Nakayama K, et al. Macrophage activation syndrome in children with systemic-onset juvenile chronic arthritis. Acta Haematol 2005; 113(2):124–9.

11. Latino GA, Manlhiot C, Yeung RS, et al. Macrophage activation syndrome in the acute phase of Kawasaki disease. J Pediatr Hematol Oncol 2010;32(7):527–31.

12. Parodi A, Davi S, Pringe AB, et al. Macrophage activation syndrome in juvenile systemic lupus erythematosus: a multinational multicenter study of thirty-eight patients. Arthritis Rheum 2009;60(11):3388–99.

13. Castillo L, Carcillo J. Secondary hemophagocytic lymphohistiocytosis and severe sepsis/systemic inflammatory response syndrome/multiorgan dysfunction syndrome/macrophage activation syndrome share common intermediate phenotypes on a spectrum of inflammation. Pediatr Crit Care Med 2009;10(3):387–92.

14. Henter JI, Horne A, Arico M, et al. HLH-2004: diagnostic and therapeutic guidelines for hemophagocytic lymphohistiocytosis. Pediatr Blood Cancer 2007;48(2): 124–31.

15. Ost A, Nilsson-Ardnor S, Henter JI. Autopsy findings in 27 children with haemophagocytic lymphohistiocytosis. Histopathology 1998;32(4):310–6.

16. Allen M, De Fusco C, Legrand F, et al. Familial hemophagocytic lymphohistiocytosis: how late can the onset be? Haematologica 2001;86(5):499–503.

17. Zhang K, Jordan MB, Marsh RA, et al. Hypomorphic mutations in PRF1, MUNC13-4, and STXBP2 are associated with adult-onset familial hemophagocytic lymphohistiocytosis. Blood 2011;118(22):5794–8.

18. Emmenegger U, Frey U, Reimers A, et al. Hyperferritinemia as indicator for intravenous immunoglobulin treatment in reactive macrophage activation syndromes. Am J Hematol 2001;68(1):4–10.

19. Miettunen PM, Narendran A, Jayanthan A, et al. Successful treatment of severe paediatric rheumatic disease-associated macrophage activation syndrome with interleukin-1 inhibition following conventional immunosuppressive therapy: case series with 12 patients. Rheumatology (Oxford) 2011;50(2):417–9.

20. Mouy R, Stephan JL, Pillet P, et al. Efficacy of cyclosporine A in the treatment of macrophage activation syndrome in juvenile arthritis: report of five cases. J Pediatr 1996;129(5):750–4.

21. Akikusa JD, Schneider R, Harvey EA, et al. Clinical features and outcome of pediatric Wegener's granulomatosis. Arthritis Rheum 2007;57(5):837–44.

22. Gallagher H, Kwan JT, Jayne DR. Pulmonary renal syndrome: a 4-year, single-center experience. Am J Kidney Dis 2002;39(1):42–7.

23. von Vigier RO, Trummler SA, Laux-End R, et al. Pulmonary renal syndrome in childhood: a report of twenty-one cases and a review of the literature. Pediatr Pulmonol 2000;29(5):382–8.

24. Williamson SR, Phillips CL, Andreoli SP, et al. A 25-year experience with pediatric anti-glomerular basement membrane disease. Pediatr Nephrol 2011;26(1):85–91.

25. Shen M, Zeng X, Tian X, et al. Diffuse alveolar hemorrhage in systemic lupus erythematosus: a retrospective study in China. Lupus 2010;19(11):1326–30.
26. Cabral DA, Uribe AG, Benseler S, et al. Classification, presentation, and initial treatment of Wegener's granulomatosis in childhood. Arthritis Rheum 2009; 60(11):3413–24.
27. Jayne DR, Gaskin G, Rasmussen N, et al. Randomized trial of plasma exchange or high-dosage methylprednisolone as adjunctive therapy for severe renal vasculitis. J Am Soc Nephrol 2007;18(7):2180–8.
28. Asherson RA, Cervera R, Piette JC, et al. Catastrophic antiphospholipid syndrome: clues to the pathogenesis from a series of 80 patients. Medicine (Baltimore) 2001; 80(6):355–77.
29. Cervera R. Catastrophic antiphospholipid syndrome (CAPS): update from the CAPS Registry. Lupus 2010;19(4):412–8.
30. Cervera R, Bucciarelli S, Plasin MA, et al. Catastrophic antiphospholipid syndrome (CAPS): descriptive analysis of a series of 280 patients from the CAPS Registry. J Autoimmun 2009;32(3–4):240–5.
31. Asherson RA, Cervera R, de Groot PG, et al. Catastrophic antiphospholipid syndrome: international consensus statement on classification criteria and treatment guidelines. Lupus 2003;12(7):530–4.
32. Cervera R, Font J, Gomez-Puerta JA, et al. Validation of the preliminary criteria for the classification of catastrophic antiphospholipid syndrome. Ann Rheum Dis 2005;64(8):1205–9.
33. Asherson RA, Espinosa G, Cervera R, et al. Disseminated intravascular coagulation in catastrophic antiphospholipid syndrome: clinical and haematological characteristics of 23 patients. Ann Rheum Dis 2005;64(6):943–6.
34. Mok GC, Menahem S. Large pericardial effusions of inflammatory origin in childhood. Cardiol Young 2003;13(2):131–6.
35. Roodpeyma S, Sadeghian N. Acute pericarditis in childhood: a 10-year experience. Pediatr Cardiol 2000;21(4):363–7.
36. Sagrista-Sauleda J, Merce AS, Soler-Soler J. Diagnosis and management of pericardial effusion. World J Cardiol 2011;3(5):135–43.
37. Beresford MW, Cleary AG, Sills JA, et al. Cardio-pulmonary involvement in juvenile systemic lupus erythematosus. Lupus 2005;14(2):152–8.
38. Goldenberg J, Pessoa AP, Roizenblatt S, et al. Cardiac tamponade in juvenile chronic arthritis: report of two cases and review of publications. Ann Rheum Dis 1990;49(7):549–53.
39. Gulati S, Kumar L. Cardiac tamponade as an initial manifestation of systemic lupus erythematosus in early childhood. Ann Rheum Dis 1992;51(2):279–80.
40. Parvez N, Carpenter JL. Cardiac tamponade in still disease: a review of the literature. South Med J 2009;102(8):832–7.
41. Rudra T, Evans PA, O'Brien EN. Systemic lupus erythematosus presenting with cardiac tamponade due to a haemorrhagic pericardial effusion. Postgrad Med J 1987;63(741):567–8.
42. Rosenbaum E, Krebs E, Cohen M, et al. The spectrum of clinical manifestations, outcome and treatment of pericardial tamponade in patients with systemic lupus erythematosus: a retrospective study and literature review. Lupus 2009;18(7):608–12.

Juvenile Idiopathic Arthritis

Peter J. Gowdie, MBBS, FRACP, Shirley M.L. Tse, MD, FRCPC*

KEYWORDS

- Juvenile idiopathic arthritis • Epidemiology • Classification
- Treatment

Key Points

- Juvenile idiopathic arthritis (JIA) is defined as arthritis ≥6 weeks duration in child ≤16 years old without other known cause.

- Juvenile idiopathic arthritis is a diagnosis of exclusion; it is important to consider the potential mimickers of JIA.

- Early referral to pediatric rheumatology should be considered.

- Use of nonsteroidal antinflammatory drugs is appropriate before review with a pediatric rheumatology specialist.

- Surveillance for and prevention of complications of JIA is critical (eg, uveitis and growth disturbance).

- Aim for early detection and treatment of flares of disease.

- In patients on immune-modulatory and biologic medication:

  ○ Monitor for side effects

  ○ Beware of infections

  ○ Avoid live vaccines.

- Goals of therapy: achieve remission, minimize medication toxicity, maximize function, optimize growth and development and improve quality of life.

Juvenile idiopathic arthritis (JIA) encompasses a complex group of disorders comprising several clinical entities with the common feature of arthritis. Each subtype of JIA is characterized by a different mode of presentation, disease course, and outcome.

An increased understanding of the underlying pathogenesis of JIA, the development of targeted biologic therapies and rigorous clinical trials studying these new therapies

---

Division of Rheumatology, The Hospital for Sick Children, University of Toronto, Toronto, Ontario, Canada
* Corresponding author.
E-mail address: shirley.tse@sickkids.ca

Pediatr Clin N Am 59 (2012) 301–327
doi:10.1016/j.pcl.2012.03.014
0031-3955/12/$ – see front matter © 2012 Elsevier Inc. All rights reserved.

as well as increasing international collaborative efforts have seen major advances in the management and outcome of children with JIA.

EPIDEMIOLOGY

JIA remains an uncommon, but by no means rare, condition affecting children world-wide.[1] It is the most common rheumatic disease of childhood. Estimates of incidence and prevalence have been difficult to ascertain because of variations in diagnostic criteria, differences in data ascertainment or study design, low disease frequency, and small study numbers.[2]

Epidemiologic studies report prevalence rates between 0.07 and 4.01 per 1000 children and annual incidence between 0.008 and 0.226 per 1000 children.[2–5] The large difference in reported rates is likely because of varying study characteristics. The highest prevalence was reported in community-based studies, in which children were examined in classrooms or homes.[3] On the other hand, clinic-based studies seem to report lower prevalence rates, perhaps reflecting that many clinicians fail to recognize JIA and that these children therefore do not come to the attention of clinicians in large study centers, hence the true prevalence is underestimated.[6]

There are few data outlining the prevalence of JIA in populations other than those of European descent. In the most heavily populated areas of the world, epidemiologic data are scarce. Lower frequencies of JIA have been reported in children in Japan and Costa Rica (annual incidence 0.0083 and 0.068 per 10000, respectively).[7–9] Many of these studies are limited by small sample size and selection bias. One retrospective study reported lower frequency of JIA in Hawaiians of Filipino, Japanese, and Samoan descent compared with White Hawaiians.[10]

One questionnaire-based study addressed ethnicity in a large multiethnic single-center cohort.[11] European descent appeared to be an important predisposing factor for oligoarticular JIA and psoriatic JIA. Black and native North American patients were less likely to have oligoarticular JIA and more likely to have rheumatoid factor (RF)-positive polyarthritis.[11]

CAUSE AND PATHOGENESIS

The underlying cause and pathogenesis of JIA remain unclear. JIA is a heterogeneous disorder, and the subtypes have varying clinical and laboratory features that may reflect distinct immunopathogenic processes. The pathogenesis for each subtype is undoubtedly multifactorial and likely triggered by environmental stimuli in genetically susceptible individuals.

Oligoarticular and RF-positive polyarticular JIA seem to be autoimmune diseases of the adaptive immune system. Positive antinuclear antibody (ANA) and RF are common and these subtypes are consistently associated with HLA genes.

Identified genetic susceptibility genes include genes in the HLA group and also non-HLA-related genes such as genes related to cytokines and other immune functions. The association of HLA class I and II alleles with JIA is well established and suggests the likely involvement of T cells and antigen presentation in the pathogenesis of JIA.

In the genetically susceptible individual, environmental triggers are considered important in the pathogenetic process of JIA. This trigger may cause an uncontrolled innate and adaptive immune response toward self-antigen, resulting in inflammation and disease. Autoantigens from cartilage and other joint tissues are believed to play important roles and to contribute to the activation of CD4+ T cells, leading to proliferation and the production of proinflammatory cytokines.

By contrast, there is increasing evidence to suggest that systemic JIA (sJIA) may be an autoinflammatory disease, primarily involving the innate immune system. sJIA does not have HLA gene associations and is not associated with autoantibodies. sJIA is characterized by uncontrolled activation of phagocytes (including macrophages, monocytes, and neutrophils) caused by unknown triggers and leads to increase of phagocyte secreted inflammatory cytokines such as interleukin 1 (IL-1), IL-6, and IL-18.

Distinct pathogenic processes seem to be involved within the subtypes of JIA, and further definition of these immunogenetic and inflammatory pathways may help explain the considerable clinical heterogeneity seen in patients with JIA and importantly help direct therapy.

DIAGNOSIS AND CLASSIFICATION

The diagnosis of JIA requires the persistence of arthritis for more than 6 weeks in a child less than 16 years of age in whom there is no other identified cause for arthritis. The differential diagnosis for inflammatory arthritis is broad and should be considered in all patients presenting with arthritis. This subject is discussed by Roberta Berrard in detail elsewhere in this issue.

JIA is a complex, heterogeneous group of disorders without clearly defined cause; classifying the various subtypes in to distinct homogeneous groups has been problematic. The International League of Associations for Rheumatology (ILAR) criteria for classification of JIA were first proposed in 1993 and are now the commonly agreed on terminology.[12,13] The aim of this classification system is to attempt to create homogeneous subtypes of JIA. The ILAR classification divides JIA into 7 subtypes: oligoarticular JIA, seropositive polyarticular JIA, seronegative polyarticular JIA, systemic-onset JIA (sJIA), enthesitis-related arthritis (ERA), psoriatic JIA (PsJIA), and undifferentiated JIA (**Table 1**).

There continues to be much debate in the literature about the classification of JIA. The current classification criteria have allowed for international consistency; however, some problems continue to arise in assigning patients to particular subtypes, resulting in a substantial proportion of patients designated as undifferentiated. Advances in the understanding of the immunogenetic pathogenesis of JIA may help refine this classification further.

CLINICAL MANIFESTATIONS OF JIA

Arthritis is clinically characterized by joint effusion, joint line tenderness and warmth, restricted range of movement, and limitation of movement secondary to pain.

The common feature of all the subtypes of JIA is arthritis. Joint inflammation results in pain, loss of function, and morning stiffness. The distribution of joint involvement varies between subtypes of JIA. Systemic symptoms typically occur in systemic and polyarticular subtypes and can include fatigue, weight loss, anemia, anorexia, or fever. Growth abnormalities can complicate JIA and result in short stature or localized growth disturbance such as bony overgrowth, prematurely fused epiphyses, and limb length discrepancies. **Table 1** describes the common features of the subtypes of JIA.

OLIGOARTICULAR JIA

Oligoarticular JIA is defined as JIA involving 4 or fewer joints in the first 6 months of disease. This subgroup is further divided into persistent and extended disease based on the number of additional joints involved beyond the first 6 months. Children with persistent oligoarthritis often enter remission, although they remain at risk for disease

Table 1
Characteristics of JIA

ILAR JIA Subtype	Age, Sex, and % Total Patients with JIA	Typical Joint Involvement	Occurrence of Uveitis	Other Features
Oligoarticular • Persistent • Extended	F>M Early childhood 40%–50%	≤4 joints Large joints: knees, ankles, wrist affected Persistent disease: never >4 joints Extended disease: involves >4 joints after first 6 mo of disease	Common (30%) especially if ANA-positive Usually asymptomatic	ANA 60%–80% positive
Polyarticular (RF-negative)	F>M 2 peaks: 2–4 y and 6–12 y 20%–25%	≥5 joints Symmetric	Common (15%)	ANA 25% positive ± C spine and TMJ
Polyarticular (RF-positive)	F>M Late childhood/early adolescence 5%	Symmetric small and large joints Erosive joint disease	Rare (<1%)	ANA 75% positive Rheumatoid nodules
Systemic	M = F Throughout childhood 5%–10%	Poly or oligoarticular	Rare (<1%)	Daily (quotidian) fever for ≥2 weeks Evanescent rash Lymphadenopathy Hepatosplenomegaly Serositis
Enthesitis-related arthritis	M>F Late childhood/adolescence 5%–10%	Weight-bearing joint especially hip and intertarsal joints History of inflammatory back pain or sacroiliac joint tenderness	Symptomatic acute uveitis (~7%)	Enthesitis HLA-B27-positive Axial involvement (including sacroiliitis) Family history of HLA-B27-associated disease
Psoriatic arthritis	F>M 2 peaks: 2–4 y and 9–11 y 5%–10%	Asymmetric or symmetric small or large joints	Common (10%)	Nail pits, onycholysis Dactylitis Psoriasis Family history psoriasis
Undifferentiated	10%			Does not fulfill criteria for any above category or fulfills criteria for >1 category

Abbreviations: F, female; M, male.

flares. Approximately 50% of patients with oligoarthritis progress to develop extended disease and within 2 years of disease onset have polyarthritis. This group have a more guarded prognosis, because fewer children with extended oligoarthritis enter remission.

Oligoarticular JIA predominantly affects the large joints, most commonly the knees, ankles, wrists, and elbows (**Fig. 1**). Uveitis may occur in up to 30% of children with oligoarthritis. Other extra-articular symptoms rarely occur.

POLYARTICULAR JIA

Polyarticular JIA is defined as JIA involving 5 or more joints and is further divided into RF-positive and RF-negative polyarthritis, based on the presence or absence of RF.

RF-negative patients have a variable disease onset and course, which contribute to the heterogeneity in this JIA subgroup. The onset of joint involvement can be acute or insidious, and large or small joints may be involved. Other than the number of inflamed joints, patients with RF-negative ANA-positive polyarticular JIA are often difficult to distinguish clinically from patients with ANA-positive extended oligoarticular JIA. According to current ILAR criteria, these 2 groups of patients are classified separately. However, the joint count and the timing of joint involvement may not be the most appropriate criteria to aid in defining homogeneous groups of JIA, and future refinement of the classification criteria may be needed.

RF-positive patients share many clinical and immunogenetic characteristics with adult patients with rheumatoid arthritis. The disease onset occurs typically in adolescence and the arthritis is often erosive and symmetric, involving the wrists and small joints of the hands and feet (**Fig. 2**). Systemic features such as fever and constitutional upset may occur at onset, and patients may have rheumatoid nodules.

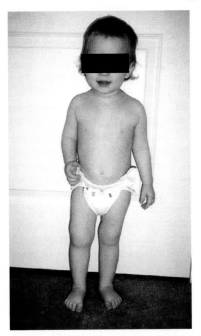

Fig. 1. Patient with oligoarticular JIA. Note the swollen right knee and limited extension.

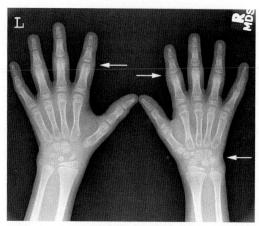

Fig. 2. Radiograph of the hands and wrist in a patient with RF-negative polyarticular JIA. Note: soft tissue swelling around proximal interphalangeal joints and wrist; periarticular osteopenia; joint space narrowing at the wrist joint; and premature maturation of the carpal bones on the right side.

Polyarticular JIA is a chronic disease, with many patients entering adulthood with active disease or functional disability.

sJIA

sJIA is characterized by arthritis and systemic features such as fever and rash. The arthritis is frequently polyarticular but can be limited to few joints, and large or small joints can be involved. The arthritis may be preceded by the systemic symptoms by months. The fever is typically high, spiking daily or twice daily, with rapid return to normal or subnormal temperatures in between (**Fig. 3**). The fever is often accompanied by a well-circumscribed evanescent salmon-pink macular rash commonly present on the trunk and proximal extremities (see **Fig. 3**). Lymphadenopathy and hepatospleno-megaly are common features of sJIA. Cardiac disease is well described, and pericar-dial effusions occur in approximately 10% of children with sJIA.[14] Myocarditis is less common.

Laboratory findings in sJIA reflect systemic inflammation and include leukocytosis, thrombocytosis, anemia, increased transaminase levels, and increased inflammatory markers. ANA is positive in only 5% to 10%, and RF is rarely seen.

In the absence of arthritis, the clinician should remain cognizant of the broad differential diagnosis of sJIA, including infection, malignancy, inflammatory bowel disease, acute rheumatic fever, and other rheumatic diseases such as vasculitis and systemic lupus erythematosus. Leukemia frequently presents with musculoskeletal symptoms at diagnosis and may mimic JIA.[15–17] Information that may differentiate leukemia from sJIA includes low white cell count, low or normal platelet count, and the presence of nighttime pain.[18] In contrast, positive ANA, high lactate dehydrogenase level, rash, and fever may not be helpful in discriminating between leukemia and JIA.[18] See article elsewhere in this issue for a review of the differential diagnosis.

Heterogeneity also is evident amongst patients with sJIA as seen by the different disease course and severity. Approximately 40% of patients have a monophasic illness, whereas more than half have a chronically persistent disease course. A small group of patients have a relapsing polycyclic course. In general, systemic features subside over the initial months to years; however, they may recur with disease

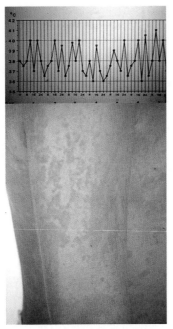

Fig. 3. Fever chart showing spiking fever pattern in patient with sJIA. Typical systemic rash composed of salmon-pink macules. Also note Koebner phenomenon.

exacerbations. In many patients, the progressive and destructive arthritis is the most significant complication, leading to significant morbidity and functional impairment. Early predictors of destructive arthritis include polyarthritis, hip involvement, thrombocytosis, or presence of active systemic disease (fever or need for systemic corticosteroids) at 6 months after diagnosis.[19–21]

Macrophage activation syndrome (MAS, see article elsewhere in this issue) is a potentially life-threatening complication of sJIA characterized by activation of T cells and macrophages, leading to an overwhelming inflammatory response. It is thought by some to be integral to the pathogenesis of sJIA.[22] MAS can be difficult to distinguish from sJIA because it shares some features. MAS is characterized by sustained fever (compared with the quotidian fever of sJIA), hepatosplenomegaly, anemia, liver function abnormalities, rash, coagulopathy, and central nervous system dysfunction. Several laboratory features suggestive of MAS include decreasing white cell count and platelets, decreasing erythrocyte sedimentation rate, increased ferritin level, hypertriglyceridemia, hypofibrinogenemia, and evidence of hemophagocytosis on bone marrow aspirate. Preliminary guidelines for the diagnosis of MAS in association with sJIA have been suggested but are yet to be validated.[23] Early diagnosis and aggressive treatment of MAS are necessary to avoid significant morbidity and mortality. High-dose corticosteroids and supportive care are the first-line therapies; however, agents such as cyclosporin, etoposide, and intravenous immunoglobulin have also been used.

ENTHESITIS-RELATED JIA

As defined by the ILAR classification, ERA is characterized by the presence of arthritis or enthesitis. The arthritis in ERA typically involves the lower limb, especially the hip and intertarsal joints. The sacroiliac joint is frequently involved, although often not until later in the clinical course. ERA represents the undifferentiated forms of spondyloarthritis in children.

Enthesitis is the term used to describe inflammation at the insertion of tendons, ligaments, or joint capsules to the bone. It is characterized by tenderness, warmth, and swelling. The typical locations for enthesitis in ERA are in the lower limbs, in particular at the iliac crest, posterior and anterior superior iliac spine, femoral greater trochanter, ischial tuberosity, patella, tibial tuberosity, Achilles, and plantar fascia insertions. ERA should be considered in patients presenting with significant heel or foot pain. Other features of this category are outlined in **Table 1**. Another unique feature of this subtype of JIA is the involvement of the axial skeleton, especially in the sacroiliac joints, with some children developing ankylosing spondylitis within 10 to 15 years of disease onset.

PsJIA

PsJIA is characterized by the presence of arthritis and psoriasis. Other common features (**Fig. 4**) include dactylitis (defined as sausagelike swelling of the involved digits), nail changes (pitting or onycholysis), or a family history of relatives with psoriasis. PsJIA further clusters into 1 of 2 subgroups. The first group has similar characteristics to oligoarticular JIA, occurring typically in young ANA-positive girls with a high risk of asymptomatic anterior uveitis. However, unlike oligoarticular JIA, dactylitis and involvement of the small joints may occur. The second group, resembling ERA, occurs in older children and adolescents, has a male predominance, and has an increased risk of spondyloarthritis.[24,25]

Psoriasis and arthritis may not occur concurrently, and arthritis may precede the development of psoriasis by many years. The psoriasis may be subtle and mandates a careful examination in children, in whom it may involve the extensor surfaces in the limbs, scalp, posterior auricular, axilla, umbilicus, or gluteal fold.

COMPLICATIONS OF JIA
Uveitis

One of the most significant complications of JIA is anterior uveitis. This is a chronic nongranulomatous inflammation of the anterior chamber of the eye, affecting the iris and ciliary body. It is usually insidious in onset and asymptomatic, mandating frequent ophthalmologic surveillance. However, patients with ERA are more likely to present

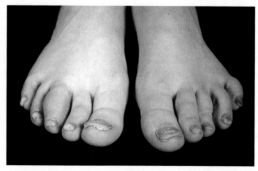

Fig. 4. Dactylitis involving the third right toe and onycholysis in patient with psoriatic arthritis.

with acute symptomatic uveitis. The risk of uveitis is based on the JIA subtype, age at disease onset, and ANA status. The highest risk group of patients is oligoarticular JIA, especially if the patient is female, ANA-positive, and less than 4 years of age. **Table 2** summarizes the recommended frequency of ophthalmologic screening in children with JIA.[26] Uveitis disease activity does not necessarily correlate with the course of arthritis.

The management of uveitis should be supervised by an eye care expert (ophthalmologist or optometrist) in conjunction with a pediatrician or pediatric rheumatologist. Uveitis is usually managed with topical corticosteroids and a mydriatic agent. Oral, periocular, or intravenous corticosteroids may be required to achieve relief of inflammation, and children with disease that is difficult to control may require additional immunomodulatory medication such methotrexate or biologic agents. Complications of uveitis include band keratopathy and cataracts (occurring in 42%–58% patients), glaucoma (19%–22% patients),[27] and blindness.

Abnormalities of Growth

JIA may be complicated by linear or localized growth disturbance. Linear growth abnormalities are particularly observed in patients with chronic active disease and are therefore most common in children with polyarticular or sJIA.

The mechanisms of poor linear growth in children with JIA are likely multifactorial. Chronic inflammation and high levels of circulating proinflammatory cytokines may play a role in growth suppression through effects on the growth plate[28] and impairment on insulinlike growth factor 1 (IGF-1).[29,30] Overexpression of IL-6, in particular, may play an important role in abnormal skeletal development, as shown in the murine model via several possible mechanisms such as a reduction of circulating IGF-1 levels, growth plate and ossification center abnormalities, and induction of osteoclast activity.[30] Severe growth restriction is now uncommon, possibly as a result of more aggressive immunomodulatory therapy with disease-modifying antirheumatic drugs (DMARDs) and biologic agents (**Tables 3** and **4**). When severe growth retardation does occur, growth hormone may be considered.

Localized growth abnormalities are more commonly observed and are likely a direct result of active arthritis. Accelerated growth at the ossification center because of inflammation may result in overgrowth of the affected limb and longer limb on the affected side. However, premature epiphyseal fusion later in the course caused by persistent inflammation may result in a shortened limb on the affected side. Uncontrolled or untreated arthritis of the temporomandibular joint (TMJ) may cause considerable micrognathia, hypoplasia, and asymmetry (**Fig. 5**). Early recognition of TMJ

Table 2
Modified recommended guidelines for ophthalmologic screening in JIA

ILAR JIA Subtype	ANA	Age at Onset of Disease	Duration of Disease ≤4 y	>4 y
Oligoarticular JIA,	Positive	≤6 y	3 monthly	6 monthly
Polyarticular JIA, and		>6 y	6 monthly	12 monthly
ERA	Negative	≤6 y	6 monthly	12 monthly
		>6 y	12 monthly	12 monthly
sJIA	Not applicable	Not applicable	12 monthly	12 monthly

Data from American Academy of Pediatrics Section on Rheumatology and Section on Ophthalmology: guidelines for ophthalmologic examinations in children with juvenile rheumatoid arthritis. Pediatrics 1993;92(2):295–6.

Table 3
DMARDs

DMARD	Action/Mechanism	Dosing	Common Side Effects	Precautions	Monitoring	Other Comments
Methotrexate	Inhibits purine synthesis. Multiple possible sites of action, including inhibition of dihydrofolate reductase and AICAR transformylase, adenosine deaminase	Weekly PO or SC	GI upset, mouth ulceration Transient liver enzyme abnormalities, hematologic abnormalities (rare)	Avoid sulfamethoxazole and trimethoprim (bone marrow suppression) Avoid pregnancy (fetal death and congenital abnormalities) Avoid alcohol consumption	CBC and LFTs 4-weekly to 12-weekly	Folate supplementation important to alleviate GI side effects and mouth ulcers Avoid live vaccines
Sulfasalazine	Not clearly understood, possibly multiple immunomodulatory and antiinflammatory effects	Twice a day PO	Rash, GI upset, myelosuppression, liver function abnormalities, hypersensitivities Hypogammaglobulinemia	Safe in pregnancy	CBC and LFTs 4-weekly to 12-weekly	Beware possible additive hepatotoxicity in conjunction with MTX
Leflunomide	Inhibits pyrimidine synthesis through inhibition of dihydro-orotate dehydrogenase	Daily PO	GI upset, rash Hypertension Liver enzyme abnormalities	Teratogenic	CBC and LFTs 4-weekly to 12-weekly	Cholestyramine can be used to enhance elimination

Abbreviations: AICAR, 5-aminoimidazole-4-carboxamide ribonucleotide; CBC, complete blood count; GI, gastrointestinal; LFT, liver function tests; MTX, methotrexate; NSAIDs, nonsteroidal antiinflammatory drugs; PO, by mouth; SC, subcutaneously.

Table 4
Biologic medications

Biologic Class	Example of Drug	Administration	Common Side Effects	Precautions	Monitoring
TNF inhibitors	Etanercept Adalimumab Infliximab	Etanercept SC every week, adalimumab SC every 2 wk, infliximab IV every 2 wk to 8 wk	Hypersensitivity infusion reactions	For all biologic medication: Avoid in patients with active infection and hold biologic in event of active infection requiring treatment Avoid in presence of TB infection	For all biologic medication: Ensure negative TB test before commencement and annually Routine laboratory investigations including CBC, LFT, renal function
IL inhibition	Anakinra (IL-1) Canakinumab (IL-1β) Tocilizumab (IL-6) Rilonacept (IL-1)	Anakinra daily Canakinumab every 4 wk Rilonacept every week Tocilizumab every 2 wk	Injection site or infusion reactions	Avoid live vaccines	For rituximab consider measurement of B-cell subsets
B-cell depletion	Rituximab	Every week × 2 doses	Infusion reactions		Consider concomitant use of methotrexate to prevent development of immunogenicity
T-cell costimulatory modulator	Abatacept	Weeks 0, 2, 4 then every 4 wk	Infusion reaction uncommon		

Abbreviations: CBC, complete blood count; LFT, liver function tests; TB, tuberculosis; TNF, tumor necrosis factor.

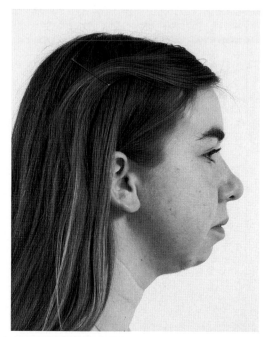

Fig. 5. Chronic arthritis of the TMJs resulting in micrognathia.

involvement is important, and patients presenting with jaw pain, jaw deviation, or limited jaw opening may warrant further investigation. The mechanism of growth retardation at the TMJ is caused by destruction of the joint and the mandibular condyle. Reduced masseter muscle development as a result of pain may also play an important role in the shortening of the mandibular ramus seen in patients with TMJ disease.

Bone Health

Children with JIA are at risk of osteopenia and osteoporosis, leading to an increased risk of fracture. Risk factors for reduced bone mineral density include chronic active arthritis and persistent inflammation, decreased physical activity, poor sunlight exposure, and exposure to corticosteroids. Strategies for the prevention of osteopenia and osteoporosis should include optimal control of inflammatory disease, encouragement of weight-bearing exercise, minimization of steroid exposure, and nutritional support. Bisphosphonates may be considered in the treatment of osteoporosis-related fractures.

TREATMENT

The care of patients with arthritis requires a family-centered approach and should be provided by a multidisciplinary team familiar with the complexities of these diseases and their treatment. The British Society of Pediatric and Adolescent Rheumatology (BSPAR) recently published guidelines defining the minimum standards of care for children with arthritis. These standards include an emphasis on: (1) early recognition of JIA and access to specialist and multidisciplinary care; (2) access to information, treatment options, and support; (3) empowering patients and care givers; and (4) a planned, coordinated transition to adult care.[31]

The goal of treatment in JIA is disease remission. With the introduction of many new JIA therapies, complete disease remission and normalization of physical and psychosocial development are now achievable objectives.

NONPHARMACOLOGIC THERAPY

Occupational and physical therapy are integral in the management of JIA. They aim to help manage pain, improve mobility and range of joint motion, and to prevent deformity. Techniques may include strength and stretching exercises, serial casting, splints, pain management techniques, orthotics, and shoe lifts to correct leg length discrepancy.

Children with JIA and particularly those children on long-term corticosteroids are at risk of osteopenia and osteoporosis. Children should be encouraged to optimize their calcium intake, and consideration should be given to the use of calcium and vitamin D supplementation, especially at times of corticosteroid administration. Calcium supplementation has been shown to be effective in improving bone mineral density in a randomized controlled study.[32] Increasing weight-bearing exercise may also be beneficial in improving bone mineral density.

Studies have suggested that physical activity may result in improved physical function and quality of life in children with JIA.[33–36] Exercise within the individual's capacity and the limitations of their disease should generally be encouraged in children with JIA. Involvement in aerobic-based exercise regimes is safe in children with JIA and may result in improved physical function.[33]

Consideration should be given to the child's general nutrition, growth, and development. The psychosocial impact of this chronic illness must also be addressed, and social work, mental health, and adolescent medicine are frequently engaged as important members of the management team.

Pain may significantly affect the physical and psychosocial quality of life of children with JIA. Increasing pain may reflect active disease; however, there are many other determinants that influence the individual's experience of pain. In addition to the pharmacologic approach, nonpharmacologic techniques and supports are an important part of the self-management of pain in JIA.

PHARMACOLOGIC THERAPY
Nonsteroidal Antiinflammatory Drugs

Nonsteroidal antiinflammatory drugs (NSAIDs) are used in JIA for the symptomatic management of joint pain and stiffness. There are no randomized controlled trials (RCTs) assessing efficacy; however, it seems that 25% to 33% of patients respond to NSAIDs as monotherapy.[37] NSAIDs require 4 to 6 weeks of therapy for beneficial therapeutic effects.[38]

It does not seem that any particular NSAID is more efficacious than the others, and the choice of NSAID is therefore often directed by other determinants such as dosing frequency, availability in liquid or pill form, cost, tolerability, and individual patient response. Naproxen is the most commonly used NSAID in many centers because it has a favorable dosing regimen and toxicity profile. Indomethacin is often favored in ERA and also in the treatment of fever and serositis in sJIA. The use of multiple NSAIDs concurrently is not recommended. Indomethacin seems to have the least favorable toxicity profile and ibuprofen the most favorable.[37]

Gastrointestinal upset is common with NSAID use, and serious gastrointestinal adverse events are rare but possible.[39,40] Pseudoporphyria is a photodermatitis associated with naproxen that may cause skin scarring but mostly resolves with discontinuation. Pseudoporphyria is most commonly seen in fair-skinned children. Renal complications (renal insufficiency, acute interstitial nephritis, nephrotic syndrome, and papillary necrosis) are rare but all children requiring long-term use of NSAIDs should have routine renal monitoring. Increased transaminase levels may also occur, and liver function should be monitored in those patients administered long-term NSAIDs.

CORTICOSTEROIDS
Oral

Systemic oral and parenteral corticosteroid therapy may be used in the treatment of patients with JIA; however, attempts are made to minimize exposure given the potential side effects encountered with prolonged steroid used. Furthermore, they do not induce disease remission. Corticosteroids are particularly used in the treatment of sJIA, especially in the setting of fever, serositis, and MAS. Oral steroid therapy is also administered in the treatment of severe polyarthritis, with the goal of using the steroids as a bridging therapy while other steroid-sparing treatment regimes take effect.

Intra-articular Steroid Injections

The benefits of intra-articular steroid (IAS) injections are well established. Studies have reported sustained remission after IAS.[41–43] IAS injections performed under general anesthesia along with concomitant use of weekly systemic methotrexate may be predictive factors for sustained remission.[42] Choice of steroid used in IAS is important, and triamcinolone hexacetonide is believed to be superior to triamcinolone acetonide.[43] There is some evidence in the adult literature to suggest that 24 hours' bed rest after IAS improves efficacy.[44]

Young children often require the use of general anesthetic or sedation. IAS injections are generally well tolerated. Subcutaneous atrophy is reported to occur at approximately 2% of injection sites[41–43,45] and other complications such as infection are rarely seen.

DMARDs

DMARDs are used for their long-term beneficial effects in controlling disease activity. These medications also play an important role in reducing the long-term exposure to medications such as prednisone and NSAIDs. Historically, DMARDs were used late in the course of disease because there were initial concerns regarding toxicity and safety. Moreover, the illnesses treated were not often considered life threatening and therefore DMARD therapy was considered unwarranted. However, it is now recognized that not only are many of these medications safe and effective for use in children but also that their use early in the disease course may prevent irreversible damage and decrease the burden of disease.

Methotrexate

Methotrexate is the most widely used DMARD in the treatment of JIA and is given either orally or by subcutaneous injections. The significant therapeutic benefit of methotrexate has been shown in RCTs[46,47] and also a Cochrane meta-analysis.[48] Benefit has also been shown in many retrospective and uncontrolled studies. The appropriate dose is approximately 15 mg/m^2 and full therapeutic effect may be appreciated only after 6 to 12 months of therapy.[49]

Differential responses to methotrexate may be seen amongst the various subtypes of JIA. Woo and colleagues[47] found a significant better response to methotrexate therapy in patients with extended oligoarticular JIA compared with patients with sJIA. Ravelli and colleagues[50] reported similar findings in patients with extended oligoarticular JIA treated with methotrexate compared with patients with sJIA and polyarticular JIA.

The optimal time to discontinue methotrexate after disease remission is also unclear. Gottleib and colleagues[51] found that after a mean of 8 months of sustained remission before methotrexate discontinuation, relapses occurred in 52% at a mean of 11 months. Most patients responded when methotrexate was restarted.[51] A recent study did not show a difference between continuous methotrexate therapy for 6 or 12 months before discontinuation and rates of sustained disease remission, implying weaning and discontinuation of methotrexate is possible after at least 6 months of no disease activity.[52]

Oral methotrexate is absorbed by the gastrointestinal tract by a saturable process and subcutaneous administration may increase the bioavailability of methotrexate. Subcutaneous dosing should be considered in patients with poor response to oral methotrexate, gastrointestinal side effects, or poor adherence to oral therapy. The initiation of subcutaneous methotrexate requires patient and family education to ensure that the delivery and handling of the medication are appropriate. Live vaccines should be avoided in patients on methotrexate, and, although there are no consensus guidelines, varicella immunization may be considered before commencing therapy for susceptible patients.

Methotrexate is generally well tolerated in children. The most common side effect is gastrointestinal upset. Nausea and vomiting can be distressing and result in poor adherence or stopping of the medication. Subcutaneous administration may overcome this symptom. Folic acid has been shown to be beneficial in reducing adverse events. Mild liver function abnormalities occur in approximately 9% of children on low-dose therapy.[53] These changes are usually transient and improve with a period of cessation. There are only a few reports of hepatic fibrosis in children and no reports of cirrhosis secondary to methotrexate. Increased risk of developing hepatic fibrosis in patients with inflammatory disorders treated with methotrexate has been associated with alcohol consumption, hepatitis, obesity, or diabetes. Screening for these associated diseases before the start of methotrexate and ongoing counseling about alcohol consumption should be part of routine care in the prevention of hepatic toxicity arising from methotrexate. Oral ulceration, alopecia, hematologic abnormalities, mood changes, rash, diarrhea, and headache have been reported to occur. Because of the risk of fetal abnormalities, methotrexate must be avoided in pregnancy and patients should be counseled about the appropriate use of contraception.

Long-term methotrexate use requires regular clinical and laboratory monitoring both for the response to the medication and for its potential toxicities, including screening of liver function and complete blood count.

Leflunomide

Leflunomide is effective in the treatment of polyarticular JIA. However, when compared with methotrexate in an RCT, the rate of clinical improvement was not as high as that seen with methotrexate.[54] The role of leflunomide in the management of JIA is not clearly defined. In many centers it is used when methotrexate is not tolerated or is considered in combination with methotrexate.

Common side effects include gastrointestinal upset, headache, rash, and alopecia. Liver function abnormalities are less frequently reported[54] but increase with concomitant use of methotrexate.[55] Regular blood pressure monitoring is also recommended for patients. Leflunomide is teratogenic. As with methotrexate, surveillance with complete blood count and liver function test (LFT) is recommended on a regular basis. In the event of toxicity, cholestyramine can be used to enhance elimination.

Sulfasalazine

Sulfasalazine has shown efficacy in a double-blind, placebo RCT of patients with oligoarticular and polyarticular JIA.[56] Adverse events were more frequent but tended to be transient and reversible.[56] In a placebo RCT with patients with ERA, the response rates were similar, with significant improvement confined to the physician and patient global assessment of disease activity in the sulfasalazine-treated patients.[57] Uncontrolled studies have shown additional benefit of sulfasalazine.[58–60]

Sulfasalazine seems most effective in polyarticular and oligoarticular disease and perhaps ERA. Current evidence suggests that sulfasalazine is not effective in the management of sJIA and its use may contribute to increased risk of toxicity in these patients.[61]

Adverse effects resulting from sulfasalazine leading to discontinuation have been reported in approximately 30% of patients.[56] Gastrointestinal intolerance is the most frequently reported side effect. Liver function abnormalities occur in approx 4% patients. More severe, and potentially fatal, hepatotoxicity has been reported in association with DRESS (drug reaction with eosinophilia and systemic symptoms) syndrome (a hypersensitivity reaction believed to be caused by the sulfapyridine metabolite). Hematologic side effects such as leukopenia have an incidence across the literature of 3%.[61] Although leukopenia is reversible with cessation of the drug, other more rare but severe hematologic side effects such as agranulocytosis have been reported.[62] Routine monitoring should include complete blood counts and LFTs.

BIOLOGIC AGENTS

Despite the increasingly aggressive approach to therapy over the past 20 years with early use of DMARDs such as methotrexate, many children continue to have chronically active disease into adulthood. The introduction of biologic agents has added to the treatment options for children with JIA and offers an opportunity to decrease the rates of chronic debilitating disease and aim for complete disease remission.

Biologic agents targeting different pathogenic pathways are now available. The choice of agent depends largely on the JIA subtype, but patient preference must also be considered with respect to the route and frequency of administration. Although there seems to be vast enthusiasm regarding the biologic medications and their application in pediatric rheumatology, there remain limited long-term safety data. In addition, all of these medications come with a significant financial burden to families and health care systems.

TUMOR NECROSIS FACTOR α INHIBITORS

Tumor necrosis factor α (TNF-α) is a proinflammatory cytokine believed to play an important role in the inflammatory pathogenesis of JIA and high levels have been found in both the synovial fluid and serum in children with JIA. Moreover, the serum level of soluble TNF receptors has also been shown to correlate with disease activity.[63,64]

Etanercept

Etanercept is a fully humanized soluble TNF receptor. Etanercept was approved in 1999 by the US Food and Drug Administration (FDA) for use in children with polyarticular course JIA.

The efficacy of etanercept in the treatment of JIA was first reported by Lovell and colleagues[65] in a multicenter RCT in children with polyarticular course disease resistant to methotrexate. All patients received 0.4 mg/kg of etanercept subcutaneously twice weekly for up to 3 months. The responders were then randomized to either continuing etanercept or switching to placebo. Patients assigned to the etanercept group had significantly fewer disease flares and the median time to flare was longer.[65] Several other studies have shown the safety and effectiveness of weekly double dosing of etanercept (0.8 mg/kg per week) instead of the traditional biweekly dosing (0.4 mg/kg).[66,67]

There have subsequently been several observational studies and patient registries that have also supported the effectiveness of etanercept in JIA. A multicenter open-label North American registry found etanercept to be efficacious and safe over the 3 years of the study.[68] This study also found that combination therapy with methotrexate was safe and effective. An open-label extension study of the multicenter RCT enrolled 58 patients and followed patients for 8 years. Only 26 (45%) patients entered the eighth year of the study. Reasons for withdrawal included lack of efficacy in 7 patients (12%), adverse events in 4 (7%), physician decision in 5 patients (9%), parent or guardian refusal in 5 (9%), and 3 patients (5%) each for patient refusal, lost to follow-up, and protocol issues. There were no reports in this study of malignancy or demyelinating disorders and etanercept was considered to be safe when used long-term.[69] Etanercept has also been found to improve quality of life and functional ability in children with JIA.[70,71]

Although etanercept has been shown to be of benefit in different JIA subtypes, many observational and uncontrolled studies have observed etanercept to be less effective in sJIA.[72–75] The use of etanercept in ERA is based on evidence from uncontrolled studies and observational cohort studies that report its safety and also rapid and sustained response to therapy.[76–79]

In general, TNF-α inhibitors are recommended for patients with arthritis refractory to standard therapy and in patients with clinical and radiologic evidence of active sacroiliac disease after an adequate trial of NSAIDs.[80] Few studies have examined guidelines about the discontinuation of etanercept. It has been suggested that careful weaning off etanercept could be considered after 1.5 years of remission.[81]

Infliximab

Infliximab is a human-derived and mouse-derived chimeric anti-TNF-α antibody with cytotoxic properties. It binds to both soluble and membrane-bound TNF-α. Infliximab has been shown to be beneficial in the treatment of JIA. As opposed to etanercept, it must be administered intravenously every 4 to 8 weeks. A placebo RCT of infliximab and methotrexate in the treatment of polyarticular JIA showed efficacy at 1 year of treatment.[82] However, there was no significant difference between infliximab and placebo for the primary efficacy end point at 16 weeks. This trial did show important side effects with infliximab. In particular, a higher incidence of infusion reactions and anti-infliximab antibody formation was noted in patients who received 3 mg/kg of infliximab compared with 6 mg/kg.[82] The open-label extension of this trial reported efficacy and safety data for up to 4 years.[83] Because of the large discontinuation rates in this trial, comments on efficacy and safety are difficult to interpret. The rate of infusion reactions occurred in up to one-third of patients and more frequently in patients with anti-infliximab antibodies. Many centers advocate the use of higher-dose infliximab (>5–6 mg/kg) or concomitant low-dose methotrexate to reduce the risk of antibody formation.

The efficacy of infliximab has been examined in children with ERA and juvenile spondyloarthropathies. Efficacy, including remission of the arthritis and enthesitis, was shown in a double-blind, placebo RCT[84,85] and from observational studies and case series.[78,79,86,87]

Adalimumab

Adalimumab is a fully humanized chimeric anti-TNF-α antibody that also has cytotoxic properties. The benefit of adalimumab with or without concomitant methotrexate has been shown in a randomized placebo-controlled withdrawal trial.[88] During the 16-week open-label phase of this trial, 74% patients on adalimumab alone and 94% of patients on combination therapy (methotrexate and adalimumab) improved. Responders were then randomized to receive placebo or to continue on adalimumab. At the 48-week assessment, response rates were significantly better in the group receiving adalimumab and methotrexate compared with methotrexate and placebo.[88]

Other case series and case reports have documented the benefit of adalimumab. In 1 series of 6 patients with disease refractory to methotrexate, etanercept, or infliximab, adalimumab was beneficial in 3 patients and no adverse effects were observed. This finding shows the possible benefit of switching TNF-α inhibitors despite previously documented nonresponse to other TNF-α inhibition.[89]

Several trials are addressing the efficacy and long-term safety of adalimumab in children with JIA. A double-blind, placebo RCT of adalimumab in polyarticular JIA has recently ceased recruitment and results are pending (clinicaltrials.gov NCT00048542).

IL INHIBITORS
Anakinra

Anakinra is an IL-1 receptor antagonist and there has been much interest in its use in the management of sJIA. IL-1 is believed to be an important cytokine involved in the pathogenesis of sJIA.

A recent retrospective review examined the efficacy and safety of anakinra in 46 newly diagnosed patients with sJIA treated with anakinra alone or in combination (corticosteroids or DMARDs). Resolution of fever and rash was seen in 86% within 1 week and 97% within 1 month. Complete remission was observed in 59% of patients.[90]

A small multicenter double-blind RCT comparing anakinra with placebo in 24 patients with sJIA reported that 83% of patients on anakinra met the definition of response at 1 month. However, reduced response to anakinra was observed over time, possibly explained by the high numbers of patients with diffuse polyarthritis without systemic symptoms. Also, patients included in this trial had disease for more than 6 months and were steroid dependent, perhaps representing a group of patients with more severe disease.[91]

Differential responses to anakinra have been observed in patients with sJIA refractory to other DMARDs. One study reported approximately 40% response rate to anakinra in this group of patients.[92] The nonresponsive group had improved systemic features; however, arthritis and inflammation was not controlled. The group of patients that responded to anakinra had lower joint count and higher neutrophil count at baseline, suggesting that early treatment may be most beneficial.[92]

Anakinra is generally well tolerated and serious adverse events are uncommon. An erythematous pruritic rash at the injection site is frequently observed. This rash tends to improve with time and can be relieved with ice packs. Opportunistic infections have not been reported.

Canakinumab

Canakinumab is a newer biologic agent with fewer studies in patients with JIA. It is a fully humanized IL-1β antibody. A recent phase II study of canakinumab addressing dosing and safety in children with sJIA has revealed promising preliminary safety and efficacy data.[93]

Rilonacept

Rilonacept is a human dimeric protein that binds to IL-1 inhibiting IL-1 signaling. A double-blind, placebo-controlled trial in 21 patients with sJIA showed improvement.[94] Further studies are needed to clarify the role of rilonacept in the management of JIA.

Tocilizumab

Tocilizumab is a monoclonal anti-IL-6 receptor antibody that binds to IL-6 receptors, inhibiting the formation of IL6-IL6R complex.

Results from a phase III double-blind, placebo RCT of tocilizumab in 56 patients with sJIA showed an excellent response rate, with 91% of patients meeting the primary end point after 6 weeks.[95] Forty-three patients, deemed to be responders, entered the double-blind, randomized phase, and after a further 6 weeks of therapy, 80% of the tocilizumab group maintained a clinical response compared with only 17% of the placebo group. In the open-label extension, 90% of patients achieved good disease control (American College of Rheumatology Pediatric 70 criteria) and 98% had total absence of systemic features. Common adverse events included upper respiratory tract infection, nasopharyngitis, bronchitis, and gastroenteritis. An anaphylactoid reaction occurred in 1 patient. LFT abnormalities were also noted and tended to subside during continuation of treatment. There were no reports of tuberculosis.

T-CELL AND B-CELL TARGETED THERAPY
Abatacept

Abatacept is a T-cell costimulatory pathway inhibitor approved by the FDA for use in children older than 6 years with polyarticular JIA. The evidence for its use is based on the results of a multicenter international randomized, double-blind withdrawal trial of children with polyarticular JIA refractory or intolerant to at least 1 DMARD including biologic agents such as TNF inhibitors.[96] Patients first entered a 4-month open-label lead-in phase (n = 190), with responders (n = 122) randomized to continue abatacept monthly or to receive placebo for 6 months. At 6 months, the rate of flares between the groups was significantly different, favoring treatment with abatacept (control group 53% compared with treatment group 20%). No serious adverse events were described in the abatacept group. A long-term open-label extension phase of this trial reported ongoing clinically significant efficacy.[97] Some patients who failed to respond initially during the open-label phase were noted to have responded at follow-up, suggesting that a long-term trial of abatacept may be necessary before treatment is considered to be a failure. Abatacept was generally well tolerated. There were no cases of malignancy or tuberculosis attributed to abatacept. However, 6 serious infections were seen and 1 patient developed multiple sclerosis.[97]

Health-related quality-of-life measures have also been shown to improve with the use of abatacept.[98]

Rituximab

Rituximab is a monoclonal mouse antibody that induces B-cell apoptosis and causes CD20 B-cell depletion. Antibody production is not entirely depleted because plasma cells are not removed. There is little evidence for the use of rituximab in children with JIA. The best evidence for its use is provided by an observational study and several case reports.

A recent observational study reviewed the use of rituximab in 55 patients with severe refractory polyarticular or sJIA and reported significant improvement in disease activity and remission in many patients.[99] Other case reports have supported the improvement with rituximab in JIA but the exact role of rituximab remains unclear.

Rituximab is administered intravenously in 2 doses 2 weeks apart for the treatment of JIA and RA. It is generally well tolerated and side effects are unusual. Infusion reactions such as flushing and itch may be observed and are generally avoided with premedication.

ADVERSE EFFECTS OF BIOLOGIC AGENTS

In 2008, the FDA reported several cases of malignancy in patients with JIA receiving biologic therapy. There has been much controversy about the implication of this warning and how to apply this information in the clinical setting, especially given that the background incidence of malignancy in JIA is unknown and the role of concomitant immunosuppressive medications is also unclear. Although some studies have suggested a possible link between JIA treatment and cancer occurrence, a direct causal relationship between biologic agents and cancer has not been established.[100–102]

Reported serious infections include opportunistic infection and tuberculosis. In general, patients do not require treatment with prophylactic antibiotics while on biologic therapy. Tuberculosis screening with Mantoux skin test is recommended before commencing any biologic medication and repeating on an annual basis.

Other side effects include the development of autoimmune disorders such as demyelinating disorders (multiple sclerosis), inflammatory bowel disease, psoriasis, systemic lupus erythematosus, vasculitic rashes, and uveitis. The safety data suggest that these medications are safe, but long-term safety data in children are not available. Clinicians must remain vigilant in the monitoring of adverse effects in any patient on biologic therapy.

Outcome

The disease outcome and prognosis in JIA are variable and to some degree predictable based on the different disease subtypes. Many children with JIA have an excellent prognosis and for the most part remain free from significantly debilitating disease. However, a considerable proportion of children with JIA have chronic disease activity. Rates of remission are highest in persistent oligoarticular JIA and lower in polyarticular JIA (RF-positive and RF-negative), ERA, and PsJIA.[103] Active disease continues into adulthood in 50% to 70% of patients with systemic and polyarticular disease and 40% to 50% of oligoarticular arthritis.[103–107] Functional disability is estimated in up to 20% of children transitioning to adulthood[107] and 30% to 40% have other long-term disabilities, including unemployment.[108] Major surgery, including joint replacement, is required in 25% to 50%.[108] Delay in referral and initiation of acceptable therapy is associated with poorer outcome.[1]

There remains considerable difficulty in acquiring data relating to estimates of the global burden of JIA. The impact of juvenile arthritis on disability and handicap, the educational and vocational disadvantages, life expectancy, and quality of life as well as the cost of medical care have yet to be evaluated.

SUMMARY

JIA encompasses a diverse group of disorders with a complex multifactorial pathogenesis and cause. Considerable advances have been made in understanding the pathogenesis of JIA; however, further definition of the underlying immunogenetic mechanisms is required. This knowledge may enable more refined homogeneous classification of JIA and allow the clinician to individualize therapy based on each patient's unique biologic and genetic parameters.

In recent years, new biologic medications have added significantly to the management of children with JIA. Despite this situation, many children with JIA continue to have persistently active arthritis into adulthood. Sustained and multinational collaborative efforts addressing disease manifestations and outcome, as well as treatment efficacy and safety surveillance, are central to future advances in the management of children with JIA.

REFERENCES

1. Cassidy JT, Laxer RM, Petty RE, et al. Textbook of pediatric rheumatology. 6th Edition. Philadelphia (PA): Elsevier Saunders; 2011. [Chapter: 13].
2. Manners PJ, Bower C. Worldwide prevalence of juvenile arthritis why does it vary so much? J Rheumatol 2002;29(7):1520–30.
3. Manners PJ, Diepeveen DA. Prevalence of juvenile chronic arthritis in a population of 12-year-old children in urban Australia. Pediatrics 1996;98(1):84–90.
4. Mielants H, Veys EM, Maertens M, et al. Prevalence of inflammatory rheumatic diseases in an adolescent urban student population, age 12 to 18, in Belgium. Clin Exp Rheumatol 1993;11(5):563–7.
5. Tayel MY, Tayel KY. Prevalence of juvenile chronic arthritis in school children aged 10 to 15 years in Alexandria. J Egypt Public Health Assoc 1999;74(5–6):529–46.
6. Petty RE. Frequency of uncommon diseases: is juvenile idiopathic arthritis underrecognized? J Rheumatol 2002;29(7):1356–7.
7. Arguedas O, Fasth A, Andersson-Gare B. A prospective population based study on outcome of juvenile chronic arthritis in Costa Rica. J Rheumatol 2002;29(1):174–83.
8. Arguedas O, Fasth A, Andersson-Gäre B, et al. Juvenile chronic arthritis in urban San Jose, Costa Rica: a 2 year prospective study. J Rheumatol 1998; 25(9):1844–50.
9. Fujikawa S, Okuni M. A nationwide surveillance study of rheumatic diseases among Japanese children. Acta Paediatr Jpn 1997;39(2):242–4.
10. Kurahara D, Tokuda A, Grandinetti A, et al. Ethnic differences in risk for pediatric rheumatic illness in a culturally diverse population. J Rheumatol 2002;29(2): 379–83.
11. Saurenmann RK, Rose JB, Tyrrell P, et al. Epidemiology of juvenile idiopathic arthritis in a multiethnic cohort: ethnicity as a risk factor. Arthritis Rheum 2007; 56(6):1974–84.
12. Petty RE, Southwood TR, Manners P, et al. International League of Associations for Rheumatology classification of juvenile idiopathic arthritis: second revision, Edmonton, 2001. J Rheumatol 2004;31(2):390–2.
13. Petty RE, Southwood TR, Baum J, et al. Revision of the proposed classification criteria for juvenile idiopathic arthritis: Durban, 1997. J Rheumatol 1998;25(10): 1991–4.
14. Goldenberg J, Ferraz MB, Pessoa AP, et al. Symptomatic cardiac involvement in juvenile rheumatoid arthritis. Int J Cardiol 1992;34(1):57–62.
15. Cabral DA, Tucker LB. Malignancies in children who initially present with rheumatic complaints. J Pediatr 1999;134(1):53–7.

16. Ostrov BE, Goldsmith DP, Athreya BH. Differentiation of systemic juvenile rheumatoid arthritis from acute leukemia near the onset of disease. J Pediatr 1993; 122(4):595–8.

17. Schaller J. Arthritis as a presenting manifestation of malignancy in children. J Pediatr 1972;81(4):793–7.

18. Jones OY, Spencer CH, Bowyer SL, et al. A multicenter case-control study on predictive factors distinguishing childhood leukemia from juvenile rheumatoid arthritis. Pediatrics 2006;117(5):e840–4.

19. Schneider R, Lang BA, Reilly BJ, et al. Prognostic indicators of joint destruction in systemic-onset juvenile rheumatoid arthritis. J Pediatr 1992;120(2 Pt 1): 200–5.

20. Spiegel LR, Schneider R, Lang BA, et al. Early predictors of poor functional outcome in systemic-onset juvenile rheumatoid arthritis: a multicenter cohort study. Arthritis Rheum 2000;43(11):2402–9.

21. Modesto C, Woo P, García-Consuegra J, et al. Systemic onset juvenile chronic arthritis, polyarticular pattern and hip involvement as markers for a bad prognosis. Clin Exp Rheumatol 2001;19(2):211–7.

22. Behrens EM, Beukelman T, Paessler M, et al. Occult macrophage activation syndrome in patients with systemic juvenile idiopathic arthritis. J Rheumatol 2007;34(5):1133–8.

23. Ravelli A, Magni-Manzoni S, Pistorio A, et al. Preliminary diagnostic guidelines for macrophage activation syndrome complicating systemic juvenile idiopathic arthritis. J Pediatr 2005;146(5):598–604.

24. Stoll ML, Zurakowski D, Nigrovic LE, et al. Patients with juvenile psoriatic arthritis comprise two distinct populations. Arthritis Rheum 2006;54(11):3564–72.

25. Stoll ML, Punaro M. Psoriatic juvenile idiopathic arthritis: a tale of two subgroups. Curr Opin Rheumatol 2011;23(5):437–43.

26. American Academy of Pediatrics Section on Rheumatology and Section on Ophthalmology: opthalmologic examination in children with juvenile rheumatoid arthritis. Pediatrics 2006;117(5):1843–5.

27. Kanski JJ, Shun-Shin GA. Systemic uveitis syndromes in childhood: an analysis of 340 cases. Ophthalmology 1984;91(10):1247–52.

28. Wong SC, MacRae VE, Gracie JA, et al. Inflammatory cytokines in juvenile idiopathic arthritis: effects on physical growth and the insulin-like-growth factor axis. Growth Horm IGF Res 2008;18(5):369–78.

29. Davies UM, Jones J, Reeve J, et al. Juvenile rheumatoid arthritis. Effects of disease activity and recombinant human growth hormone on insulin-like growth factor 1, insulin-like growth factor binding proteins 1 and 3, and osteocalcin. Arthritis Rheum 1997;40(2):332–40.

30. De Benedetti F. The impact of chronic inflammation on the growing skeleton: lessons from interleukin-6 transgenic mice. Horm Res 2009;72(Suppl 1): 26–9.

31. Davies K, Cleary G, Foster H, et al. BSPAR Standards of Care for children and young people with juvenile idiopathic arthritis. Rheumatology (Oxford) 2010; 49(7):1406–8.

32. Lovell DJ, Glass D, Ranz J, et al. A randomized controlled trial of calcium supplementation to increase bone mineral density in children with juvenile rheumatoid arthritis. Arthritis Rheum 2006;54(7):2235–42.

33. Singh-Grewal D, Schneiderman-Walker J, Wright V, et al. The effects of vigorous exercise training on physical function in children with arthritis: a randomized, controlled, single-blinded trial. Arthritis Rheum 2007;57(7):1202–10.

34. Takken T, van der Net J, Helders PJ. Relationship between functional ability and physical fitness in juvenile idiopathic arthritis patients. Scand J Rheumatol 2003; 32(3):174–8.
35. Takken T, van der Net J, Kuis W, et al. Physical activity and health related physical fitness in children with juvenile idiopathic arthritis. Ann Rheum Dis 2003; 62(9):885–9.
36. Takken T, Van Der Net J, Kuis W, et al. Aquatic fitness training for children with juvenile idiopathic arthritis. Rheumatology (Oxford) 2003;42(11):1408–14.
37. Giannini EH, Cawkwell GD. Drug treatment in children with juvenile rheumatoid arthritis. Past, present, and future. Pediatr Clin North Am 1995;42(5):1099–125.
38. Lovell DJ, Giannini EH, Brewer EJ Jr. Time course of response to nonsteroidal antiinflammatory drugs in juvenile rheumatoid arthritis. Arthritis Rheum 1984; 27(12):1433–7.
39. Keenan GF, Giannini EH, Athreya BH. Clinically significant gastropathy associated with nonsteroidal antiinflammatory drug use in children with juvenile rheumatoid arthritis. J Rheumatol 1995;22(6):1149–51.
40. Dowd JE, Cimaz R, Fink CW. Nonsteroidal antiinflammatory drug-induced gastroduodenal injury in children. Arthritis Rheum 1995;38(9):1225–31.
41. Lanni S, Bertamino M, Consolaro A, et al. Outcome and predicting factors of single and multiple intra-articular corticosteroid injections in children with juvenile idiopathic arthritis. Rheumatology (Oxford) 2011;50(9):1627–34.
42. Marti P, Molinari L, Bolt IB, et al. Factors influencing the efficacy of intra-articular steroid injections in patients with juvenile idiopathic arthritis. Eur J Pediatr 2008;167(4):425–30.
43. Zulian F, Martini G, Gobber D, et al. Triamcinolone acetonide and hexacetonide intra-articular treatment of symmetrical joints in juvenile idiopathic arthritis: a double-blind trial. Rheumatology (Oxford) 2004;43(10):1288–91.
44. Chakravarty K, Pharoah PD, Scott DG. A randomized controlled study of post-injection rest following intra-articular steroid therapy for knee synovitis. Br J Rheumatol 1994;33(5):464–8.
45. Wallen M, Gillies D. Intra-articular steroids and splints/rest for children with juvenile idiopathic arthritis and adults with rheumatoid arthritis. Cochrane Database Syst Rev 2006;1:CD002824.
46. Giannini EH, Brewer EJ, Kuzmina N, et al. Methotrexate in resistant juvenile rheumatoid arthritis. Results of the U.S.A.-U.S.S.R. double-blind, placebo-controlled trial. The Pediatric Rheumatology Collaborative Study Group and The Cooperative Children's Study Group. N Engl J Med 1992;326(16):1043–9.
47. Woo P, Southwood TR, Prieur AM, et al. Randomized, placebo-controlled, cross-over trial of low-dose oral methotrexate in children with extended oligoarticular or systemic arthritis. Arthritis Rheum 2000;43(8):1849–57.
48. Takken T, Van Der Net J, Helders PJ. Methotrexate for treating juvenile idiopathic arthritis. Cochrane Database Syst Rev 2001;4:CD003129.
49. Ruperto N, Murray KJ, Gerloni V, et al. A randomized trial of parenteral methotrexate comparing an intermediate dose with a higher dose in children with juvenile idiopathic arthritis who failed to respond to standard doses of methotrexate. Arthritis Rheum 2004;50(7):2191–201.
50. Ravelli A, Viola S, Migliavacca D, et al. The extended oligoarticular subtype is the best predictor of methotrexate efficacy in juvenile idiopathic arthritis. J Pediatr 1999;135(3):316–20.
51. Gottlieb BS, Keenan GF, Lu T, et al. Discontinuation of methotrexate treatment in juvenile rheumatoid arthritis. Pediatrics 1997;100(6):994–7.

52. Foell D, Wulffraat N, Wedderburn LR, et al. Methotrexate withdrawal at 6 vs 12 months in juvenile idiopathic arthritis in remission: a randomized clinical trial. JAMA 2010;303(13):1266–73.

53. Singsen BH, Goldbach-Mansky R. Methotrexate in the treatment of juvenile rheumatoid arthritis and other pediatric rheumatoid and nonrheumatic disorders. Rheum Dis Clin North Am 1997;23(4):811–40.

54. Silverman E, Mouy R, Spiegel L, et al. Leflunomide or methotrexate for juvenile rheumatoid arthritis. N Engl J Med 2005;352(16):1655–66.

55. Cannon GW, Kremer JM. Leflunomide. Rheum Dis Clin North Am 2004;30(2): 295–309, vi.

56. van Rossum MA, Fiselier TJ, Franssen MJ, et al. Sulfasalazine in the treatment of juvenile chronic arthritis: a randomized, double-blind, placebo-controlled, multi-center study. Dutch Juvenile Chronic Arthritis Study Group. Arthritis Rheum 1998;41(5):808–16.

57. Burgos-Vargas R, Vázquez-Mellado J, Pacheco-Tena C, et al. A 26 week randomised, double blind, placebo controlled exploratory study of sulfasalazine in juvenile onset spondyloarthropathies. Ann Rheum Dis 2002;61(10):941–2.

58. Imundo LF, Jacobs JC. Sulfasalazine therapy for juvenile rheumatoid arthritis. J Rheumatol 1996;23(2):360–6.

59. Joos R, Veys EM, Mielants H, et al. Sulfasalazine treatment in juvenile chronic arthritis: an open study. J Rheumatol 1991;18(6):880–4.

60. Ozdogan H, Turunç M, Deringöl B, et al. Sulphasalazine in the treatment of juvenile rheumatoid arthritis: a preliminary open trial. J Rheumatol 1986;13(1): 124–5.

61. Brooks CD. Sulfasalazine for the management of juvenile rheumatoid arthritis. J Rheumatol 2001;28(4):845–53.

62. Marouf ES, Morris IM. Neutropenia in patients with rheumatoid arthritis, treated with sulphasalazine. Br J Rheumatol 1990;29(5):407–9.

63. Gattorno M, Picco P, Buoncompagni A, et al. Serum p55 and p75 tumour necrosis factor receptors as markers of disease activity in juvenile chronic arthritis. Ann Rheum Dis 1996;55(4):243–7.

64. Mangge H, Gallistl S, Schauenstein K. Long-term follow-up of cytokines and soluble cytokine receptors in peripheral blood of patients with juvenile rheumatoid arthritis. J Interferon Cytokine Res 1999;19(9):1005–10.

65. Lovell DJ, Giannini EH, Reiff A, et al. Etanercept in children with polyarticular juvenile rheumatoid arthritis. Pediatric Rheumatology Collaborative Study Group. N Engl J Med 2000;342(11):763–9.

66. Horneff G, Ebert A, Fitter S, et al. Safety and efficacy of once weekly etanercept 0.8 mg/kg in a multicentre 12 week trial in active polyarticular course juvenile idiopathic arthritis. Rheumatology (Oxford) 2009;48(8):916–9.

67. Prince FH, Twilt M, Jansen-Wijngaarden NC, et al. Effectiveness of a once weekly double dose of etanercept in patients with juvenile idiopathic arthritis: a clinical study. Ann Rheum Dis 2007;66(5):704–5.

68. Giannini EH, Ilowite NT, Lovell DJ, et al. Long-term safety and effectiveness of etanercept in children with selected categories of juvenile idiopathic arthritis. Arthritis Rheum 2009;60(9):2794–804.

69. Lovell DJ, Reiff A, Ilowite NT, et al. Safety and efficacy of up to eight years of continuous etanercept therapy in patients with juvenile rheumatoid arthritis. Arthritis Rheum 2008;58(5):1496–504.

70. Halbig M, Horneff G. Improvement of functional ability in children with juvenile idiopathic arthritis by treatment with etanercept. Rheumatol Int 2009;30(2):229–38.

71. Prince FH, Geerdink LM, Borsboom GJ, et al. Major improvements in health-related quality of life during the use of etanercept in patients with previously refractory juvenile idiopathic arthritis. Ann Rheum Dis 2010;69(1):138–42.
72. Katsicas MM, Russo RA. Use of infliximab in patients with systemic juvenile idiopathic arthritis refractory to etanercept. Clin Exp Rheumatol 2005;23(4):545–8.
73. Kimura Y, Pinho P, Walco G, et al. Etanercept treatment in patients with refractory systemic onset juvenile rheumatoid arthritis. J Rheumatol 2005;32(5):935–42.
74. Prince FH, Twilt M, ten Cate R, et al. Long-term follow-up on effectiveness and safety of etanercept in juvenile idiopathic arthritis: the Dutch national register. Ann Rheum Dis 2009;68(5):635–41.
75. Quartier P, Taupin P, Bourdeaut F, et al. Efficacy of etanercept for the treatment of juvenile idiopathic arthritis according to the onset type. Arthritis Rheum 2003;48(4):1093–101.
76. Henrickson M, Reiff A. Prolonged efficacy of etanercept in refractory enthesitis-related arthritis. J Rheumatol 2004;31(10):2055–61.
77. Sulpice M, Deslandre CJ, Quartier P. Efficacy and safety of TNFalpha antagonist therapy in patients with juvenile spondyloarthropathies. Joint Bone Spine 2009;76(1):24–7.
78. Tse SM, Burgos-Vargas R, Laxer RM. Anti-tumor necrosis factor alpha blockade in the treatment of juvenile spondylarthropathy. Arthritis Rheum 2005;52(7):2103–8.
79. Otten MH, Prince FH, Twilt M, et al. Tumor necrosis factor-blocking agents for children with enthesitis-related arthritis–data from the Dutch Arthritis and Biologicals in Children Register, 1999-2010. J Rheumatol 2011;38(10):2258–63.
80. Beukelman T, Patkar NM, Saag KG, et al. 2011 American College of Rheumatology recommendations for the treatment of juvenile idiopathic arthritis: initiation and safety monitoring of therapeutic agents for the treatment of arthritis and systemic features. Arthritis Care Res (Hoboken) 2011;63(4):465–82.
81. Prince FH, Twilt M, Simon SC, et al. When and how to stop etanercept after successful treatment of patients with juvenile idiopathic arthritis. Ann Rheum Dis 2009;68(7):1228–9.
82. Ruperto N, Lovell DJ, Cuttica R, et al. A randomized, placebo-controlled trial of infliximab plus methotrexate for the treatment of polyarticular-course juvenile rheumatoid arthritis. Arthritis Rheum 2007;56(9):3096–106.
83. Ruperto N, Lovell DJ, Cuttica R, et al. Long-term efficacy and safety of infliximab plus methotrexate for the treatment of polyarticular course juvenile rheumatoid arthritis: findings from an open-label treatment extension. Ann Rheum Dis 2010;69:718–22.
84. Burgos-Vargas R, Gutierrez-Suarez R. A 3-month, double-blind, placebo-controlled, randomized trial of infliximab in juvenile-onset spondyloarthritis (SpA) and a 52-week open extension. Clin Exp Rheumatol 2008;26:745.
85. Burgos-Vargas R, Gutierrez-Suarez R, Vazquez-Mellado J. Efficacy, safety, and tolerability of Infliximab in Juvenile-onset Spondyloarthropathies (JO-SpA): results of the three month, randomized, double-blind, placebo-controlled trial phase. Arthritis Rheum 2007;56:319.
86. Schmeling H, Horneff G. Infliximab in two patients with juvenile ankylosing spondylitis. Rheumatol Int 2004;24(3):173–6.
87. Tse SM, Laxer RM, Babyn PS, et al. Radiologic Improvement of juvenile idiopathic arthritis-enthesitis-related arthritis following anti-tumor necrosis factor-alpha blockade with etanercept. J Rheumatol 2006;33(6):1186–8.
88. Lovell DJ, Ruperto N, Goodman S, et al. Adalimumab with or without methotrexate in juvenile rheumatoid arthritis. N Engl J Med 2008;359(8):810–20.

89. Katsicas MM, Russo RA. Use of adalimumab in patients with juvenile idiopathic arthritis refractory to etanercept and/or infliximab. Clin Rheumatol 2009;28(8): 985–8.

90. Nigrovic PA, Mannion M, Prince FH, et al. Anakinra as first-line disease modifying therapy in systemic juvenile idiopathic arthritis. Arthritis Rheum 2011; 63(2):545–55.

91. Quartier P, Allantaz F, Cimaz R, et al. A multicentre, randomised, double-blind, placebo-controlled trial with the interleukin-1 receptor antagonist anakinra in patients with systemic-onset juvenile idiopathic arthritis (ANAJIS trial). Ann Rheum Dis 2011;70(5):747–54.

92. Gattorno M, Piccini A, Lasigliè D, et al. The pattern of response to anti-interleukin-1 treatment distinguishes two subsets of patients with systemic-onset juvenile idiopathic arthritis. Arthritis Rheum 2008;58(5):1505–15.

93. Ruperto N, Quartier P, Wulffraat N, et al. A phase II study to evaluate dosing and preliminary safety and efficacy of canakinumab in systemic juvenile idiopathic arthritis with active systemic features. Arthritis Rheum 2012;64(2):557–67.

94. Lovell DJ, Giannini EH, Kimura Y, et al. Preliminary evidence for sustained bioactivity of IL-1 Trap (rilonacept), a long acting IL-1 inhibitor, in systemic juvenile idiopathic arthritis (SJIA). Arthritis Rheum 2007;56:S515.

95. Yokota S, Imagawa T, Mori M, et al. Efficacy and safety of tocilizumab in patients with systemic-onset juvenile idiopathic arthritis: a randomised, double-blind, placebo-controlled, withdrawal phase III trial. Lancet 2008;371(9617):998–1006.

96. Ruperto N, Lovell DJ, Quartier P, et al. Abatacept in children with juvenile idiopathic arthritis: a randomised, double-blind, placebo-controlled withdrawal trial. Lancet 2008;372(9636):383–91.

97. Ruperto N, Lovell DJ, Quartier P, et al. Long-term safety and efficacy of abatacept in children with juvenile idiopathic arthritis. Arthritis Rheum 2010;62(6): 1792–802.

98. Ruperto N, Lovell DJ, Li T, et al. Abatacept improves health-related quality of life, pain, sleep quality, and daily participation in subjects with juvenile idiopathic arthritis. Arthritis Care Res (Hoboken) 2010;62(11):1542–51.

99. Alexeeva EI, Valieva SI, Bzarova TM, et al. Efficacy and safety of repeat courses of rituximab treatment in patients with severe refractory juvenile idiopathic arthritis. Clin Rheumatol 2011;30(9):1163–72.

100. Cron RQ, Beukelman T. Guilt by association–what is the true risk of malignancy in children treated with etanercept for JIA? Pediatr Rheumatol Online J 2010;8:23.

101. Horneff G, Foeldvari I, Minden K, et al. Report on malignancies in the German juvenile idiopathic arthritis registry. Rheumatology (Oxford) 2011;50(1):230–6.

102. Simard JF, Neovius M, Hagelberg S, et al. Juvenile idiopathic arthritis and risk of cancer: a nationwide cohort study. Arthritis Rheum 2010;62(12):3776–82.

103. Nordal E, Zak M, Aalto K, et al. Ongoing disease activity and changing categories in a long-term nordic cohort study of juvenile idiopathic arthritis. Arthritis Rheum 2011;63(9):2809–18.

104. Fantini F, Gerloni V, Gattinara M, et al. Remission in juvenile chronic arthritis: a cohort study of 683 consecutive cases with a mean 10 year followup. J Rheumatol 2003;30(3):579–84.

105. Minden K, Niewerth M, Listing J, et al. Long-term outcome in patients with juvenile idiopathic arthritis. Arthritis Rheum 2002;46(9):2392–401.

106. Packham JC, Hall MA. Long-term follow-up of 246 adults with juvenile idiopathic arthritis: functional outcome. Rheumatology (Oxford) 2002;41(12):1428–35.

107. Zak M, Pedersen FK. Juvenile chronic arthritis into adulthood: a long-term follow-up study. Rheumatology (Oxford) 2000;39(2):198–204.
108. Hashkes PJ, Laxer RM. Medical treatment of juvenile idiopathic arthritis. JAMA 2005;294(13):1671–84.

Making Sense of the Cytokine Storm: A Conceptual Framework for Understanding, Diagnosing, and Treating Hemophagocytic Syndromes

Scott W. Canna, MD, Edward M. Behrens, MD*

KEYWORDS

- Cytokine storm • Macrophage activation syndrome
- Hemophagocytic lymphohistiocytosis • Sepsis

OBJECTIVES

After reading this article, the reader should be able to:

1. Identify clinical similarities and differences between the variety of cytokine storm syndromes
2. Describe the clinical and immunologic hallmarks of macrophage activation syndrome and hemophagocytic lymphohistiocytosis
3. Describe a pathoetiologic framework for understanding cytokine storm syndromes.

THE FINAL COMMON PATHWAY
History

In the days before germ theory, the term sepsis (from the Greek *sepo*, "I rot") was applied to all states of uncontrolled inflammation. Today, sepsis is reserved to refer to overwhelming inflammation in the context of a systemic infection (although even this definition can be ambiguous). The term cytokine storm syndrome (CSS) was developed to accommodate the observation that multiple inflammatory causes can result in a disease that appears similar to sepsis. The unifying feature of CSS is

Drs Canna and Behrens have no significant financial disclosures pertaining to this article.
Division of Rheumatology, The Children's Hospital of Philadelphia, 3615 Civic Center Boulevard, Philadelphia, PA 19104, USA
* Corresponding author.
E-mail address: behrens@email.chop.edu

Pediatr Clin N Am 59 (2012) 329–344
doi:10.1016/j.pcl.2012.03.002
0031-3955/12/$ – see front matter © 2012 Elsevier Inc. All rights reserved.

a clinical and laboratory phenotype suggestive of massive inflammation, progressing to multiple organ dysfunction syndrome (MODS) and eventually death, a final common pathway.

Examination and Laboratory Findings

The clinical constituents of this pathway can include fever, tachycardia, tachypnea, hypotension, malaise, generalized swelling, altered mental status, diffuse lymphoadenopathy, organomegaly (particularly of the liver and spleen), and often erythematous or purpuric rash. In response to the desire by intensive care practitioners to standardize hemodynamic management of CSS, criteria for systemic inflammatory response syndrome (SIRS) were proposed in 1992[1] and have been amended several times, notably to accommodate pediatric practice (**Table 1**).[2]

CSS also have several common laboratory abnormalities. Hematologic parameters like leukocytosis or thrombocytosis can indicate the acute phase response. Alternatively, increased cell counts can decrease precipitously as a feature of nearly all CSS, suggesting consumption. Clinicians can also take advantage of a host of nonspecific acute phase reactants, including erythrocyte sedimentation rate (ESR), C-reactive protein, procalcitonin, serum amyloid A, ferritin, and fibrinogen among others. Akin to acute cytopenias, an acute decrease in ESR and fibrinogen is most associated with macrophage activation syndrome (MAS), but can be seen in any CSS and often suggests active disseminated intravascular coagulopathy (DIC). Screens for coagulopathy such as fibrin split products and d-dimer are often increased in CSS even in the absence of overt DIC, suggesting subclinical endothelial activation. Likewise, hypoalbuminemia is frequently observed and likely represents systemic capillary leak. Routine testing often reflects various organs in distress, including the liver, pancreas, and kidneys. Such tests are rarely capable of distinguishing direct inflammatory damage from that induced by insufficient oxygen delivery.

The Elusive Hemophagocyte

Hemophagocytes are activated macrophages seen histologically to be have engulfed other hematopoietic elements (erythrocytes, leukocytes, or platelets (**Fig. 1**)).

Table 1
Pediatric SIRS criteria

SIRS	
Presence of at least 2 of the following 4 criteria Must include abnormal temperature or leukocyte count	
Core temperature	>38.5°C or <36°C
Abnormal heart rate	>2SD more than normal for age[a] or unexplained persistent increase over 0.5-h to 4-h period, or for children <1 year old: heart rate <10th percentile for age[a] or unexplained persistent heart rate depression over a 0.5-h period
Respiratory rate	>2SD more than normal for age or acute requirement for mechanical ventilation
Leukocyte count	Increased or depressed[b] for age or >10% immature neutrophils

[a] Not explained by external stimuli or drugs.
[b] Not caused by chemotherapy-induced leukopenia.
Adapted from Goldstein B, Giroir B, Randolph A. International pediatric sepsis consensus conference: definitions for sepsis and organ dysfunction in pediatrics. Pediatr Crit Care Med 2005;6(1):4; with permission.

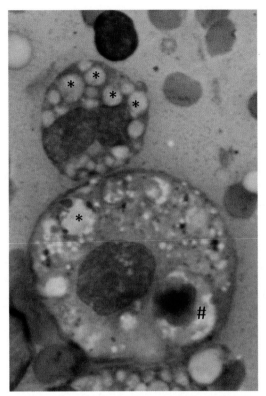

Fig. 1. Hemophagocyte seen in the spleen of a WT mouse treated with TLR9 stimulation and IL-10 blockade. *, engulfed red blood cell (so-called ghost cell); #, engulfed leukocyte.

Hemophagocytes are the pathologic hallmark of hemophagocytic lymphohistiocytosis (HLH) and MAS. However, hemophagocytes are not essential to the diagnosis of HLH[3] and can be seen in juvenile patients with arthritis without overt MAS.[4] In addition, hemophagocytes are found commonly in a host of other inflammatory states including sepsis[5] and after bone marrow transplant.[6] Whether hemophagocytes are inflammatory, antiinflammatory, or serve different roles in differing diseases is a matter of ongoing study.

CAUSES

An analysis of the underlying pathoetiology of all CSS supports this simple but essential postulate: cytokine storm results from excessive proinflammatory stimuli, inadequate regulation of inflammation, or elements of both. Proinflammatory stimuli can include antigens, superantigens (compounds that trigger nonspecific but massive activation of T-cell receptors), adjuvants (such as toll-like receptor [TLR] ligands; for an excellent review of TLRs in infection and autoimmunity see Ref.[7]), allergens (antigens triggering an allergic response), and proinflammatory cytokines themselves. Antiinflammatory mechanisms can be humoral or cellular and seek to dampen or terminate a proinflammatory pathway. **Table 2** provides several examples of both proinflammatory stimuli and antiinflammatory mechanisms. Defects leading to

Table 2	
Common examples of proinflammatory and antiinflammatory contributors to CSS	
Proinflammatory Agents	
Antigens	Antibody or B-cell receptor epitopes
	Peptides presented on MHC
Adjuvants	TLR ligands
	LPS, bacterial DNA, dsRNA, flagellin, etc
	Other PRR ligands
	Microbial nucleic acids
	Inflammasome triggers
	Uric acid crystals, hyperglycemia, ATP
Cytokines/chemokines	IL-1β, IL-6, IL-12, IL-18, TNFα, IFNγ,...
Antiinflammatory Agents	
Cells	Regulatory T cells
	Alternatively activated macrophages
	B10 B cells
Cytokines	IL-10, TGFβ, IL-1ra
Molecules	Antimicrobial peptides

Abbreviations: ATP, adenosine triphosphate; IL-1ra, IL-1 receptor antagonist; LPS, lipopolysaccharide; MHC, major histocompatibility complex; PRR, pattern recognition receptors; TGFβ, Transforming growth factor β.

excessive proinflammatory or inadequate antiinflammatory responses can be host-derived or environmental.

Host Factors

Conventional immunodeficiencies

Because sepsis is common among otherwise immunologically normal hosts, it is easy to forget that there are likely hundreds of genetic and epigenetic risk factors for the development of sepsis. Patients with immunodeficiencies should be considered at risk for CSS by virtue of their inability to effectively clear the proinflammatory elements of an infection. Persistent infection provides a rich source of both antigen and adjuvant, which, as the infection worsens, can quickly overwhelm the ability of the body to regulate inflammation.

The primary immunodeficiencies encompass defects in both innate and adaptive immunity and include entities such as severe combined immunodeficiency (SCID), X-linked agammaglobulinemia, common variable immunodeficiency, chronic granulomatous disease, and complement component deficiencies (see http://www. immunodeficiencysearch.com/ for a thorough, searchable review of immunodeficiency syndromes[8]). Other host-derived immunodeficiency states such as extremes of age and malnutrition can contribute to the inability to effectively clear inflammatory stimuli.

Familial HLH

Familial HLH (fHLH) is a CSS usually occurring in younger children who present with immense inflammation, pancytopenias, and other features of the final common pathway. Such patients' disease is usually triggered by viral infection, and patients are unable to effectively clear the virus. fHLH, by definition, occurs in individuals with little to no ability of their natural killer (NK) cells and cytotoxic T cells to kill targeted cells.[3] The genetic defects associated with fHLH all relate to the packaging, exocytosis, or function of cytotoxic granules (**Table 3**),[9] with perforin gene defects being

Table 3
Genetic disorders associated with the occurrence of HLH

	FHLH2	FHLH3	FHLH4	FHLH5	GS2	CHS	HPSII
Gene	PRF1	UNC13D	STX11	STXBP2	RAB27A	CHSI/LYST	AP3BI
Protein/function	Perforin/pore-forming protein	Munc12–14/priming factor	Syntaxin11/membrane fusion	Munc18-2/membrane fusion	Rab27a/tethering	Lyst/lysosomal fission-protein sorting	Ap3β1/sorting of lysosomal protein
Murine model	Prf1–/–	Jinx	None	None	Ashen	Beige	Pearl
HLH	+	+	+	+	+	+	1 case report
Cytotoxic activity	–	–	±	±	–	–	–

Abbreviations: CHS, Chediak-Higashi syndrome; GS, Griscelli syndrome; HPS, Hermansky-Pudlak syndrome.
Data from Pachlopnik Schmid J, Cote M, Menager MM, et al. Inherited defects in lymphocyte cytotoxic activity. Immunol Rev 2010;235(1):10–23; and Jyonouchi S. Immunodeficiency Search. 2011. Available at: http://www.immunodeficiencysearch.com. Accessed November 1, 2011.

the most common and best studied. Similar to patients with SCID, children with fHLH eventually succumb to their illness without allogeneic bone marrow transplantation.[3] Animal models of HLH suggest that uncontrolled activation of cytotoxic T cells by antigen-presenting cells (APCs) drives the disease, with interferon-γ (IFN-γ) being the primary pathogenic cytokine.[10–12] Other inflammatory pathways are also involved in these models, as recently illustrated by the crucial role of MyD88 in disease development.[13] MyD88 is a critical signaling molecule downstream of interleukin 1 (IL-1) receptor and TLR signaling, and as discussed later, may provide some common inflammatory link to MAS.

The absence of functional cytotoxicity makes it impossible for T cells to terminate the stimulatory responses they receive from APCs. In this way, HLH may rightly be viewed as a primary immunodeficiency: these patients' genetic defect makes it impossible for them to clear infection and terminate T-cell stimulation by APCs. Similar to sepsis, in fHLH it is the uncontrolled immune response to infection that causes the cytokine storm.

The limited studies in patients with HLH have not yet borne out a major role for IFN-γ. Microarray of RNA from peripheral blood mononuclear cells (PBMCs) of patients with HLH did not show induction or suppression of IFN-γ–inducible genes.[14] Rather, signaling downstream of various inflammatory cytokines such as IL-6, IL-1, and IL-8 was upregulated. Accordingly, IL-10 (a potent antiinflammatory cytokine) signaling was highly upregulated. Genes governing NK cell activities, T-cell differentiation, and TLR signaling were also downregulated.[14] Such genes downregulated in sick patients support a possible pathogenic role for these pathways. Only some patients in this study had identified mutations,[14] suggesting that our knowledge of all of the genetic defects that lead to fHLH is incomplete.

X-linked lymphoproliferative syndromes and Epstein-Barr virus-related HLH

While in fHLH, there is a genetic defect in the ability to kill infected cells, other genetic defects have been associated with HLH as well. The X-linked lymphoproliferative syndromes XLP1 and XLP2 are both marked by a susceptibility to Epstein-Barr virus (EBV) infection, often resulting in an HLH phenotype.[15] XLP1 is caused by a mutation in SAP, an intracellular protein important for regulating IFN-γ signaling. XLP2 is caused by mutations in XIAP, a protein known to inhibit apoptosis. How XIAP mutations contribute to HLH is unknown. Nonetheless, HLH in patients with XLP nearly always occurs in the context of EBV infection.[15]

Even in the absence of a known mutation, chronic EBV infection is a risk factor for the development of HLH. In EBV-related HLH, viral loads correlate with the progression or improvement of disease,[16] suggesting that persistent proinflammatory stimulation is important for disease maintenance. The association of EBV with various other lymphoproliferative diseases and hematologic malignancies suggests that this virus has a propensity for uncontrolled immune activation and proliferation.[16]

MAS

The nomenclature among CSS does not lend itself to clear delineations. For the purposes of this review, MAS is defined as a CSS occurring in the context of a rheumatic disease and not otherwise associated with severe infection. Others have referred to hemophagocytic syndromes not associated with fHLH mutations as secondary or reactive HLH.[3,17] MAS occurs in between 10% and 50% of patients with systemic juvenile idiopathic arthritis (sJIA) depending on its definition.[4] MAS also complicates systemic lupus erythematosus (SLE), Kawasaki disease, and more rarely a host of other rheumatic conditions.[18,19] That MAS seems to occur more commonly in some rheumatic illnesses than others suggests that MAS-prone diseases may share a similar mechanistic propensity for cytokine storm. In addition, the fact that MAS occurs only rarely amongst patients with inflammasome disorders (illnesses associated with genetic defects known to cause excessive cytokine activation[20]) suggests that proinflammatory conditions alone are not sufficient to result in MAS.

Efforts to understand the pathogenesis of MAS have focused on patients with sJIA, because this seems to be the most susceptible population. Several studies have suggested that, like in fHLH, a defect in cytotoxic function plays a role in the development of MAS.[21,22] More recent studies have even found an increased risk of developing MAS in patients with sJIA harboring polymorphisms associated with fHLH genes.[23,24] However, because many patients with sJIA with NK dysfunction do not develop MAS, it is possible that cytotoxic cell dysfunction may be a nonspecific finding in sJIA that correlates with MAS.

Like in fHLH, IL-1/TLR signaling may be important for the development of MAS. Studies looking at PBMC RNA microarrays from newly diagnosed, untreated patients with sJIA identified regulation of the IL-1 and TLR pathways in those patients at higher risk for MAS.[25] In addition, polymorphisms in a gene critical for TLR signaling (IFN regulatory factor 5) are associated with a 4-fold higher risk of MAS among patients with sJIA.[26]

The only animal model of MAS uses repeated TLR9 stimulation in otherwise genetically normal mice.[27] TLR9 is a bacterial and viral DNA sensor implicated in bacterial and EBV infection and SLE.[28,29] As in HLH models, the TLR9 model supports an important role for IFN-γ in the development of disease.[27] IL-10 is critical in this model for protection from severe disease and hemophagocytosis. Further supporting a protective role for IL-10 in MAS, 2 genomic studies have associated low IL-10–expressing polymorphisms with sJIA.[30,31] In contrast, IL-10 inhibition in an fHLH model did not seem to hasten disease,[10] suggesting that this regulatory mechanism may be more important in some CSS than others.

Measurements of serum cytokines from patients with MAS have done little to clarify a single pathogenic pathway. IL-18, macrophage colony-stimulating factor (M-CSF), neopterin, and IL-6 have all been shown to be increased in patients with MAS, but variably depending on the underlying disease.[32,33] This finding suggests that different rheumatic conditions exploit different pathways to arrive at an MAS phenotype.

Malignancy-associated hemophagocytic syndromes

Hemophagocytic syndromes occur in the context of malignancy under 2 circumstances: first, malignancy-associated hemophagocytic syndromes (MAHS) can occur as a masking feature of the presentation of various hematolymphoid malignancies, and second, they may complicate the initial course.[34] The types of malignancies in each group are different. T-cell leukemias and lymphomas are often masked by a hyperinflammatory MAHS state, whereas B-cell leukemias and germ cell tumors are often complicated by MAHS.[34] When MAHS masks a malignancy, it is often the case that neoplastic cells are producing macrophage-activating cytokines such as IFN-γ and CD25, whereas HLH complicating a malignancy usually occurs when severe infection complicates an intrinsically or iatrogenically immunocompromised state.[34]

Environmental Factors

We have described that infection plays a key role in the induction of genetic causes of CSS like fHLH and XLP. However, even in normal hosts, environmental agents frequently provide sufficient proinflammatory stimuli (or inhibition of regulatory processes) to drive a CSS. Anyone can get septic.

Infection

Infection provides (at least) 2 important proinflammatory stimuli: antigen and adjuvant. Antigenic stimulation is necessary for a specific response as well as generation of memory, whereas adjuvant provides the first stimulus to cells of the innate immune system. Although theoretically any infection can provide sufficient stimulation to generate cytokine storm, this section focuses on infections commonly associated with hemophagocytic syndromes.

Bacteria

It was previously held that bacterial infections were uncommon causes of hemophagocytic syndromes. A review spanning 1979 to 1996 identified only 11 cases of bacterial-induced HLH, but 149 cases of viral-induced HLH.[34] However, this understanding preceded widespread testing for mutations associated with XLP and fHLH, and thus many viral-associated HLH cases would now be classified as primarily genetic. In addition, there is an increasing appreciation for consumption, cytopenias, and hemophagocytosis in severe infection.[5,16,17]

Bacterial infection provides a rich source of antigenic as well as TLR stimulation. However, if host defects in cellular cytotoxicity are critical to the development of hemophagocytic syndromes, it may be that most bacteria do not require this mechanism for their efficient clearance. A model of secondary HLH uses the intracellular bacteria *Salmonella enterica* to drive disease,[35] suggesting that perhaps viruses and intracellular bacteria exploit a common immunologic weakness in driving hemophagocytic syndromes.

Viruses

It is not clear why viral infections are especially predisposed to hemophagocytic CSS. IFN-γ is made in abundance by a variety of hematopoietic cells in response to viral infection, and may be particularly important in facilitating hemophagocytosis.[36] EBV, cytomegalovirus, and other γ-herpesviruses are the infections most commonly associated with HLH,[34] and this may have to do with their predilection for triggering TLR9, which has been associated in animal models with MAS.[27,28] In addition, certain viruses alter the immune response to infection and may predispose to cytokine storm. The EBV genome encodes an IL-10 homolog that may alter the host immune response to infection.[37] In addition, there are numerous case reports of HLH complicating both the presentation of and opportunistic infections in human immunodeficiency virus infections.[38]

Other infectious agents

Fungal and parasitic infections are also capable of inducing a robust immune response. Again, it may be instructive that there are only rare case reports of hemophagocytic disease complicating highly cytokine-driven infections such as *Plasmodium falciparum*.[39] Alternatively, it may be that fungal and malarial sepsis are common enough causes of cytokine storm that a thorough evaluation for defective cytotoxicity or hemophagocytosis is rarely undertaken.

Immunosuppressive therapy

As suggested in relation to MAHS, chemotherapy not only inhibits the ability to clear infections but may alter the regulatory machinery necessary for modulating the immune response to infection.

Allergens

Allergens are a potent source of antigenic stimulation without infection. Prolonged exposure to high doses of the allergy-associated cytokine IL-4 resulted in hemophagocytosis in mice.[40] However, this model of hemophagocytic disease occurs independent of IFN-γ. Data regarding hemophagocytosis in human anaphylaxis or other severe allergic reactions, such as DRESS (drug reaction with eosinophilia and systemic symptoms) are lacking.

DISTINGUISHING CSSs

The authors and others have supported the notion that the CSS share a similar final phenotype.[17] In addition, we have shown that a variety of host-derived and environmental insults can result in this phenotype. We later show that optimal treatment varies widely between CSS. Thus, distinguishing among these syndromes is critically important if one wishes to interrupt the final common pathway and restore inflammatory homeostasis.

The workup of any CSS must begin with an assessment of hemodynamic stability and appropriate intensive care intervention. Next, an assessment of organ dysfunction and coagulopathy is critical, but rarely provides specific diagnostic information. A thorough evaluation for infection or malignancy should preempt a diagnosis of HLH or MAS.

Cytopenias and Macrophage Activation

Diagnostically, the pattern or trend of hematologic and immunologic values can be useful. Although sometimes observed in severe sepsis, acute decreases in all 3 cell lines are characteristic of the hemophagocytic syndromes. Pancytopenia occurring before the onset of systemic inflammation should raise concern for malignancy. Increased triglycerides may be a serum marker for HLH and MAS.

As its name implies, MAS is accompanied by markers of macrophage activation. Ferritin levels in MAS and HLH are often more than 10,000 ng/mL, although such values are in the range of a few hundred ng/mL in sepsis.[3,41] Other markers of macrophage activation, such as neopterin, soluble CD163, and soluble CD25 (also known as soluble IL-2 receptor α [sIL2R-α]), may show more clinical usefulness as they become available outside reference laboratories.[42,43]

Tests of Cytotoxic Dysfunction

As mentioned earlier, fHLH is characterized by the paralysis of cellular cytotoxicity, and this mechanism may be important in MAS as well. Such cytotoxicity is mediated through the exocytosis of preformed lytic granules within cytotoxic cells.[9] Increasing arrays of tests are available to assess this exocytic and cytotoxic function. Many centers are able to perform a standardized assay of NK cell cytotoxic function, which assesses the ability of NK cells to lyse a tumor cell line that lacks major histocompatibility complex type I. This ex vivo assay is useful in screening for CSS associated with cytotoxic dysfunction, but impaired NK function in this assay is frequently described in sepsis and MODS as well.[17]

Other assays of cytotoxic dysfunction are increasingly available in reference laboratories. The presence of the perforin protein in cytotoxic cells can be tested through flow cytometric assays. In addition, screening for a defect in fusion of cytotoxic vesicles to the cell membrane can be accomplished by evaluating for mobilization of CD107a (also known as lysosomal-associated membrane protein 1).[44] Once a defect of cellular cytotoxicity is strongly suspected, genetic testing for fHLH-associated mutations should proceed (see **Table 3**).

Diagnostic Criteria

In 2004, the Histiocyte Society revised criteria for the diagnosis of both familial and reactive HLH (HLH-04, **Box 1**).[3] Although the performance of these criteria against other CSS has not been formally evaluated, increasing data suggest that they do not offer a high degree of specificity for fHLH.[17]

In recognition that distinction of MAS from a flare of its underlying disease presented a diagnostic challenge, Ravelli and colleagues have created criteria for the distinction of MAS from a flare of sJIA (**Box 2**).[41,45] These criteria were based on retrospective evidence of features that may distinguish sJIA from MAS and have yet to be prospectively validated.

CAUSE-BASED TREATMENT

As with diagnosis, treatment of CSS must begin by addressing the final common pathway: intensive care of hemodynamic instability, support of specific organ dysfunction, and correction of coagulopathy. However, such supportive measures are unlikely to be sufficient to reestablish homeostasis without also addressing the factors driving cytokine production and effect.

Box 1
Diagnostic guidelines for HLH

The diagnosis of HLH is suggested by one of either 1 or 2 below

1. A molecular diagnosis consistent with HLH (see **Table 3**)

2. Five of 8 of the following criteria

    a. Fever

    b. Splenomegaly

    c. Cytopenias affecting at least 2 lineages

        i. Hemoglobin <90 g/L (in infants <4 weeks: hemoglobin <100 g/L)

        ii. Platelets <100 $\times$ 10^9/L

        iii. Neutrophils <1.0 $\times$ 10^9/L

    d. Hypertriglyceridemia or hypofibrinogenemia:

        i. Fasting triglycerides $\geq$3.0 mmol/L ($\geq$265 mg/dL)

        ii. Fibrinogen $\leq$1.5 g/L

    e. Hemophagocytosis in spleen, lymph node, or bone marrow

    f. Low or absent NK cell activity (per performing laboratory range)

    g. Ferritin $\geq$500 μg/L

    h. Soluble CD25 (sIL2R-α) >2400 U/mL

Guidelines assume no evidence of malignancy.

Adapted from Henter JI, Horne A, Arico M, et al. HLH-2004: diagnostic and therapeutic guidelines for hemophagocytic lymphohistiocytosis. Pediatr Blood Cancer 2007;48(2):124–31; with permission.

Box 2
Preliminary diagnostic criteria for MAS complicating SJIA

Laboratory criteria

1. Decreased platelet count ($\leq$262 $\times$ 10^9/L)

2. Increased levels of aspartate aminotransferase (>59 U/L)

3. Decreased white blood cell count ($\leq$4.0 $\times$ 10^9/L)

4. Hypofibrinogenemia ($\leq$2.5 g/L)

Clinical criteria

1. Central nervous system dysfunction (irritability, disorientation, lethargy, headache, seizures, coma)

2. Hemorrhages (purpura, easy bruising, mucosal bleeding)

3. Hepatomegaly ($\geq$3 cm below the costal arch)

Histopathologic criterion

1. Evidence of macrophage hemophagocytosis in the bone marrow aspirate

The diagnosis of MAS requires the presence of any 2 or more laboratory criteria or of any 2 or 3 or more clinical and/or laboratory criteria. A bone marrow aspirate for the demonstration of hemophagocytosis may be required only in doubtful cases. These criteria are likely more valuable for classification rather than diagnosis, given many items occur late in the course of disease.

Data from Lykens JE, Terrell CE, Zoller EE, et al. Perforin is a critical physiologic regulator of T-cell activation. Blood 2011; and Ravelli A, Magni-Manzoni S, Pistorio A, et al. Preliminary diagnostic guidelines for macrophage activation syndrome complicating systemic juvenile idiopathic arthritis. J Pediatr 2005;146(5):598–604.

Altering the Environment

For CSS of primarily environmental cause, elimination of the offending microbe, allergen, or cytotoxic agent when possible may be all that is needed to allow restoration of homeostasis. An assessment for underlying immunodeficiency should help guide empiric treatment of suspected sepsis. MAHS, although of intrinsic origin, requires a similar strategy: clear the source of inflammatory stimulation, in this case neoplastic cells.

Although supportive care and antimicrobials may be sufficient to treat sepsis, antimicrobial use is indicated in any CSS in which a contributing treatable pathogen is suspected. For example, a patient with a known defect in cytotoxicity infected with a herpesvirus would likely benefit from appropriate antiviral therapy.

In addition to clearing proinflammatory stimuli, treatments that alter immune response to such stimuli are emerging as potentially beneficial. Agents such as hydroxychloroquine, which are purported to act through inhibition of TLR signaling, are useful in treating SLE. More specific inhibitors of TLR signaling are now being considered for use in autoinflammatory disorders.[46]

Managing the Host Defect

Conventional immunodeficiency

Although elimination of the opportunistic pathogen is critical, supplementation of immune responses may be beneficial. In conventional immunodeficiency, this supplementation is best achieved preventatively with intravenous immunoglobulin (IVIg), granulocyte M-CSF, or appropriate vaccination. Acute supplementation of the immune response may also be beneficial, and it is unclear to what extent IVIg treatment successes in hemophagocytic syndromes are attributable to clearance of infection versus direct antiinflammatory effects.[17,39]

HLH

HLH-04 provided treatment recommendations for both fHLH and reactive HLH that use corticosteroids, cyclosporine, and etoposide as a bridge to transplant.[3] The goals of acute treatment of fHLH are to manage the immune response and preserve organ function in anticipation of allogeneic bone marrow transplantation. Although some alterations in this protocol have been proposed,[47] HLH-04 remains the foundation of fHLH treatment.

However, it is increasingly recognized that most disorders meeting HLH-04 criteria do not require such aggressive immunosuppression.[17] In addition, chemotherapeutic strategies similar to HLH-04 carry a high risk for iatrogenic infection and hematologic malignancy.[17,48] This concern for excessive toxicity has led to the use of more specific cytotoxic treatments in diseases with more discret target populations. For example, rituximab has been shown to be effective in EBV-related HLH, potentially because of cytotoxic effects on infected cells,[49] and IVIg may be effective in secondary HLH and MAS.[17,50]

MAS

The management of MAS is far from standardized and remains controversial. Most agree that high doses of corticosteroids are useful, but the mechanisms by which corticosteroids exert this beneficial effect are unclear. One postulated mechanism is that they help skew macrophages away from an M1, or proinflammatory differentiation state, toward a more regulatory or scavenger state.[51] In this case, one may expect corticosteroids to be effective in the treatment of any CSS showing significant macrophage activation.

Although many practitioners treat MAS with an HLH-04-like approach, less toxic strategies targeted at specific inflammatory defects have emerged. Accumulating evidence suggests that anakinra, a recombinant IL-1 receptor antagonist, may be beneficial in MAS. The successful treatment of sJIA with anakinra,[51–53] coupled with evidence that IL-1 receptor signaling may be implicated in MAS,[25] support IL-1 inhibition as a viable strategy. Several practitioners have reported successful treatment of MAS with only corticosteroids and anakinra.[54,55] It is unclear if IL-1 inhibition is a viable strategy for MAS in general, or whether it is uniquely suited to a potentially IL-1–mediated disease such as sJIA.

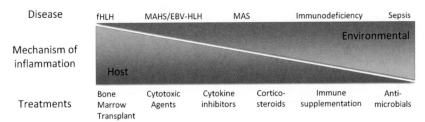

Fig. 2. Conceptual model of various CSSs on a spectrum based on the nature of their mechanism of inflammation.

SUMMARY

The hemophagocytic syndromes MAS and HLH overlap considerably with other CSS and share a final common pathway with them. Laboratory findings such as decreasing cell counts, decreasing ESR, increased ferritin level, NK dysfunction, and hemophago-cytosis, which were once believed to be unique to hemophagocytic disorders, are increasingly recognized in a host of infectious and possibly even allergic CSS. However, because addressing the primary defect(s) driving CSS is crucial to restoring immunologic balance, it is critical to understand and differentiate the mechanisms by which various CSS arrive at their final common pathway.

We propose a framework for understanding CSS wherein a careful assessment for the presence of host and environmental contributors to CSS guides a rational thera-peutic approach (**Fig. 2**). A greater understanding of the mechanisms by which host and environmental factors contribute to CSS, as well as more precise knowledge of how our therapeutics alter those mechanisms, will allow even more precise direction of treatment.

REFERENCES

1. American College of Chest Physicians/Society of Critical Care Medicine Consensus Conference: definitions for sepsis and organ failure and guidelines for the use of innovative therapies in sepsis. Crit Care Med 1992;20(6):864–74.
2. Goldstein B, Giroir B, Randolph A. International pediatric sepsis consensus conference: definitions for sepsis and organ dysfunction in pediatrics. Pediatr Crit Care Med 2005;6(1):2–8.
3. Henter JI, Horne A, Arico M, et al. HLH-2004: diagnostic and therapeutic guide-lines for hemophagocytic lymphohistiocytosis. Pediatr Blood Cancer 2007;48(2): 124–31.
4. Behrens EM, Beukelman T, Paessler M, et al. Occult macrophage activation syndrome in patients with systemic juvenile idiopathic arthritis. J Rheumatol 2007;34(5):1133–8.
5. Kuwata K, Yamada S, Kinuwaki E, et al. Peripheral hemophagocytosis: an early indicator of advanced systemic inflammatory response syndrome/hemophago-cytic syndrome. Shock 2006;25(4):344–50.
6. Imahashi N, Inamoto Y, Ito M, et al. Clinical significance of hemophagocytosis in BM clot sections during the peri-engraftment period following allogeneic hemato-poietic SCT. Bone Marrow Transplant 2011;47(3):387–94.
7. Marshak-Rothstein A. Toll-like receptors in systemic autoimmune disease. Nat Rev Immunol 2006;6(11):823–35.
8. Jyonouchi S. Immunodeficiency Search. 2011. Available at: http://www. immunodeficiencysearch.com. Accessed November 1, 2011.
9. Pachlopnik Schmid J, Cote M, Menager MM, et al. Inherited defects in lympho-cyte cytotoxic activity. Immunol Rev 2010;235(1):10–23.
10. Jordan MB, Hildeman D, Kappler J, et al. An animal model of hemophagocytic lymphohistiocytosis (HLH): CD8+ T cells and interferon gamma are essential for the disorder. Blood 2004;104(3):735–43.
11. Lykens JE, Terrell CE, Zoller EE, et al. Perforin is a critical physiologic regulator of T-cell activation. Blood 2011;118(3):618–26.
12. Crozat K, Hoebe K, Ugolini S, et al. Jinx, an MCMV susceptibility phenotype caused by disruption of Unc13d: a mouse model of type 3 familial hemophago-cytic lymphohistiocytosis. J Exp Med 2007;204(4):853–63.

13. Krebs P, Crozat K, Popkin D, et al. Disruption of MyD88 signaling suppresses hemophagocytic lymphohistiocytosis in mice. Blood 2011;117(24):6582–8.

14. Sumegi J, Barnes MG, Nestheide SV, et al. Gene expression profiling of peripheral blood mononuclear cells from children with active hemophagocytic lymphohistiocytosis. Blood 2011;117(15):e151–60.

15. Pachlopnik Schmid J, Canioni D, Moshous D, et al. Clinical similarities and differences of patients with X-linked lymphoproliferative syndrome type 1 (XLP-1/SAP deficiency) versus type 2 (XLP-2/XIAP deficiency). Blood 2011;117(5):1522–9.

16. Imashuku S. Clinical features and treatment strategies of Epstein-Barr virus-associated hemophagocytic lymphohistiocytosis. Crit Rev Oncol Hematol 2002;44(3): 259–72.

17. Castillo L, Carcillo J. Secondary hemophagocytic lymphohistiocytosis and severe sepsis/systemic inflammatory response syndrome/multiorgan dysfunction syndrome/macrophage activation syndrome share common intermediate phenotypes on a spectrum of inflammation. Pediatr Crit Care Med 2009;10(3): 387–92.

18. Avcin T, Tse SM, Schneider R, et al. Macrophage activation syndrome as the presenting manifestation of rheumatic diseases in childhood. J Pediatr 2006;148(5): 683–6.

19. Sawhney S, Woo P, Murray KJ. Macrophage activation syndrome: a potentially fatal complication of rheumatic disorders. Arch Dis Child 2001;85(5):421–6.

20. Hoffman HM, Brydges SD. Genetic and molecular basis of inflammasome-mediated disease. J Biol Chem 2011;286(13):10889–96.

21. Grom AA, Villanueva J, Lee S, et al. Natural killer cell dysfunction in patients with systemic-onset juvenile rheumatoid arthritis and macrophage activation syndrome. J Pediatr 2003;142(3):292–6.

22. Villanueva J, Lee S, Giannini EH, et al. Natural killer cell dysfunction is a distinguishing feature of systemic onset juvenile rheumatoid arthritis and macrophage activation syndrome. Arthritis Res Ther 2005;7(1):R30–7.

23. Vastert SJ, van Wijk R, D'Urbano LE, et al. Mutations in the perforin gene can be linked to macrophage activation syndrome in patients with systemic onset juvenile idiopathic arthritis. Rheumatology (Oxford) 2010;49(3):441–9.

24. Zhang K, Biroschak J, Glass DN, et al. Macrophage activation syndrome in patients with systemic juvenile idiopathic arthritis is associated with MUNC13-4 polymorphisms. Arthritis Rheum 2008;58(9):2892–6.

25. Fall N, Barnes M, Thornton S, et al. Gene expression profiling of peripheral blood from patients with untreated new-onset systemic juvenile idiopathic arthritis reveals molecular heterogeneity that may predict macrophage activation syndrome. Arthritis Rheum 2007;56(11):3793–804.

26. Yanagimachi M, Naruto T, Miyamae T, et al. Association of IRF5 polymorphisms with susceptibility to macrophage activation syndrome in patients with juvenile idiopathic arthritis. J Rheumatol 2011;38(4):769–74.

27. Behrens EM, Canna SW, Slade K, et al. Repeated TLR9 stimulation results in macrophage activation syndrome-like disease in mice. J Clin Invest 2011; 121(6):2264–77.

28. Guggemoos S, Hangel D, Hamm S, et al. TLR9 contributes to antiviral immunity during gammaherpesvirus infection. J Immunol 2008;180(1):438–43.

29. Santiago-Raber ML, Baudino L, Izui S. Emerging roles of TLR7 and TLR9 in murine SLE. J Autoimmun 2009;33(3–4):231–8.

30. Fife MS, Gutierrez A, Ogilvie EM, et al. Novel IL10 gene family associations with systemic juvenile idiopathic arthritis. Arthritis Res Ther 2006;8(5):R148.

31. Moller JC, Paul D, Ganser G, et al. IL10 promoter polymorphisms are associated with systemic onset juvenile idiopathic arthritis (SoJIA). Clin Exp Rheumatol 2010; 28(6):912–8.

32. Maruyama J, Inokuma S. Cytokine profiles of macrophage activation syndrome associated with rheumatic diseases. J Rheumatol 2010;37(5):967–73.

33. Shimizu M, Yokoyama T, Yamada K, et al. Distinct cytokine profiles of systemic-onset juvenile idiopathic arthritis-associated macrophage activation syndrome with particular emphasis on the role of interleukin-18 in its pathogenesis. Rheumatology 2010;49(9):1645–53.

34. Janka G, Imashuku S, Elinder G, et al. Infection- and malignancy-associated hemophagocytic syndromes. Secondary hemophagocytic lymphohistiocytosis. Hematol Oncol Clin North Am 1998;12(2):435–44.

35. Brown DE, McCoy MW, Pilonieta MC, et al. Chronic murine typhoid fever is a natural model of secondary hemophagocytic lymphohistiocytosis. PLoS One 2010;5(2):e9441.

36. Zoller EE, Lykens JE, Terrell CE, et al. Hemophagocytosis causes a consumptive anemia of inflammation. J Exp Med 2011;208(6):1203–14.

37. Moore KW, de Waal Malefyt R, Coffman RL, et al. Interleukin-10 and the interleukin-10 receptor. Annu Rev Immunol 2001;19:683–765.

38. Doyle T, Bhagani S, Cwynarski K. Haemophagocytic syndrome and HIV. Curr Opin Infect Dis 2009;22(1):1–6.

39. Veerakul G, Sanpakit K, Tanphaichitr VS, et al. Secondary hemophagocytic lymphohistiocytosis in children: an analysis of etiology and outcome. J Med Assoc Thai 2002;85(Suppl 2):S530–41.

40. Milner JD, Orekov T, Ward JM, et al. Sustained IL-4 exposure leads to a novel pathway for hemophagocytosis, inflammation, and tissue macrophage accumulation. Blood 2010;116(14):2476–83.

41. Ravelli A, Magni-Manzoni S, Pistorio A, et al. Preliminary diagnostic guidelines for macrophage activation syndrome complicating systemic juvenile idiopathic arthritis. J Pediatr 2005;146(5):598–604.

42. Ibarra MF, Klein-Gitelman M, Morgan E, et al. Serum neopterin levels as a diagnostic marker of hemophagocytic lymphohistiocytosis syndrome. Clin Vaccine Immunol 2011;18(4):609–14.

43. Bleesing J, Prada A, Siegel DM, et al. The diagnostic significance of soluble CD163 and soluble interleukin-2 receptor alpha-chain in macrophage activation syndrome and untreated new-onset systemic juvenile idiopathic arthritis. Arthritis Rheum 2007;56(3):965–71.

44. Wheeler RD, Cale CM, Cetica V, et al. A novel assay for investigation of suspected familial haemophagocytic lymphohistiocytosis. Br J Haematol 2010; 150(6):727–30.

45. Davi S, Consolaro A, Guseinova D, et al. An international consensus survey of diagnostic criteria for macrophage activation syndrome in systemic juvenile idiopathic arthritis. J Rheumatol 2011;38(4):764–8.

46. Sun S, Rao NL, Venable J, et al. TLR7/9 antagonists as therapeutics for immune-mediated inflammatory disorders. Inflamm Allergy Drug Targets 2007;6(4):223–35.

47. Marsh RA, Jordan MB, Filipovich AH. Reduced-intensity conditioning haematopoietic cell transplantation for haemophagocytic lymphohistiocytosis: an important step forward. Br J Haematol 2011;154(5):556–63.

48. Henter JI, Samuelsson-Horne A, Arico M, et al. Treatment of hemophagocytic lymphohistiocytosis with HLH-94 immunochemotherapy and bone marrow transplantation. Blood 2002;100(7):2367–73.

49. Balamuth NJ, Nichols KE, Paessler M, et al. Use of rituximab in conjunction with immunosuppressive chemotherapy as a novel therapy for Epstein Barr virus-associated hemophagocytic lymphohistiocytosis. J Pediatr Hematol Oncol 2007;29(8):569–73.

50. Gupta AA, Tyrrell P, Valani R, et al. Experience with hemophagocytic lymphohistiocytosis/macrophage activation syndrome at a single institution. J Pediatr Hematol Oncol 2009;31(2):81–4.

51. Gordon S. Alternative activation of macrophages. Nat Rev Immunol 2003;3(1): 23–35.

52. Pascual V, Allantaz F, Arce E, et al. Role of interleukin-1 (IL-1) in the pathogenesis of systemic onset juvenile idiopathic arthritis and clinical response to IL-1 blockade. J Exp Med 2005;201(9):1479–86.

53. Nigrovic PA, Mannion M, Prince FH, et al. Anakinra as first-line disease-modifying therapy in systemic juvenile idiopathic arthritis: report of forty-six patients from an international multicenter series. Arthritis Rheum 2011;63(2):545–55.

54. Behrens EM, Kreiger PA, Cherian S, et al. Interleukin 1 receptor antagonist to treat cytophagic histiocytic panniculitis with secondary hemophagocytic lymphohistiocytosis. J Rheumatol 2006;33(10):2081–4.

55. Bruck N, Suttorp M, Kabus M, et al. Rapid and sustained remission of systemic juvenile idiopathic arthritis-associated macrophage activation syndrome through treatment with anakinra and corticosteroids. J Clin Rheumatol 2011;17(1):23–7.

Systemic Lupus Erythematosus in Children and Adolescents

Deborah M. Levy, MD, MS, FRCPC[a],*, Sylvia Kamphuis, MD, PhD[b]

KEYWORDS

- Pediatric • Clinical features • Neuropsychiatric • Nephritis
- Diagnosis • Treatment • Complications

Key Points

- cSLE is a rare but severe autoimmune disease with multisystem involvement and wide heterogeneity of disease manifestations.
- Making the diagnosis of cSLE can be difficult, but early recognition of the disease is important to limit adverse outcomes.
- cSLE follows a more severe disease course than adult-onset SLE, with higher frequency of morbidity and lower survival rates.
- Dealing with the diagnosis of a lifelong, unpredictable, and relapsing-remitting disease in adolescence is challenging for cSLE patients, and recognition of the specific needs of this age group is important for optimal outcome.

Systemic lupus erythematosus (SLE) is a chronic autoimmune disease that can involve any organ system, and may lead to significant morbidity and even mortality. This article reviews the epidemiology, common clinical features, and complications of this disease, and briefly addresses available treatment options. Important medical and psychosocial issues relevant to the pediatrician caring for children and adolescents with SLE are discussed.

EPIDEMIOLOGY

Childhood-onset SLE (cSLE) is a rare disease with an incidence of 0.3 to 0.9 per 100,000 children-years and a prevalence of 3.3 to 8.8 per 100,000 children.[1] A higher

---

[a] Division of Rheumatology, Hospital for Sick Children, University of Toronto, 555 University Avenue, Toronto, ON M5G 1X8, Canada; [b] Divisions of Infectiology/Immunology/Rheumatology, Sophia Children's Hospital, Erasmus University MC, SP 3429, PO Box 2060, 3000 CB Rotterdam, The Netherlands
* Corresponding author. Division of Rheumatology, Hospital for Sick Children, 555 University Avenue, Toronto, ON M5G 1X8, Canada.
E-mail address: deborah.levy@sickkids.ca

Pediatr Clin N Am 59 (2012) 345–364
doi:10.1016/j.pcl.2012.03.007
0031-3955/12/$ – see front matter © 2012 Elsevier Inc. All rights reserved.

frequency of cSLE is reported in Asians, African Americans, Hispanics, and Native Americans.[2,3] When compared with 2 more common childhood autoimmune diseases, juvenile idiopathic arthritis (JIA) and type 1 diabetes, cSLE is approximately 10 to 15 times less common in White children.[4,5] However, in Asian children, cSLE is reported to be equally as common as JIA.[6] Most studies report a median age of onset of cSLE between 11 and 12 years; the disease is rare in children younger than 5 years. As in adult-onset SLE, approximately 80% of patients with cSLE are female.[7,8]

CLASSIFICATION AND DIAGNOSIS OF cSLE

SLE is called the great mimicker, as the disease shares characteristics with many other (autoimmune) diseases. Especially when the classic malar rash is absent, diagnosing SLE can be a challenge. However, the astute pediatrician who considers SLE when presented with an unusual constellation of symptoms can recognize important patterns of disease manifestations crucial for the diagnosis. Most patients who are diagnosed with cSLE fulfill 4 or more of the American College of Rheumatology classification criteria for SLE (**Table 1**).[9,10] The criteria were designed for use in research studies, and it must be cautioned that the diagnosis of SLE should not solely be based on fulfilling these criteria. Although not rigorously studied in cSLE, the criteria have a greater than 95% sensitivity and specificity for the diagnosis of cSLE.[11]

CLINICAL FEATURES

This review does not attempt to describe all possible clinical manifestations but instead focuses on specific features that may be crucial for immediate recognition. **Table 2** summarizes the frequencies of the common manifestations of cSLE.[7,12–17] SLE can affect any organ system, and leads to glomerulonephritis and central nervous system (CNS) involvement arguably more often in cSLE than in adults with SLE.

Constitutional Symptoms

Patients ultimately diagnosed with cSLE frequently recount nonspecific constitutional symptoms that include fever, fatigue, anorexia, weight loss, alopecia, and arthralgias.[7,12] These and other signs of diffuse generalized inflammation, including lymphadenopathy and hepatosplenomegaly, may occur both at onset and during disease flares.

Mucocutaneous

The hallmark of SLE is the malar, or butterfly, rash. Seen in 60% to 85% of children with SLE, the rash is generally described as erythematous, raised, nonpruritic, and nonscarring. It often extends over the nasal bridge, affects the chin and ears, but spares the nasolabial folds (**Fig. 1**). It is photosensitive in more than one-third of patients, and exacerbation of the photosensitive rash frequently heralds the onset of a systemic flare. Therefore, sunscreen with a high sun-protection factor, as well as hats and protective clothing, are recommended year-round for all individuals with SLE.

Discoid rash, unlike in adult-onset SLE, is a rare manifestation of cSLE, occurring in fewer than 10% of patients.[7] This scarring rash most frequently occurs on the forehead and scalp, and its scaly appearance may be mistaken as a tinea lesion.[18] **Box 1** summarizes the spectrum of dermatologic involvement, illustrating the diverse range of skin manifestations. Children and adolescents with SLE can develop a rash of (almost) any morphology, location, and distribution, often presenting a diagnostic challenge to the primary care physician. A skin biopsy for histology aids in making the correct diagnosis, although biopsies of facial skin should be avoided. Nonscarring

Table 1
Classification criteria for SLE

Criterion	Definition
1. Malar rash	Flat or raised erythema over the malar eminences, spares the nasolabial folds
2. Discoid rash	Erythematosus raised patches with adherent keratotic scaling and follicular plugging; atrophic scarring may occur
3. Photosensitivity	Rash following sunlight exposure, by history or physician observation
4. Oral ulcers	Oral or nasopharyngeal ulceration, usually painless
5. Arthritis	Nonerosive arthritis involving 2 or more peripheral joints, characterized by tenderness, swelling, or effusion
6. Serositis	Pleuritis—convincing history of pleuritic pain or rub on auscultation or evidence of pleural effusion or Pericarditis—documented by electrocardiogram, echocardiogram or rub
7. Renal disorder	Persistent proteinuria >0.5 g/d or Cellular casts—may be red cell, hemoglobin, granular, tubular, or mixed
8. Neurologic disorder	Seizures in the absence of offending drugs or metabolic derangements or Psychosis in the absence of offending drugs or metabolic derangements
9. Hematologic disorder	Hemolytic anemia with reticulocytosis or Leukopenia <4000/μL on 2 or more occasions, or Lymphopenia <1500/μL on 2 or more occasions, or Thrombocytopenia <100,000/μL
10. Immunologic disorder	Antibody to native DNA, or Antibody to Sm protein, or Antiphospholipid antibodies—either anticardiolipin antibodies, presence of the lupus anticoagulant, or false-positive serologic test for syphilis
11. Antinuclear antibody	Presence of antinuclear antibody by immunofluorescence or an equivalent assay

Data from Tan EM, Cohen AS, Fries JF, et al. The 1982 revised criteria for the classification of systemic lupus erythematosus. Arthritis Rheum 1982;25:1271–7; and Hochberg MC. Updating the American College of Rheumatology revised criteria for the classification of systemic lupus erythematosus. Arthritis Rheum 1997;40:1725.

hair loss is common, but not specific for SLE. The alopecia is most often noted as thinning of the temporal areas of the scalp, although rarely it is more global and severe enough to require systemic immunosuppressive therapy. Nevertheless, for the affected child or adolescent even minimal hair loss can be distressing.

Involvement of the oral and nasal mucosa ranges from oral and/or nasal hyperemia to painless oral ulcers of the hard palate (**Fig. 2**) and shallow nasal septal ulcers and, rarely, nasal septal perforation. Because of both the location and painless nature of these lesions, the practitioner may overlook these findings if the degree of suspicion for SLE is low.

Musculoskeletal

The range of musculoskeletal involvement includes features that occur as a consequence of active SLE, and those that are secondary to treatment and/or chronic

Table 2
Common clinical features of cSLE

Clinical Feature	Prevalence of Involvement (%)
Constitutional and generalized symptoms	
Fever	37–100
Lymphadenopathy	13–45
Weight loss	21–32
Mucocutaneous	60–90
Musculoskeletal	60–90
Nephritis	48–78
Neuropsychiatric disease (NPSLE)	15–95
Gastrointestinal	24–40
Hematologic	50–100
Cardiovascular	25–60
Pulmonary	18–81

Data from Refs.[7,12–17]

illness. Manifestations include arthralgias and arthritis, avascular necrosis, bone-fragility fractures, and secondary pain amplification. Arthritis occurs in 80% of patients with cSLE, and although the typical description is that of a painful polyarthritis, in practice a significant proportion of children with SLE experience minimal pain. The arthritis is identical in many ways to JIA, with effusions and decreased range of motion of both small and large joints and significant morning stiffness; however; the arthritis is almost always nonerosive and nondeforming. Arthralgias also commonly occur, and can be secondary to a pain amplification syndrome that occurs during or following a disease flare with resultant poor sleep and daytime fatigue, decreased cardiovascular conditioning, and generalized pain.

Avascular necrosis can occur in patients treated with corticosteroids, and may be idiosyncratic to the dose of medication, although it occurs more frequently in patients with SLE than with other diseases that are similarly treated with corticosteroids. In

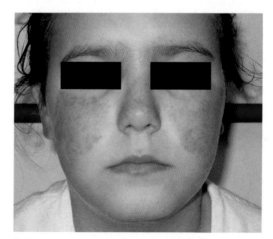

Fig. 1. Malar rash of cSLE.

Box 1
Commonest dermatologic manifestations

Rash

    Malar (butterfly) rash

    Annular erythema

    Discoid lupus erythematosus

    Maculopapular and/or linear (nonspecific) rash

    Bullous lupus (rare)

Photosensitivity

Alopecia

Raynaud phenomenon

Palmar/plantar/periungual erythema

Livedo reticularis

Vasculitis

    Petechiae

    Palpable purpura (leukocytoclastic vasculitis)

    Chilblains/nodules

    Digital ulcers

---

addition, osteoporosis is frequent, related to corticosteroid use, and associated with an increased risk of fracture.

Renal Disease

Renal involvement occurs in 50% to 75% of all cSLE patients, and more than 90% of those who develop renal disease will do so within the first 2 years after diagnosis.[7] Initial manifestations of renal disease range from minimal proteinuria and microscopic hematuria to nephrotic-range proteinuria, urinary casts, severe hypertension, peripheral edema, and renal insufficiency or acute renal failure. SLE most commonly affects the glomerulus (ie, lupus nephritis), with rare involvement of the renal interstitium. In

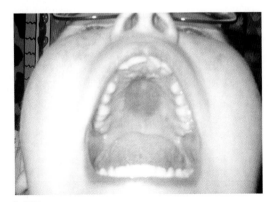

Fig. 2. Oral ulcer of cSLE.

a patient with acute renal failure, thrombotic thrombocytopenic purpura (TTP), a thrombotic microangiopathy and infrequent complication of SLE, should also be considered. As the severity of the nephritis may not correlate with the severity of the clinical signs and symptoms, a renal biopsy should be performed for any suspicion of glomerulonephritis, including persistent mild proteinuria. Histologic diagnosis using a standardized classification (**Table 3**) guides treatment and aids in determining overall prognosis.

The classification of glomerulonephritis in SLE ranges from Class I (minimal mesangial) to Class VI (advanced sclerosing lupus nephritis), and contains descriptions of the mesangial involvement, degree of renal involvement (focal vs diffuse), and degree of involvement of the affected glomeruli (segmental vs global). In general, Class I (minimal mesangial) and Class II (mesangial proliferative) nephritis are mild lesions, and often require little to no immunosuppressive treatment because their natural history is favorable. Class III (focal proliferative) and Class IV (diffuse proliferative) lesions are the most frequent and severe lesions, with more than 80% of cSLE biopsies done at the Hospital for Sick Children, Toronto demonstrating one of these lesions.[7] Patients with these proliferative lesions have the highest risk of end-stage renal disease (ESRD), and thus are treated with aggressive immunosuppression in attempts to avert this outcome. By contrast, Class V (membranous lupus nephritis), when it occurs as the exclusive lesion, rarely leads to ESRD and therefore is generally

Table 3
Classification of lupus nephritis

Lupus Nephritis Class	Description	Histology
Class I	Minimal mesangial lupus nephritis	Normal glomeruli by light microscopy, but mesangial immune deposits by immunofluorescence
Class II	Mesangial proliferative lupus nephritis	Mesangial hypercellularity or mesangial matrix expansion by light microscopy, with mesangial immune deposits by immunofluorescence
Class III	Focal lupus nephritis	Active or chronic focal, segmental, or global glomerulonephritis involving <50% of all glomeruli with diffuse subendothelial immune deposits
Class IV	Diffuse lupus nephritis	Active or chronic diffuse, segmental, or global glomerulonephritis involving >50% of all glomeruli with diffuse subendothelial immune deposits
Class V	Membranous lupus nephritis	Global or segmental subepithelial immune deposits by immunofluorescence or electron microscopy
Class VI	Advanced sclerosing lupus nephritis	≥90% glomeruli globally sclerosed without residual activity

Data from Weening JJ, D'Agati VD, Schwartz MM, et al. The classification of glomerulonephritis in systemic lupus erythematosus revisited. J Am Soc Nephrol 2004;15:241–50.

not treated with the same degree of immunosuppression as Class III or IV disease. However, Class V lesions are frequently observed in conjunction with other lesions (usually Class III or IV), and in this case the presence of the proliferative lesion directs therapy. Any patient with SLE should have regular measurements of blood pressure, serum creatinine, and urinalysis for proteinuria, hematuria, and evidence of urinary casts.

With the use of an aggressive treatment regimen, the incidence of ESRD is lower than in past decades, but still remains between 10% and 20% by 10 years from diagnosis.[19,20] Patients who develop ESRD require dialysis, and can undergo renal transplant when a donor organ is available providing their disease is stable at the time of transplant. A recent study noted that whereas one-third of cSLE patients with ESRD received a transplant within 5 years, another 22% died in that same time period.[21] Moreover, there is a risk of recurrence of nephritis in the graft kidney.[22] Overall, renal disease remains a significant cause of morbidity and mortality, with the possibility of disease flares even after years of remission.

Neuropsychiatric Involvement

SLE can involve both the central and peripheral nervous systems, with 19 distinct neuropsychiatric SLE (NPSLE) syndromes described (**Table 4**).[23] Up to 65% of cSLE patients will develop NPSLE at some time during their disease course, and up to 85% of these patients develop NPSLE within the first 2 years from diagnosis.[13,24] Because many of the syndromes are infrequent, only the commonest are briefly outlined here.

Headache
Symptoms ranging from mild intermittent tension-type headaches to daily, debilitating severe headaches that require prescription pain medication occur in 50% to 95% of patients.[13,25] Headache on its own can be a manifestation of active SLE, an indication of increased intracranial pressure, or of an intracranial abnormality such as cerebral vein thrombosis, especially in patients with antiphospholipid antibodies.[26] The occurrence of a new severe headache is a red flag in a patient with SLE, and immediate evaluation is required.[27,28]

Table 4 Neuropsychiatric syndromes observed in SLE (NPSLE)	
Central Nervous System	**Peripheral Nervous System**
Aseptic meningitis	Acute inflammatory demyelinating polyradiculoneuropathy (Guillain-Barré syndrome)
Cerebrovascular disease	Autonomic disorder
Demyelinating syndrome	Mononeuropathy, single/multiplex
Headache	Myasthenia gravis
Movement disorder (chorea)	Neuropathy, cranial
Myelopathy	Plexopathy
Seizure disorder	Polyneuropathy
Acute confusional state	
Anxiety disorder	
Cognitive dysfunction	
Mood disorder	
Psychosis	

Data from American College of Rheumatology: nomenclature and case definitions for neuropsychiatric lupus syndromes. Arthritis Rheum 1999;42:599–608.

Mood disorder

Depressive affect may be a normal and appropriate reaction for an adolescent dealing with a chronic disease, and thus attribution of depression to SLE is often challenging and requires input from psychiatry colleagues. Major depression is not as frequent, and occurs in fewer than 10% to 20% of patients.[28,29]

Cognitive dysfunction

Impairment of cognition may be manifested by declining school performance and subtle difficulties with working memory and concentration tasks. Cognitive dysfunction is diagnosed with traditional neuropsychological testing, and has been observed in more than one-third of asymptomatic cSLE patients.[29–31]

Psychosis

Hallucinations, predominantly visual but also auditory, are experienced by more than 10% of all patients with cSLE. Visual distortions are also common, with children reporting that the clock or light is distorted, or that the words on the page are "popping out." The psychosis differs from that of primary psychiatric disease in that SLE patients have preserved insight; however, evaluation by a psychiatrist is recommended to assist with the diagnosis. Psychosis is frequently concomitant with cognitive dysfunction and acute confusional state.[24] Although investigations including magnetic resonance imaging (MRI) are often normal, aggressive treatment is recommended and frequently leads to complete resolution of symptoms.[32,33]

Seizures

Seizures are rarely seen in cSLE as an isolated event, but instead are frequently observed concomitantly with other NPSLE syndromes. When they do occur, seizures are more often generalized than focal. Seizures may also occur in patients with CNS infections or severe hypertension, and in patients who have a recently recognized complication known as posterior reversible encephalopathy syndrome.[34,35]

In contrast to CNS disease, peripheral nervous system involvement is rarely observed in cSLE. Any cSLE patient presenting with new neurologic symptoms warrants consideration for a full diagnostic workup. This workup may include a lumbar puncture, MRI with MR angiography and venography, electroencephalogram (EEG), and psychiatry, psychology, and neurology evaluations as appropriate. Before attribution to SLE, other possible causes, in particular infection in the immunocompromised host, inappropriate prescription or illicit drug use, and new-onset primary psychiatric disease, must be considered in this predominantly adolescent population. Furthermore, patients rarely present with isolated features of one syndrome, and instead one may think of NPSLE as a series of overlapping symptoms, with coexistent symptoms in most patients.[24] Treatment of NPSLE depends on the clinical presentation, with psychosis and acute confusional state requiring the most aggressive immunosuppressants, whereas other NPSLE syndromes require therapies directed at the observed manifestations.

Hematologic Features

Cytopenias are common in cSLE, with more than 50% of patients presenting a decrease in at least 1 cell line.[7,12] Mild leukopenia (white blood cell count 3000–4000/mm^3) is the most common hematologic manifestation, and is usually due to lymphopenia (<1500 cells/mm^3) and, less frequently, neutropenia. Whereas persistent lymphopenia may be a feature of active disease, neutropenia is more frequently a result of treatment (eg, during treatment with cyclophosphamide). Anemia can take any form: the anemia of chronic disease that is normocytic and normochromic, iron-deficiency anemia, or a Coombs positive hemolytic anemia. In addition, coexistent hemoglobinopathies such as sickle cell anemia and thalassemia trait must be considered. The workup includes iron studies, hemoglobin electrophoresis depending on the patient's indices, and other markers of hemolysis (reticulocyte count, haptoglobin, lactate dehydrogenase). Hemolytic anemia, occurring in 10% to 15% of patients,[12] is rarely severe enough to require transfusion. The thrombocytopenia observed in cSLE patients spans the spectrum from mild (<150,000 platelets/μl) to profound (<10,000 platelets/μl). However, in the absence of excess bleeding and/or bruising, little treatment is required for patients with a stable platelet count of ≥20,000/μl. The risks of bleeding (intracranial, intraperitoneal) in SLE-related thrombocytopenia are similar to those in immune thrombocytopenic purpura (ITP), thus treatment is generally reserved for symptomatic or severe thrombocytopenia, and for patients with a history of severe thrombocytopenia who demonstrate an acute drop (ie, flare) in their platelet count. Children and adolescents with chronic ITP should be assessed for the presence of antinuclear antibodies, as they are at high risk of developing SLE.[36]

Antiphospholipid antibodies (lupus anticoagulant and/or anticardiolipin antibodies) are present in 40% of patients with cSLE and are generally associated with hypercoagulability. However, fewer than half of these patients manifest a thrombotic or thromboembolic event.[27] The most common events are deep venous thrombosis, cerebral vein thrombosis, and pulmonary embolus. Arterial events, including stroke, are less frequent.[37]

Gastrointestinal Involvement

Abdominal pain and discomfort are frequent, although not well characterized manifestations of SLE. Abdominal vessel vasculitis, with or without bowel perforation, is rare.[38] A sterile peritonitis occurs in fewer than 10% of patients, leading to abdominal pain and ascites, and is akin to pleuritis and pericarditis (ie, serositis). Pancreatitis is another well documented although infrequent manifestation of disease.[39] More often, (epigastric) abdominal pain is an adverse effect of prescribed medications including corticosteroids and nonsteroidal anti-inflammatory drugs (NSAIDs). As there is an association between cSLE and celiac disease, patients with persistent abdominal pain, diarrhea, and/or weight loss should have the appropriate testing.[40] Elevated liver enzyme tests occur in up to 25% of patients, and may be due to a medication side effect, active SLE, fatty infiltration, thrombosis, or infection. Testing for anti-liver kidney microsomal (anti-LKM) and anti–smooth muscle antibodies should be considered, as this may indicate primary autoimmune hepatitis that would require appropriate treatment.[41]

Cardiopulmonary Features

Serositis, namely pericarditis and/or pleuritis, occurs in up to 30% of cSLE patients.[7,12] Symptoms of pleuritis include shortness of breath and pleuritic chest pain, whereas pericarditis presents with tachycardia, precordial or retrosternal chest pain, and the inability to lie flat. Either pericarditis or pleuritis may present with or without associated fever. An inflammatory process, serositis is one of the few SLE manifestations that is associated with a significantly elevated C-reactive protein (CRP),[42] and this laboratory test may be a useful clue. Although large pericardial and pleural effusions are seen on chest radiograph or echocardiogram, a serositis flare can present with only pain, bloodwork indicative of disease activity, and increased CRP in the face of minimal findings on radiographic investigations.

Other infrequent cardiopulmonary manifestations of SLE include myocarditis, non-infective (Libman-Sacks) endocarditis, interstitial pneumonitis, pulmonary hemorrhage, and pulmonary hypertension. These conditions are frequently severe, and can be life-threatening complications requiring prompt and aggressive treatment.[43,44]

Vascular Manifestations

Although SLE is not generally thought of as an active vasculitis, inflammation and/or thrombosis of almost any vessel is possible. Cutaneous vasculitis may manifest as small, tender nodules of the digits, or palpable purpura (leukocytoclastic vasculitis) of the lower extremities, while retinal vasculitis (cotton-wool spots) and small-vessel CNS vasculitis are rare, but recognized. Although often clustered under the term vasculitis, neither livedo reticularis nor Raynaud phenomenon are due to inflammation within a vessel wall, but instead are a result of vasospasm that is common in SLE. Finally, TTP is an infrequent but life-threatening manifestation of SLE. TTP is a thrombotic microangiopathy that is diagnosed on observation of the triad of acute renal failure, thrombocytopenia, and CNS involvement, closely resembling atypical hemolytic uremic syndrome. Treatment involves plasmapheresis and significant immunosuppression with corticosteroids and a second-line agent.

Laboratory Findings

In the presence of suggestive clinical signs and symptoms, laboratory testing can support and confirm the diagnosis of SLE. A hallmark of SLE is the production of multiple autoantibodies. The commonest autoantibody is the antinuclear antibody (ANA), present in more than 95% of cSLE patients. In the presence of an ANA, it is appropriate to examine for specific autoantibodies including double-stranded DNA (dsDNA) and the extractable nuclear antigens, recognizing that particular autoantibodies correlate with certain disease features.[45] The test for ANA has high sensitivity (>95%), but its specificity for SLE is as low as 36%.[46] Moreover, up to 10% of healthy children demonstrate a positive ANA. In SLE, anti-dsDNA antibodies have high specificity. Anti-Smith antibodies (anti-Sm, not to be confused with anti–smooth muscle antibodies indicating autoimmune hepatitis) have the greatest specificity but low sensitivity for SLE. Both anti-dsDNA and anti-Sm antibodies are associated with renal involvement, and anti-Sm may be associated with more severe disease. Other autoantibodies observed in cSLE include anti–ribonuclear protein (anti-RNP), anti-Ro (also known as anti-SSA), and anti-La (or anti-SSB) antibodies. Offspring of females with anti-Ro antibodies are at risk for neonatal lupus erythematosus (NLE). NLE can lead to congenital heart block in these neonates, therefore any adolescent female with cSLE and anti-Ro antibodies should be informed of this risk prior to pregnancy, and referred for fetal echocardiogram monitoring by the end of the first trimester.

Other supporting features for SLE include hypocomplementemia (particularly C3 and C4, which are readily testable), cytopenia of one or more cell line as discussed earlier, and elevated erythrocyte sedimentation rate (ESR) in the face of a normal CRP level. CRP is often normal or only minimally elevated during an SLE flare except when the flare is of serositis, or in the presence of concurrent infection or macrophage activation syndrome (MAS) (see later discussion and see also the relevant article by Canna and Behrens elsewhere in this issue). Elevated liver enzymes can indicate fatty liver (secondary to corticosteroids), an adverse drug reaction, or active SLE. Less common causes in cSLE would include an intrahepatic thrombotic process, or elevated transaminases as a reflection of muscle inflammation. Routine hematology and biochemistry testing are used to monitor disease status for flare and remission, side effects of medication, and the effects of chronic disease and inflammation. Urinalysis should be done regularly for proteinuria and hematuria, and to examine for casts, while urine protein to creatinine ratios (spot or 24-hour collection) are required for monitoring response to treatment of lupus nephritis.

IS IT SLE?

The differential diagnosis of SLE is broad, and includes infection, malignancy, and other inflammatory disorders. The adolescent female patient who presents with a photosensitive malar rash, painless oral ulcer, polyarthritis, Raynaud phenomenon, and pleural effusions is not a diagnostic challenge. However, initial symptoms may be vague, and red flags for the pediatrician include an older child or adolescent with any combination of persistent fever, fatigue, anemia, leukopenia, thrombocytopenia, lymphadenopathy, malar or other rash, alopecia, Raynaud phenomenon, unexplained weight loss, arthralgia or arthritis, headaches and other neuropsychiatric symptoms, or unexplained microscopic hematuria or proteinuria. **Table 5** lists some of the

Table 5 Differential diagnosis of cSLE	
	Generalized (Systemic) Symptoms
Infection	
Viral	CMV EBV Parvovirus B19 HIV HHV-6
Bacterial	Sepsis (*Streptococcus*, *Salmonella*) Brucella Leptospira
Other	Q fever (coxiella) Tuberculosis (mycobacterial) Lyme disease (spirochetal) Toxoplasmosis (protozoan)
Malignant	Leukemia Lymphoma (Hodgkin/non-Hodgkin) Neuroblastoma Langerhans cell histiocytosis
Autoimmune or inflammatory	Antiphospholipid syndrome Juvenile idiopathic arthritis Juvenile dermatomyositis Sjögren syndrome Mixed connective tissue disease Systemic vasculitis Crohn disease Acute rheumatic fever Sarcoidosis Hemolytic uremic syndrome Antiphospholipid syndrome Autoimmune lymphoproliferative syndrome Common variable immunodeficiency Other primary immune deficiencies Hemophagocytic lymphohistiocytosis
Other	Chronic (widespread) pain syndrome

Abbreviations: CMV, cytomegalovirus; EBV, Epstein-Barr virus; HHV, human herpesvirus; HIV, human immunodeficiency virus.

more common differential diagnoses to consider in a patient presenting with systemic features. In contrast, **Table 6** reviews some of the possible presentations of SLE as isolated organ system involvement without generalized features.

COMPLICATIONS

In addition to severe disease flares and complications secondary to medications, 2 further categories warrant mention: infection and MAS.

Infection

SLE patients in general are immunocompromised because of immune dysfunction intrinsic to the disease itself as well as the frequent use of high-dose corticosteroids and other immunosuppressive treatment. Secondary infection is an important and frequent cause of morbidity, and should be included in the differential of any patient with a suspected SLE flare.[47,48] Infections are frequently bacterial (60%–80%), and one clue to their presence is an associated high CRP. Most bacterial infections require intravenous antibiotic treatment, as SLE patients are known to have impaired defenses against encapsulated bacteria including *Pneumococcus*, *Meningococcus*, *Haemophilus influenzae* type B, and *Salmonella*. The polysaccharide capsule protects against direct complement-associated lysis, and the necessary specific antipolysaccharide immunoglobulin G_2 response to the capsule is inadequately produced by SLE patients. Viral infections may mimic disease flares with normal or mildly elevated CRP. Systemic cytomegalovirus infections are recognized, and may be severe or even fatal in the immunocompromised cSLE patient; they may occur as either a primary infection, or more often as reactivation of a previous infection. Patients receiving corticosteroids are particularly at risk of herpes zoster, regardless of prior primary varicella disease or varicella vaccination. Patients receiving treatment with potent agents such as cyclophosphamide are at risk for other opportunistic infections such as *Pneumocystis jiroveci* or *Cryptococcus*.

Routine killed and recombinant vaccinations are safe, and are recommended at their usual administration time. Yearly influenza vaccination (killed injectable vaccine, not the live attenuated nasal mist vaccine) is strongly recommended.[49] Additional recommendations include meningococcal and pneumococcal vaccination, because of the specific susceptibility of SLE patients to these pathogens, as already discussed. For those who have not had either varicella disease or prior vaccination, it is recommended that this live attenuated vaccine be given 4 weeks before the start of

Table 6
Isolated or focal symptoms that may indicate an underlying or concomitant diagnosis of SLE

Organ System	
Thyroid	Hypothyroidism (Hashimoto)
Gastrointestinal	Autoimmune hepatitis
Cardiovascular	(Autoimmune) chronic pericarditis Noninfective endocarditis
Hematologic	Immune thrombocytopenic purpura (ITP) Autoimmune hemolytic anemia (AIHA) Evans syndrome (ITP plus AIHA)
Neuropsychiatric	Primary psychiatric disorders (eg, major depression, schizophrenia) Primary CNS vasculitis
Lymphoid system	Kikuchi-Fujimoto disease

immunosuppression, if at all possible. At present, there is no recommendation for herpes zoster vaccination in immunosuppressed children, and all other live attenuated vaccines (including measles, mumps, and rubella) are contraindicated in a cSLE patient receiving systemic immunosuppressive drugs.

Macrophage Activation Syndrome

MAS is an increasingly recognized complication in children and adolescents not only with SLE but also with several other rheumatic and infectious diseases. Its pathophysiology is not well understood, but reflects uncontrolled immune activation with increasing numbers of phagocytosing histiocytic cells infiltrating organs such as the liver, spleen, lymph nodes, and brain. Presentation can resemble an acute disease flare with fever and fatigue, but with some differences in bloodwork and physical findings. Significant cytopenias (any or all of the white blood cell, hemoglobin, and platelet counts), with elevated CRP, liver enzymes, bilirubin and lactate dehydrogenase, extremely elevated ferritin, and unexpectedly low (low- or normal-range) ESR, along with high serum fasting triglycerides, fibrinogen, and D-dimer should prompt rapid treatment with high-dose corticosteroid treatment and often hospitalization for this potentially life-threatening complication.[50] Intravenous immunoglobulin may also be given as part of initial therapy, although second-line immunosuppressives such as cyclosporine are frequently required if the initial treatment is insufficient. In any cSLE patient presenting with clinical signs of disease flare, MAS should be included in the differential diagnosis. Finding a normal ESR and high CRP may differentiate between MAS and flare, but all features must be considered and rapid evaluation is required.

TREATMENT

The care of a child or adolescent with SLE requires a multidisciplinary approach, and ideally involves rheumatology, a primary care physician, nephrology (for any patient with renal disease), adolescent medicine, psychiatry and psychology, nursing, social work, and physical and occupational therapy. Pharmacologic treatment is often aggressive, but tailored to the severity and extent of disease manifestations. Although few drugs are actually approved by the Food and Drug Administration (FDA) for use in patients with cSLE (only aspirin and prednisone), the use of multiple immunosuppressants on an off-label basis is the reality. All drugs have potential side effects, so the balance of risk versus benefit is always at the forefront of a treatment regimen. The antimalarials, hydroxychloroquine (Plaquenil) and chloroquine (Aralen), remain a staple for the treatment of mild symptoms, particularly rash and arthritis, and for disease maintenance therapy.[51] NSAIDs are prescribed primarily for musculoskeletal symptoms, and may also be used for serositis. Oral and intravenous corticosteroids remain the backbone of most therapeutic regimens, and are most effective for rapid disease control. More than 90% of all cSLE patients will receive corticosteroids at some point in their disease course.[52] The dose and duration of corticosteroid therapy depends on the active manifestation being treated.

Immunosuppressive agents used in cSLE are given primarily for either improved outcome of patients with glomerulonephritis and/or NPSLE, or as a steroid-sparing agent for other manifestations that are resistant to a corticosteroid taper (eg, persistent cytopenia or serositis). Methotrexate is predominantly prescribed for persistent arthritis in the absence of other systemic features, while azathioprine (Imuran) is also effective for arthritis as well as vasculitic rash, cytopenias, and/or serositis. Mycophenolate mofetil (Cellcept) is now frequently used for the induction of remission in lupus nephritis, and for maintenance therapy of other significant organ manifestations.[53] For patients with glomerulonephritis, the choice of immunosuppressant depends on the histologic classification, in addition to other patient factors including race/ethnicity (eg, Hispanic and African American patients may respond better to mycophenolate mofetil than to cyclophosphamide),[54] drug insurance coverage, and patient compliance with a treatment regimen. Concomitant control of hypertension, peripheral edema, and proteinuria with fluid restriction, low salt diet, and antihypertensives are important for optimal outcome. Angiotensin-converting enzyme inhibitors are particularly effective for reducing proteinuria. Although prescribed by some physicians, there are no recommendations for the use of lipid-lowering statins in cSLE.

Cyclophosphamide (Cytoxan), an alkylating agent, is reserved for the most severe and life-threatening symptoms because of its risk for toxicities including infertility, infection, and long-term risk of cancer. It is prescribed for severe NPSLE syndromes (psychosis, acute confusional state)[55] and in some cases for renal disease and other manifestations resistant to initial therapies, or for the patient who is noncompliant with oral medications. Management of NPSLE manifestations may also require antidepressants, psychotropic drugs, antiepileptics, and anticoagulation as appropriate.

Contraception may be an important consideration for adolescents with cSLE. While nonpharmacologic options should be discussed, estrogen-containing oral contraceptive pills, patches, intravaginal rings, or dermal implants are acceptable for patients who do not have antiphospholipid antibodies. Progesterone-only containing pills, intramuscular medroxyprogesterone, or the levonorgestrel-releasing intrauterine device are effective alternatives that will not increase the risk of thrombotic events in individuals with these antibodies.

Newer therapies are showing promise for the next generation of SLE patients. Rituximab (Rituxan), a monoclonal antibody that binds and kills active B cells, is effective for the treatment of cytopenias, and rheumatologists also use this drug in combination with other immunosuppressants for other disease manifestations.[56–58] Belimumab (Benlysta), an anti–B-lymphocyte stimulator antibody, was recently shown to be effective for treatment of mild to moderate symptoms in an adult SLE population.[59] Remarkably, belimumab is the first new drug that has been FDA approved for the treatment of SLE in the past 50 years; however, it has not yet been studied for use in cSLE. Studies are under way examining several other biologics that target specific cells and mediators of the immune system, and it is anticipated that over the next several years there will be many more effective treatments for both adults and children with SLE.[60]

ADOLESCENT ISSUES TO CONSIDER FOR OPTIMAL DISEASE MANAGEMENT

SLE is a lifelong disease, characterized by periods of flare and remission. Because the typical cSLE patient is an adolescent female, addressing the usual challenges of adolescence becomes crucial to ensuring that the adolescents are making informed and correct choices. As the onset of SLE occurs at an already challenging time in life, further stresses and comorbidities of disease should be minimized. At this age, teens are trying to exert their independence, are learning self-sufficiency skills, and are practicing adult-type problem solving. Adolescents must transition to new junior, middle, and high schools, where the ability to establish new peer relationships is frequently influenced by physical appearance. Normal peer pressures including smoking, drug and alcohol experimentation, dating and sexual relationships, along with authority challenges, are complicated by chronic disease. The opportunity for part-time employment and some financial freedom is often thwarted by their disease.

Many teens with cSLE have significant issues with school, peers, and their family relationships. Disease manifestations including malar and discoid rash, alopecia, and arthritis that can be painful or make writing difficult, along with the possibility of significant cognitive dysfunction, can make the life of a teenager even more challenging. Side effects of treatments compound these issues as high-dose systemic corticosteroids lead to weight gain, moon facies, striae, and acne, while other treatments may cause alopecia or carry a risk of infertility. Therefore, it is not surprising that many teens with SLE are noncompliant with their medications and medical care, and are reluctant to attend school. Moreover, the transition to adult care comes at 18 years in most centers, an age that frequently brings other significant transitions (eg, to postsecondary education, a move from the family home), and added stressors to independently manage medications, appointments, and their chronic disease. A comprehensive interdisciplinary clinical team that includes adolescent medicine, psychiatry, and social work, in addition to rheumatology and nephrology, is crucial in addressing many of these issues. Furthermore, issues of seamless transition to adult medical care must be addressed.

LONG-TERM OUTLOOK

Studies have shown that patients with SLE do not achieve long-lasting drug-free remission, and many patients have persistently active disease requiring long-term immunosuppressive treatment.[61,62] However, cSLE patients are younger at diagnosis and have a more severe disease course than those with adult-onset SLE, therefore they are prone to develop significant damage caused by the disease or its treatment at a relatively young age.[7,63] Nonwhite ethnicity, especially African American (or Afro-Caribbean) or Hispanic ethnicity, is associated with a worse outcome.[2,64,65] These studies need to be interpreted with caution, as the numbers of patients are frequently low, and socioeconomic status, a potential confounder, is not always taken into account. Mortality rates have decreased significantly over the past 2 decades, with 10- and 15-year survival exceeding 85%. However, with a median age of disease onset around 12 years, this means that at the age of 22 to 27 years up to 15% of cSLE patients have died.[66] Mortality in the first several years of disease is most commonly due to infection, ESRD, or severe lupus flare, while cardiovascular disease plays a significant role in late mortality.

With longer survival there has been an increase in long-term comorbidities including premature atherosclerosis, and a 50-fold increased risk of myocardial infarction in young women with SLE in their 30s and 40s.[67,68] Other long-term complications include ESRD requiring dialysis and/or renal transplant and its concomitant morbidities, osteoporosis leading to increased bone fragility and fracture risk, hip (or other joint) replacement secondary to avascular necrosis, and multiple hospitalizations because of infection and other treatment-related complications. Moreover, SLE leads to an increased risk of malignancy, particularly lymphoma.[69]

Considering the aforementioned, it is not surprising that SLE interferes with many aspects of daily life. Adult-onset SLE has been associated with suboptimal mental and physical functioning and loss of work productivity.[70] Similarly, more than one-third of cSLE patients report that the disease has negatively interfered with their education. Most adults with cSLE live on relatively low incomes, with 11% to 23% living on full-time disability support.[71,72] Assessment of health-related quality of life demonstrates significantly lower scores in cSLE patients compared with healthy controls, especially in the physical domain.[72–74]

SUMMARY

Childhood-onset SLE is a lifelong autoimmune disease that may be difficult to diagnose because of its multisystem involvement and heterogeneity of clinical manifestations. It follows a more aggressive disease course than adult-onset SLE, with greater disease activity at presentation and over time, and consequently leads to greater morbidity and mortality than adult-onset SLE. Moreover, children with SLE have to deal with this unpredictable, relapsing-remitting disease during adolescence, an already challenging time of life when physical appearance is important, self-esteem and identity are yet to be developed, and overestimation of personal skills regarding decision making and responsibility for their disease are frequent. Recognition of these cSLE-specific issues is key to optimal disease management of these patients. Long-term outcome studies of cSLE are limited, but new studies are under way to examine population-based cSLE cohorts that have reached adulthood. The results from these studies will better determine the long-term outcome of cSLE, and may form the basis of a more tailored management and treatment approach for children and adolescents with cSLE.

REFERENCES

1. Kamphuis S, Silverman ED. Prevalence and burden of pediatric-onset systemic lupus erythematosus. Nat Rev Rheumatol 2010;6:538–46.
2. Hiraki LT, Benseler SM, Tyrrell PN, et al. Ethnic differences in pediatric systemic lupus erythematosus. J Rheumatol 2009;36:2539–46.
3. Pons-Estel GJ, Alarcon GS, Scofield L, et al. Understanding the epidemiology and progression of systemic lupus erythematosus. Semin Arthritis Rheum 2009; 39:257–68.
4. Malleson PN, Fung MY, Rosenberg AM. The incidence of pediatric rheumatic diseases: results from the Canadian Pediatric Rheumatology Association Disease Registry. J Rheumatol 1996;23:1981–7.
5. Bahillo MP, Hermoso F, Ochoa C, et al. Incidence and prevalence of type 1 diabetes in children aged <15 yr in Castilla-Leon (Spain). Pediatr Diabetes 2007;8: 369–73.
6. Huang JL, Yao TC, See LC. Prevalence of pediatric systemic lupus erythematosus and juvenile chronic arthritis in a Chinese population: a nation-wide prospective population-based study in Taiwan. Clin Exp Rheumatol 2004;22:776–80.
7. Hiraki LT, Benseler SM, Tyrrell PN, et al. Clinical and laboratory characteristics and long-term outcome of pediatric systemic lupus erythematosus: a longitudinal study. J Pediatr 2008;152:550–6.
8. Pluchinotta FR, Schiavo B, Vittadello F, et al. Distinctive clinical features of pediatric systemic lupus erythematosus in three different age classes. Lupus 2007;16: 550–5.
9. Hochberg MC. Updating the American College of Rheumatology revised criteria for the classification of systemic lupus erythematosus. Arthritis Rheum 1997;40: 1725.
10. Tan EM, Cohen AS, Fries JF, et al. The 1982 revised criteria for the classification of systemic lupus erythematosus. Arthritis Rheum 1982;25:1271–7.
11. Ferraz MB, Goldenberg J, Hilario MO, et al. Evaluation of the 1982 ARA lupus criteria data set in pediatric patients. Committees of Pediatric Rheumatology of the Brazilian Society of Pediatrics and the Brazilian Society of Rheumatology. Clin Exp Rheumatol 1994;12:83–7.

12. Ramirez Gomez LA, Uribe Uribe O, Osio Uribe O, et al. Childhood systemic lupus erythematosus in Latin America. The GLADEL experience in 230 children. Lupus 2008;17:596–604.
13. Sibbitt WL Jr, Brandt JR, Johnson CR, et al. The incidence and prevalence of neuropsychiatric syndromes in pediatric onset systemic lupus erythematosus. J Rheumatol 2002;29:1536–42.
14. Wang LC, Yang YH, Lu MY, et al. Retrospective analysis of mortality and morbidity of pediatric systemic lupus erythematosus in the past two decades. J Microbiol Immunol Infect 2003;36:203–8.
15. Descloux E, Durieu I, Cochat P, et al. Influence of age at disease onset in the outcome of paediatric systemic lupus erythematosus. Rheumatology (Oxford) 2009;48:779–84.
16. Uziel Y, Gorodnitski N, Mukamel M, et al. Outcome of a national Israeli cohort of pediatric systemic lupus erythematosus. Lupus 2007;16:142–6.
17. Salah S, Lotfy HM, Sabry SM, et al. Systemic lupus erythematosus in Egyptian children. Rheumatol Int 2009;29:1463–8.
18. Sampaio MC, de Oliveira ZN, Machado MC, et al. Discoid lupus erythematosus in children—a retrospective study of 34 patients. Pediatr Dermatol 2008;25:163–7.
19. Costenbader KH, Desai A, Alarcon GS, et al. Trends in the incidence, demographics and outcomes of end-stage renal disease due to lupus nephritis in the U.S., 1995-2006. Arthritis Rheum 2011;63(6):1681–8.
20. Fiehn C, Hajjar Y, Mueller K, et al. Improved clinical outcome of lupus nephritis during the past decade: importance of early diagnosis and treatment. Ann Rheum Dis 2003;62:435–9.
21. Hiraki LT, Lu B, Alexander SR, et al. End-stage renal disease due to lupus nephritis among children in the U.S., 1995-2006. Arthritis Rheum 2011;63(7):1988–97.
22. Cochat P, Fargue S, Mestrallet G, et al. Disease recurrence in paediatric renal transplantation. Pediatr Nephrol 2009;24:2097–108.
23. The American College of Rheumatology nomenclature and case definitions for neuropsychiatric lupus syndromes. Arthritis Rheum 1999;42:599–608.
24. Benseler SM, Silverman ED. Neuropsychiatric involvement in pediatric systemic lupus erythematosus. Lupus 2007;16:564–71.
25. Brunner HI, Jones OY, Lovell DJ, et al. Lupus headaches in childhood-onset systemic lupus erythematosus: relationship to disease activity as measured by the systemic lupus erythematosus disease activity index (SLEDAI) and disease damage. Lupus 2003;12:600–6.
26. Mitsikostas DD, Sfikakis PP, Goadsby PJ. A meta-analysis for headache in systemic lupus erythematosus: the evidence and the myth. Brain 2004;127:1200–9.
27. Levy DM, Massicotte MP, Harvey E, et al. Thromboembolism in paediatric lupus patients. Lupus 2003;12:741–6.
28. Singh S, Gupta MK, Ahluwalia J, et al. Neuropsychiatric manifestations and anti-phospholipid antibodies in pediatric onset lupus: 14 years of experience from a tertiary center of North India. Rheumatol Int 2009;29:1455–61.
29. Williams TS, Aranow C, Ross GS, et al. Neurocognitive impairment in childhood-onset systemic lupus erythematosus: measurement issues in diagnosis. Arthritis Care Res (Hoboken) 2011;63(8):1178–87.
30. Brunner HI, Ruth NM, German A, et al. Initial validation of the pediatric automated neuropsychological assessment metrics for childhood-onset systemic lupus erythematosus. Arthritis Rheum 2007;57:1174–82.

31. Levy DM, Ardoin SP, Schanberg LE. Neurocognitive impairment in children and adolescents with systemic lupus erythematosus. Nat Clin Pract Rheumatol 2009;5:106–14.
32. Pego-Reigosa JM, Isenberg DA. Psychosis due to systemic lupus erythematosus: characteristics and long-term outcome of this rare manifestation of the disease. Rheumatology (Oxford) 2008;47:1498–502.
33. Fong KY, Thumboo J. Neuropsychiatric lupus: clinical challenges, brain-reactive autoantibodies and treatment strategies. Lupus 2010;19:1399–403.
34. Appenzeller S, Cendes F, Costallat LT. Epileptic seizures in systemic lupus erythematosus. Neurology 2004;63:1808–12.
35. Varaprasad IR, Agrawal S, Prabu VN, et al. Posterior reversible encephalopathy syndrome in systemic lupus erythematosus. J Rheumatol 2011;38:1607–11.
36. Schmugge M, Revel-Vilk S, Hiraki L, et al. Thrombocytopenia and thromboembolism in pediatric systemic lupus erythematosus. J Pediatr 2003;143:666–9.
37. Avcin T, Benseler SM, Tyrrell PN, et al. A followup study of antiphospholipid antibodies and associated neuropsychiatric manifestations in 137 children with systemic lupus erythematosus. Arthritis Rheum 2008;59:206–13.
38. Tu YL, Chen LC, Ou LH, et al. Mesenteric vasculitis as the initial presentation in children with systemic lupus erythematosus. J Pediatr Gastroenterol Nutr 2009; 49:251–3.
39. Richer O, Ulinski T, Lemelle I, et al. Abdominal manifestations in childhood-onset systemic lupus erythematosus. Ann Rheum Dis 2007;66:174–8.
40. Zitouni M, Daoud W, Kallel M, et al. Systemic lupus erythematosus with celiac disease: a report of five cases. Joint Bone Spine 2004;71:344–6.
41. Deen ME, Porta G, Fiorot FJ, et al. Autoimmune hepatitis and juvenile systemic lupus erythematosus. Lupus 2009;18:747–51.
42. ter Borg EJ, Horst G, Limburg PC, et al. C-reactive protein levels during disease exacerbations and infections in systemic lupus erythematosus: a prospective longitudinal study. J Rheumatol 1990;17:1642–8.
43. Beresford MW, Cleary AG, Sills JA, et al. Cardio-pulmonary involvement in juvenile systemic lupus erythematosus. Lupus 2005;14:152–8.
44. Jain D, Halushka MK. Cardiac pathology of systemic lupus erythematosus. J Clin Pathol 2009;62:584–92.
45. Jurencak R, Fritzler M, Tyrrell P, et al. Autoantibodies in pediatric systemic lupus erythematosus: ethnic grouping, cluster analysis, and clinical correlations. J Rheumatol 2009;36:416–21.
46. Copple SS, Sawitzke AD, Wilson AM, et al. Enzyme-linked immunosorbent assay screening then indirect immunofluorescence confirmation of antinuclear antibodies: a statistical analysis. Am J Clin Pathol 2011;135:678–84.
47. Ruiz-Irastorza G, Olivares N, Ruiz-Arruza I, et al. Predictors of major infections in systemic lupus erythematosus. Arthritis Res Ther 2009;11:R109.
48. Zandman-Goddard G, Shoenfeld Y. Infections and SLE. Autoimmunity 2005;38: 473–85.
49. Heijstek MW, Ott de Bruin LM, Bijl M, et al. EULAR recommendations for vaccination in paediatric patients with rheumatic diseases. Ann Rheum Dis 2011;70: 1704–12.
50. Parodi A, Davi S, Pringe AB, et al. Macrophage activation syndrome in juvenile systemic lupus erythematosus: a multinational multicenter study of thirty-eight patients. Arthritis Rheum 2009;60:3388–99.
51. Lee SJ, Silverman E, Bargman JM. The role of antimalarial agents in the treatment of SLE and lupus nephritis. Nat Rev Nephrol 2011;7(12):718–29.

52. Brunner HI, Klein-Gitelman MS, Ying J, et al. Corticosteroid use in childhood-onset systemic lupus erythematosus-practice patterns at four pediatric rheumatology centers. Clin Exp Rheumatol 2009;27:155–62.

53. Ginzler EM, Dooley MA, Aranow C, et al. Mycophenolate mofetil or intravenous cyclophosphamide for lupus nephritis. N Engl J Med 2005;353:2219–28.

54. Isenberg D, Appel GB, Contreras G, et al. Influence of race/ethnicity on response to lupus nephritis treatment: the ALMS study. Rheumatology 2009;49:128–40.

55. Trevisani VF, Castro AA, Neves Neto JF, et al. Cyclophosphamide versus methylprednisolone for treating neuropsychiatric involvement in systemic lupus erythematosus. Cochrane Database Syst Rev 2006;2:CD002265.

56. Merrill JT, Neuwelt CM, Wallace DJ, et al. Efficacy and safety of rituximab in moderately-to-severely active systemic lupus erythematosus: the randomized, double-blind, phase II/III systemic lupus erythematosus evaluation of rituximab trial. Arthritis Rheum 2010;62:222–33.

57. Kumar S, Benseler SM, Kirby-Allen M, et al. B-cell depletion for autoimmune thrombocytopenia and autoimmune hemolytic anemia in pediatric systemic lupus erythematosus. Pediatrics 2009;123:e159–63.

58. Ramos-Casals M, Soto MJ, Cuadrado MJ, et al. Rituximab in systemic lupus erythematosus: a systematic review of off-label use in 188 cases. Lupus 2009;18:767–76.

59. Navarra SV, Guzman RM, Gallacher AE, et al. Efficacy and safety of belimumab in patients with active systemic lupus erythematosus: a randomised, placebo-controlled, phase 3 trial. Lancet 2011;377:721–31.

60. Landmark lupus approval opens door for next wave of drugs. Nat Rev Drug Discov 2011;10:243–5.

61. Swaak AJ, van den Brink HG, Smeenk RJ, et al. Systemic lupus erythematosus: clinical features in patients with a disease duration of over 10 years, first evaluation. Rheumatology (Oxford) 1999;38:953–8.

62. Urowitz MB, Feletar M, Bruce IN, et al. Prolonged remission in systemic lupus erythematosus. J Rheumatol 2005;32:1467–72.

63. Brunner HI, Silverman ED, To T, et al. Risk factors for damage in childhood-onset systemic lupus erythematosus: cumulative disease activity and medication use predict disease damage. Arthritis Rheum 2002;46:436–44.

64. Baqi N, Moazami S, Singh A, et al. Lupus nephritis in children: a longitudinal study of prognostic factors and therapy. J Am Soc Nephrol 1996;7:924–9.

65. Gibson KL, Gipson DS, Massengill SA, et al. Predictors of relapse and end stage kidney disease in proliferative lupus nephritis: focus on children, adolescents, and young adults. Clin J Am Soc Nephrol 2009;4:1962–7.

66. Hersh AO, Trupin L, Yazdany J, et al. Childhood-onset disease as a predictor of mortality in an adult cohort of patients with systemic lupus erythematosus. Arthritis Care Res (Hoboken) 2010;62:1152–9.

67. Urowitz MB, Gladman D, Ibanez D, et al. Atherosclerotic vascular events in a multinational inception cohort of systemic lupus erythematosus. Arthritis Care Res (Hoboken) 2010;62:881–7.

68. Manzi S, Meilahn EN, Rairie JE, et al. Age-specific incidence rates of myocardial infarction and angina in women with systemic lupus erythematosus: comparison with the Framingham Study. Am J Epidemiol 1997;145:408–15.

69. Bernatsky S, Boivin JF, Joseph L, et al. An international cohort study of cancer in systemic lupus erythematosus. Arthritis Rheum 2005;52:1481–90.

70. Jolly M. How does quality of life of patients with systemic lupus erythematosus compare with that of other common chronic illnesses? J Rheumatol 2005;32:1706–8.

71. Tucker LB, Uribe AG, Fernandez M, et al. Adolescent onset of lupus results in more aggressive disease and worse outcomes: results of a nested matched case-control study within LUMINA, a multiethnic US cohort (LUMINA LVII). Lupus 2008;17:314–22.
72. Candell Chalom E, Periera B, Cole R, et al. Educational, vocational and socioeconomic status and quality of life in adults with childhood-onset systemic lupus erythematosus. Pediatr Rheumatol Online J 2004;2:207–26.
73. Ruperto N, Buratti S, Duarte-Salazar C, et al. Health-related quality of life in juvenile-onset systemic lupus erythematosus and its relationship to disease activity and damage. Arthritis Rheum 2004;51:458–64.
74. Brunner HI, Higgins GC, Wiers K, et al. Health-related quality of life and its relationship to patient disease course in childhood-onset systemic lupus erythematosus. J Rheumatol 2009;36:1536–45.

Idiopathic Inflammatory Myopathies in Childhood: Current Concepts

Adam M. Huber, MSc, MD

KEYWORDS

- Juvenile idiopathic myopathies • Juvenile dermatomyositis
- Juvenile polymyositis • Connective tissue myositis

The juvenile idiopathic inflammatory myopathies (JIIM) are a group of rare, chronic autoimmune diseases that have muscle involvement as a primary feature. Muscle inflammation results in muscle weakness (proximal greater than distal), reductions in endurance, and impairment of physical function. Juvenile dermatomyositis (JDM), the most common member of this group, also manifests a variety of cutaneous features. Other forms of JIIM include juvenile polymyositis (JPM) and myositis associated with another connective tissue disease (JCTM) (also called overlap myositis). Less commonly, JIIM can be associated with other organ involvement, including lung, heart, and brain.

The underlying pathogenesis of JIIM is unknown. The current state of this knowledge has been recently reviewed.[1]

Although JIIM are rare, affecting 2 to 4 per 1 million children,[2,3] they occupy an important proportion of time in pediatric rheumatology clinics because of their complexity, chronicity, and risk of mortality and morbidity. This rarity also makes it unlikely that most pediatricians or family physicians will have seen or cared for a child with JIIM, making recognition and early management challenging.

This review focuses on practical issues of relevance to the practicing pediatrician, including clinical presentation, differential diagnosis, investigation, therapy, and prognosis. The goal is to facilitate early recognition and referral for appropriate specialist care and to assist the reader in comanagement of these patients with a pediatric rheumatologist.

CLINICAL PRESENTATION AND EVALUATION

Presenting features of children with JIIM have been reported by numerous investigators. Two of the largest descriptions have included a total of 641 patients, mostly with JDM.[4,5] Their findings are summarized in **Table 1**. As expected, most patients presented with weakness and rashes. However, it should be noted that a significant

Division of Pediatric Rheumatology, IWK Health Centre, 5850 University Avenue, Halifax, NS B3K 6R8, Canada
E-mail address: adam.huber@iwk.nshealth.ca

Pediatr Clin N Am 59 (2012) 365–380
doi:10.1016/j.pcl.2012.03.006
0031-3955/12/$ – see front matter © 2012 Elsevier Inc. All rights reserved.

Table 1
Typical presenting features of children with JIIM

	McCann et al,[5] 2006	Guseinova et al,[4] 2011
Population	151 children with JIIM 120 JDM 4 JPM 27 other JIIM (most overlap)	490 JDM
Gender (F:M)	104:47	321:169
Age at diagnosis (years) (median)	7.0 (range 1–16)	7.0 (172 were <5, 211 were 5–10, 103 were 10–18)
Characteristic or Gottron rash	88%	n/a
Gottron rash	n/a	72%
Heliotrope rash	n/a	61%
Malar rash	n/a	56%
Proximal muscle weakness	82%	84%
Systemic features	81%	n/a
Myalgias	68%	n/a
Arthralgias or arthritis	66%	n/a
Arthritis	36%	35%
Edema	32%	n/a
Dysphagia	29%	18%
Contractures	27%	n/a
Skin ulcers	23%	6%
Dyspnea	18%	n/a
Dysphonia	17%	11%
Lipoatrophy	10%	n/a
Raynaud phenomenon	n/a	5%
Calcinosis	6%	4%

Abbreviation: n/a, no data available.

proportion of children were not found to be clinically weak. Many children also present with systemic features (>80% in one series)[5] including fever, fatigue, and weight loss. Other common symptoms include muscle and joint pain, subcutaneous edema, and symptoms of pharyngeal weakness (dysphonia or dysphagia).

Given that muscle involvement is common to all forms of JIIM, many children will present with complaints of weakness or changes in physical function. However, the extent of these changes may vary from nearly imperceptible to profound. Careful assessment of muscle strength is crucial, and the possibility of JIIM should not be discounted if weakness is not immediately obvious. Weakness primarily affects the proximal (shoulder and hip girdle) and axial (mainly paraspinal and abdominal) musculature. Distal muscle weakness may be present, but it should be less prominent than the proximal muscle weakness. Otherwise, alternative diagnoses should be considered.

In the clinic, muscle strength is most commonly evaluated using confrontational manual muscle testing (MMT). An abbreviated form of MMT has recently been validated in children using 8 muscle groups.[6] However, MMT can be challenging, due to a variety of factors. MMT requires cooperation, and may be difficult for young children. It also requires considerable experience to determine normal strength, particularly when a full-sized adult is examining a young child.

Other tools that may be helpful in assessing strength and physical function of the child with suspected JIIM are also available. The Childhood Myositis Assessment Scale (CMAS) is a 14-item, performance-based tool that assesses muscle strength, endurance, and physical function.[7,8] The CMAS is validated in children with JIIM, but is probably not useful in very young children.[9] The CMAS explicitly includes endurance assessment through the use of timed items (eg, keeping the leg raised off the examination table for a specified time). However, some clinicians have criticized the CMAS as taking too long to administer. The Children's Health Assessment Questionnaire (CHAQ), a 30-item self-report questionnaire commonly used in childhood arthritis, has also been validated in JIIM.[10,11] Both of these tools are recognized to have significant ceiling effects (relative insensitivity to change as patients approach normal strength), but are considered useful in baseline and longitudinal evaluation of JIIM patients.

Cutaneous involvement is a feature primarily of JDM and, to a lesser extent, is also common in JCTM. These features have been reviewed in an online pictorial atlas.[12,13] Some features are particularly common and highly suggestive of the underlying diagnosis. Gottron papules are raised, erythematous lesions with a fine, overlying silvery scale, which are found most commonly over the metacarpophalangeal and proximal interphalangeal joints, but can also be present over the elbows, knees, toes, and medial malleoli (**Fig. 1**). It is not uncommon for these lesions to be mistaken for psoriasis, which they can closely resemble. Erythema in the distribution of Gottron papules is also common, and is called the Gottron sign. The presence of either Gottron papules or sign should lead to consideration of JIIM.

The heliotrope sign is a violaceous discoloration of the upper eyelid, sometimes accompanied by fine scaling (**Fig. 2**). Accompanying localized swelling (periorbital edema or puffiness) is also common. An accentuation of blood vessels along the upper lash line (eyeliner sign), which may persist long after other acute cutaneous features have disappeared, is also commonly seen.

Abnormalities of the digital nailfold capillaries are common in JIIM, particularly JDM, and are thought to reflect the underlying vasculopathy. These changes are also commonly seen in other rheumatic disorders, particularly systemic lupus

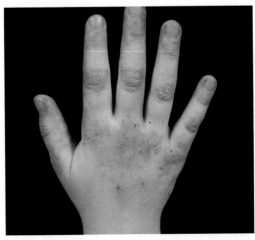

Fig. 1. Typical Gottron rash (both papules and sign) in a child with juvenile dermatomyositis.

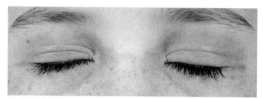

Fig. 2. Heliotrope rash in a child with juvenile dermatomyositis. Note the distribution of erythema and presence of periorbital edema.

erythematosus and scleroderma. In the literature, most studies have used photomicroscopy but when prominent, capillary changes can be seen without magnification (**Fig. 3**). In the clinic, use of a hand lens or ophthalmoscope can be very helpful. When visualizing the nailfold capillaries, abnormalities to note include dilatation, tortuosity/arborization, hemorrhage, and dropout (and resulting impact on overall capillary density). The methods for nailfold capillaroscopy are well described.[14] This assessment is valuable both in assisting with diagnosis, as many of the other illnesses under consideration will not have these changes, and in following patients. Capillary changes, particularly capillary density, have been shown to correlate well with disease activity and other clinically relevant outcomes.[15–18]

There are several tools available for assessing skin disease in children with JIIM, including the disease activity score (DAS),[19] the cutaneous assessment tool (CAT),[19–22] the cutaneous dermatomyositis disease area and severity index (CDASI),[23] and the dermatomyositis skin severity index (DSSI).[24] Some attempts have been made to compare these tools,[25] but at this time it is not clear which of these is the most useful; they are primarily useful as research tools at present.

The 2 studies of clinical features discussed previously found that 6% to 23% of children presented with skin ulcers.[4,5] The presence of skin ulceration may be suggestive of medium vessel vasculitis, and should alert the examining physician to the possibility of vasculitic involvement of the bowel. This aspect is particularly important because of the potential for a catastrophic presentation with massive gastrointestinal bleeding or perforation and infectious complications. The presence of abdominal pain (particularly if severe), hematemesis, or melena should also be considered warning signs, and warrant swift investigation and intervention.

The development of cutaneous calcium deposits in children with JIIM is an important problem. The incidence of calcinosis can vary from 20% to 40%, and increases

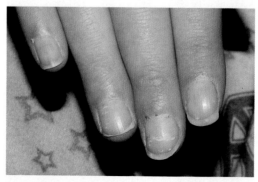

Fig. 3. Capillary changes of the digital nailbed in a child with juvenile dermatomyositis, seen without magnification.

with disease duration.[26–28] It may take a variety of forms, including small asymptomatic papules, larger superficial or deep masses that can be painful and functionally limiting, and platelike calcifications in the skin or fascial planes that can have a major impact on physical function. The underlying pathogenesis is not well understood, but calcinosis has been associated with delayed or inadequate therapy[29,30] and persistent skin inflammation.[31] Unfortunately, despite some anecdotal reports, there are no established treatments for calcinosis once it has formed. Surgery can be helpful, but the lesions have a tendency to recur at the surgical site. For these reasons, prevention through the provision of optimal medical care is crucial.

Lipodystrophy, which is a loss of adipose tissue, is also described in children with JIIM (mostly JDM).[32] It may be generalized, affecting the entire body, or localized, most commonly affecting the face or a limb. When the face is affected, this results in prominence of the masseter muscles and sunken cheeks. In the extremities, loss of fat results in a more defined appearance of the muscles. Focal depressions may also be seen. The etiology is not well understood, but in some cases is associated with inflammation of the subcutaneous tissues (panniculitis).[32] The incidence of lipodystrophy has been reported to be 10% to 40%, but the true incidence may be higher because of difficulties in recognition.[32] Various metabolic abnormalities have been associated with lipodystrophy, including impaired glucose tolerance, hypertriglyceridemia, steatohepatitis, and menstrual irregularities with increases in serum testosterone and hypertension.[32–34] The presence of lipodystrophy should lead to investigation to uncover these potentially serious problems.

Manifestations of JIIM outside the muscle and skin are less common, but may have a major impact on the disease course. In particular, involvement of the gastrointestinal tract and respiratory systems should be noted. The main concern with the bowel is the possibility of bowel vasculitis,[35] which may present with abdominal pain, upper or lower gastrointestinal bleeding, or perforation. Bleeding, when it occurs, may be massive and is a potential cause of mortality. Perforation and associated infectious complications is also serious and may be masked by the use of corticosteroids. These complications may occur at presentation or later in the disease course. The presence of bowel symptoms is a major cause for concern and should be investigated quickly.

Interstitial lung disease is rare in children with JIIM, but is a potential cause of late mortality. As described in adults, the development of lung disease is associated with the presence of anti-tRNA synthetase antibodies.[36] In addition, associations with other autoantibodies have been described in children.[37] Presentation may include cough and shortness of breath, but may also be clinically silent.[38,39] Unfortunately, once established, pulmonary disease in JIIM is frequently progressive, making early detection and aggressive therapy of utmost importance.

DIFFERENTIAL DIAGNOSIS

In the child who presents with classic proximal weakness, Gottron papules, and heliotrope rash, the diagnosis of JDM is not difficult to make. However, for many children a variety of other potential diagnoses will need to be considered; these are summarized in **Box 1**. For a more detailed listing of differential diagnoses, the reader is referred to Ref.[40]

When the presentation is one of weakness or reduction in physical function, a careful examination to determine the distribution is needed. Most patients with JIIM will present with approximately symmetric weakness of the axial and proximal muscle groups. Significant asymmetry should lead to consideration of possible local causes of weakness, such as peripheral nerve problems or structural injuries. The presence

---

Box 1
Summary of differential diagnosis of juvenile idiopathic inflammatory myopathy

Weakness With/Without Rash

Juvenile idiopathic inflammatory myopathy

Juvenile dermatomyositis

Juvenile polymyositis

Overlap myositis (including systemic lupus erythematosus, scleroderma, mixed connective tissue disease)

Focal myositis

Granulomatous myositis

Orbital myositis

Eosinophilic myositis

Malignancy-associated/paraneoplastic myositis

Infection-associated

Viral—influenza, Coxsackie, echovirus, parvovirus, hepatitis B, human immunodeficiency virus, human T lymphotropic virus

Bacterial (pyomyositis)—staphylococcal and streptococcal species most common

Parasitic—*Toxoplasma*, *Trichinella*

Postinfectious—influenza B

Weakness only (usually)[a]

Muscular dystrophies—eg, Duchenne, Becker

Myopathies—eg, myotubular myopathy, nemaline rod disease

Myotonic disorders

Metabolic myopathies—eg, glycogen storage diseases, respiratory chain defects, mitochondrial disorders

Endocrine disorders—eg, thyroid, adrenal

Drug induced—eg, corticosteroids, HMG-CoA reductase inhibitors

Neurogenic—both congenital (eg, spinal muscular atrophy) and acquired (eg, Guillain-Barré)

Neuromuscular junction—eg, myasthenia gravis

Rash only

Amyopathic juvenile dermatomyositis

Mimicking cutaneous disease (psoriasis, eczema)

[a] It is possible to see some cutaneous features, although usually not classic Gottron lesions or heliotrope.
Data from Cassidy JT, Petty RE, Laxer RM, et al. Textbook of pediatric rheumatology. 6th edition. Philadelphia: Saunders Elsevier; 2011. p. 394–5.

---

of distal muscle weakness, particularly if it is similar to or greater than the corresponding proximal weakness, should lead to consideration of alternate diagnoses, such as myopathies or dystrophies. Involvement of a neuromuscular specialist early in the evaluation process is advisable.

The absence of cutaneous features in the patient presenting with weakness is also a warning signal. Although the underlying diagnosis may be JPM, this diagnosis is very rare and may be made in error in patients with other underlying muscle problems. For this reason, careful investigation is needed before committing to a diagnosis of JPM.

Measurement of serum levels of muscle enzymes (see later discussion) may also provide some guidance regarding diagnosis. While muscle enzyme levels are frequently elevated in JIIM, extreme elevations should prompt consideration of an infectious or postinfectious cause when symptoms are acute and a myopathy or dystrophy when the symptoms are more chronic.

The association of inflammatory myositis with malignancy in adults is well established. However, whether a similar association exists in children is much less clear. There have been rare cases of malignancy-associated JIIM.[41] It is likely wise to keep this possibility in mind, particularly when there are unusual features present, such as splenomegaly or marked lymphadenopathy.

INVESTIGATION

Most of the JIIM literature uses the Bohan and Peter criteria to classify patients as having definite, probable, and possible disease (**Box 2**).[42] These criteria use the presence of proximal muscle weakness, cutaneous features, elevations in muscle enzymes, and abnormalities on muscle biopsy and electromyography (EMG) typical for an inflammatory myopathy. However, these criteria were never intended to be diagnostic criteria for pediatric disease. Furthermore, current approaches in most centers have resulted in many patients with suspected JIIM never receiving either a biopsy or EMG. For example, in a registry of 151 children with JIIM in the United Kingdom, only 36% had a muscle biopsy documented and only 8% had EMG results documented. Similar trends have been documented in North America and elsewhere.[43] Work is currently being done to establish new classification and diagnostic criteria for JIIM.

Biopsy and EMG have fallen out of favor, largely because they are painful and invasive. In addition, depending on the center, local expertise in performing or reading the test may be lacking. Finally, muscle disease in JIIM is patchy, which may result in

---

Box 2
Bohan and Peter criteria for diagnosis of dermatomyositis

Symmetric weakness of the limb-girdle muscles and neck flexors

Muscle-biopsy evidence of necrosis, phagocytosis, regeneration, perifascicular atrophy, fiber size variation, perivascular inflammation

Elevation of serum muscle enzymes

Electromyography showing short, small, polyphasic motor units, fibrillations, positive sharp waves and insertional irritability, and bizarre, high-frequency, repetitive discharges

Typical cutaneous features—heliotrope rash, Gottron papules/sign

Patients are said to have "definite" JDM if they have rash + 3 other criteria

Patients are said to have "probable" JDM if they have rash + 2 other criteria

Patients are said to have "possible" JDM if they have rash + 1 other criteria

Data from Bohan A, Peter JB. Polymyositis and dermatomyositis (first of two parts). N Engl J Med 1975;292(7):344–7.

false-negative results. Despite these concerns, there are some recent data suggesting that muscle biopsy, when specific evaluations are included, may be predictive of course and outcome.[44] These data may lead to muscle biopsy becoming more commonly used again. It should be noted that some specialized pathologic assessments are not universally available.

While it is true that muscle biopsies are performed less often than in the past, it is important to recognize that muscle biopsy remains an important part of evaluation of many suspected JIIM patients. A biopsy may not be necessary in patients presenting with typical rash, classic proximal weakness, and an absence of unusual features. However, a muscle biopsy is advisable before initiating treatment when there is no rash; if weakness is asymmetric, localized, or has a prominent distal component; if there are unusual features of presentation, such as marked muscle atrophy, prominent involvement of bulbar muscles, muscle fasciculations, or myotony; or if there is a family history of a potentially heritable muscle disease. Once again, involvement of a neuromuscular specialist is advised to ensure that appropriate testing of the biopsy specimen is obtained.

Documentation of muscle involvement is clearly important in JIIM. Magnetic resonance imaging (MRI) has been become a key investigative tool (**Fig. 4**). In studies of pediatric rheumatologists, MRI has been shown to be the preferred test to identify the presence of myositis.[43,45] MRI evaluation has been shown to identify muscle inflammation and subcutaneous edema, and correlates well with other measures of disease activity.[46,47] Further discussion of the use of MRI in JIIM can be found in the article by Gardner-Medwin and colleagues.[48]

Muscle enzymes are part of a routine evaluation of all suspected JIIM patients at diagnosis. Such enzymes include alanine aminotransferase, aspartate aminotransferase, lactic acid dehydrogenase, creatinine kinase, and aldolase. Any one of these enzymes is elevated in up to 75% of patients,[5] therefore several or all of these enzymes should be checked to increase the likelihood of finding an abnormality. It also means that a small percentage of patients (around 5%–10%) may have entirely

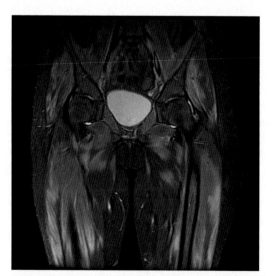

Fig. 4. Magnetic resonance imaging of the pelvic and thigh muscles in a child with juvenile dermatomyositis. Sequence is a coronal, single-tau inversion recovery (STIR) sequence with fat suppression. Note the marked increase in signal intensity, with muscle having similar intensity to the fluid-filled bladder, and the overall patchy nature of the changes.

normal muscle enzymes, despite having clear muscle disease. It should also be noted that muscle enzymes have been shown to correlate poorly with disease activity and, outside initial evaluation, should not be relied on to identify patients who are flaring or doing poorly.[5,10]

Several possible biomarkers thought to be helpful in evaluating JIIM patients have been identified, including $CD3^-CD56^+/CD16^+$ cell counts,[49,50] serum neopterin,[51,52] and serum quinolinic acid.[52] However, their role in routine clinical care remains unclear, and they should be considered research tools at this time. Serum levels of von Willebrand factor (Factor VIII-related antigen) have also been associated with disease activity, but most investigators have not found the association to be consistent in all patients.[53,54]

Other initial evaluations will depend on the clinical situation. Given the potential importance of pulmonary involvement, most clinicians would agree that a baseline chest radiograph and possibly pulmonary function testing was appropriate. Some centers would also obtain a baseline electrocardiogram and echocardiogram, although cardiac involvement is very rare. A recent study has shown that children with JDM are at increased risk of bone-fragility fractures, with up to 10% having vertebral compression fractures before initiating therapy.[55] Given this research, and treatment with corticosteroids, consideration of a lateral radiograph of the spine and baseline bone mineral density would be reasonable, particularly in the presence of back pain. Finally, appropriate investigations for alternative diagnoses should be conducted as indicated (such as genetic evaluations, thyroid function tests, or evaluation for infectious agents).

THERAPY

At the time of writing, there have been no clinical trials published concerning the treatment of children with JIIM (a study of rituximab will be published soon). As a result, there are few data on which to base treatment decisions. Virtually all recommendations and descriptions of treatment in JIIM are based on expert opinion. More recently, attempts have been made to formally describe what constitutes typical care in JDM.[56,57] Members of the Children's Arthritis and Rheumatology Research Alliance (CARRA) have used surveys and expert consensus to develop 3 treatment plans. These plans do not describe standard of care or treatment recommendations, but reflect approaches that are typically taken in treating JDM. In the future it is hoped that these treatment plans will be compared, allowing truly evidence-based recommendations to be made.

Corticosteroids remain a mainstay of therapy in JIIM. A CARRA-sponsored survey of treatment of JDM documented that more than 95% of pediatric rheumatologists included corticosteroids as part of initial management of typical, moderate JDM.[43] Similar rates of corticosteroid use have been reported by other investigators.[5] Most investigators recommend starting at 2 mg/kg/d of prednisone equivalent. However, there is some controversy regarding whether initial therapy should be with intravenous therapy. Rouster-Stevens and colleagues[58] have presented data suggesting that many patients with JDM have impaired gastrointestinal absorption of corticosteroid, and benefit from initial intravenous administration. Other investigators have not found this to be necessary in most patients.[59] This issue remains unresolved; however, changing from oral to intravenous corticosteroids in circumstances whereby clinical response is thought to be inadequate is likely reasonable.

The duration of corticosteroid therapy has also been controversial. During the consensus process discussed, the CARRA group found the anticipated corticosteroid courses for patients with moderate JDM ranged from 4 to 24 months.[57] Although this group established consensus at weaning over 12 months, there is no clear evidence on which to base this recommendation. Furthermore, this consensus assumed a typical patient with moderate disease and no complications. Decisions regarding duration of therapy must be made with the clinical state of the patient held foremost in mind. It is also pertinent to recognize that poorer outcomes have been associated with inadequate corticosteroid courses (low initial steroid dose, short duration).[29]

Until relatively recently, initial therapy for children with JIIM consisted only of corticosteroids, with other agents added if complications developed or if response to therapy was considered inadequate. More recently, methotrexate has become commonly used at treatment initiation. Ramanan and colleagues[59] described their experience using methotrexate with corticosteroids as part of initial therapy. Although this was not a randomized or blinded study, they found that patients receiving methotrexate had equivalent outcomes with fewer side effects and a shorter duration of corticosteroid use. This study has had a major impact on practice. The CARRA treatment survey indicated that more than 80% of North American pediatric rheumatologists would use methotrexate as part of initial therapy for moderate JDM.[43] Furthermore, all 3 of the CARRA JDM consensus treatment plans include methotrexate.[56,57]

Given the predictable side effects associated with prolonged courses of corticosteroid, it is reasonable to consider supportive measures. Although there is no specific evidence to support it, most pediatric rheumatologists would prescribe calcium and vitamin D supplementation at the time of corticosteroid initiation.[43,56] Appropriate sun protection (including clothing and sunblock) is also recommended, given the recognized propensity for photosensitive rashes in JIIM. Dietary counseling, to minimize weight gain and assist with control of blood pressure, is also appropriate.

Physiotherapists play an important role in the care of the child with JIIM. Their expertise is valuable in the ongoing assessment of strength and functional ability. In addition, the role of exercise and rehabilitation in the recovery of children with JIIM is becoming increasingly important. Historically, children with JIIM were prohibited from vigorous exercise, because of concerns that exercise would lead to increased muscle inflammation. Recent research suggests that this may not be the case,[60] and several investigators are currently evaluating the benefits of resistive and aerobic exercise programs in the management of JIIM. It is too early to make specific recommendations regarding exercise prescriptions, but they are likely to be important in the future.[61]

Occupational therapists also play an important role in the care of the child with JIIM. Their expertise is necessary to help the child and family negotiate any limitations the illness may impose on his or her activities, which may become particularly apparent in the home and school. Many of these limitations may be short lived, but remain relevant factors in affecting quality of life and overall functioning. Occupational therapists also have specific expertise in the assessment of the swallowing function, which may be compromised in JIIM. This function may be clinically silent, so involvement of occupational therapy is recommended early in the disease course.[62]

A variety of other medications may play an important role in the treatment of children with JIIM, including intravenous gammaglobulin, hydroxychloroquine, cyclosporin, mycophenylate mofetil, and cyclophosphamide. Discussion of these medications is beyond the scope of this review. However, their use should be limited to those specialists with experience on the care of children with JIIM. There are several excellent reviews of therapy in juvenile dermatomyositis.[63,64]

PROGNOSIS AND OUTCOME

Before the introduction of corticosteroids to the treatment of children with JIIM, the prognosis was poor, with up to one-third dying and another one-third experiencing significant permanent physical limitations.[65] Fortunately, advances in diagnosis and care have resulted in striking improvements in this sobering statistic.

Given that the JIIM are rare illnesses, it is difficult to estimate the mortality rate. One study of mortality of several different rheumatic illnesses in the United States for children diagnosed between 1992 and 2001 found that there was a standardized mortality ratio of 2.64 for children with JDM (2.64 times more likely to die that their age-mates).[66] This figure represented 5 deaths among 662 children (0.8%). Two recent large cohort studies reported deaths in 1 of 151 (0.6%)[5] and 15 of 490 (3.1%).[4] The latter study was international, and included patients from Argentina, Brazil, Italy, Mexico, and the United Kingdom. Most reviews of JDM suggest that the death rate is less than 2%.[67] It is likely true that death in JIIM is uncommon, although it remains an important consideration in the care of these children.

Considerable literature documents that the overall functional outcomes of children with JIIM are excellent. A Canadian study of medium-term and long-term outcomes of 65 children with JDM found that at a median of 7.2 years of follow-up, most children had a CHAQ score of 0, indicating near-normal physical function, and had similar educational and vocational outcomes to the healthy population.[27] Ravelli and colleagues[68] have also documented low rates of major functional limitation in a large international cohort of children with JDM followed for a median of 7.7 years, although 40% had CHAQ scores greater than 0.

Despite these good functional outcomes, there do appear to be significant long-term morbidities for children with JIIM. The Canadian study referenced previously found that 40% of children continued to have active rash, 23% had muscle weakness, and 35% remained on medications at 3.2 to 13.9 (median 7.2) years after diagnosis.[27] Ravelli and colleagues[68] reported persistent rash in 37.5% and persistent weakness in 40% to 50% (depending on method of assessment) when assessed 2 to 25.2 (median 7.7) years after diagnosis.

Recently it has been shown that there are adverse effects on bone health and fragility in children with JDM before corticosteroid initiation, with 10% having vertebral compression fractures within 30 days of steroid onset.[55] This situation is compounded by the need for prolonged courses of high-dose corticosteroid. Subsequently, children with JDM have reductions in bone mineral density and increased vertebral compression fracture rates 1 year after starting corticosteroid therapy.[69] It is possible that these factors will result in poor accrual of peak bone mass and subsequent problems with osteoporosis and bone fragility in adulthood, although this remains unproven.

Given these documented long-term health issues, it is not surprising that it has also been shown that children with JIIM have impairments in quality of life. Ravelli and colleagues[68] found that 9% and 13% had Child Health Questionnaire scores more than 1 standard deviation below the normal for healthy controls for the physical and psychosocial summary scores, respectively. Other investigators have also shown reductions in the same domains compared with healthy children.[70] These changes have been associated with increases in disease activity,[70] reductions in physical function,[70] and fatigue.[71] These results emphasize the importance of long-term follow-up and provision of appropriate support for children with JIIM, and highlight the importance of a multidisciplinary team to care for children with JIIM, including social work and/or psychology specialists.

SUMMARY

The JIIM are rare and serious chronic illnesses. Awareness and careful clinical evaluation are necessary to recognize these illnesses and to distinguish them from other muscle problems, such as dystrophies and myopathies, and from other mimicking illnesses. Clinical features, such as proximal muscle weakness, Gottron lesions, and heliotrope rash can provide important diagnostic clues. In patients with atypical presentations, additional investigations, including muscle biopsy, are warranted. Current treatment includes high-dose corticosteroids and methotrexate, which in most patients results in good clinical outcomes, although significant morbidities are not uncommon. Given the rarity and complexity of these illnesses, it is recommended that patients with suspected JIIM are referred for multidisciplinary specialist care to maximize the likelihood of the best outcomes possible.

REFERENCES

1. Feldman BM, Rider LG, Reed AM, et al. Juvenile dermatomyositis and other idiopathic inflammatory myopathies of childhood. Lancet 2008;371:2201–12.
2. Mendez EP, Lipton R, Ramsey-Goldman R, et al. US incidence of juvenile dermatomyositis, 1995-1998: results from the National Institute of arthritis and musculoskeletal and skin diseases registry. Arthritis Rheum 2003;49(3):300–5.
3. Symmons D, Sills J, Davis S. The incidence of juvenile dermatomyositis: results from a nation-wide study. Br J Rheumatol 1995;34:732–6.
4. Guseinova D, Consolaro A, Trail L, et al. Comparison of clinical features and drug therapies among European and Latin American patients with juvenile dermatomyositis. Clin Exp Rheumatol 2011;29(1):117–24.
5. McCann L, Juggins A, Maillard S, et al. The Juvenile Dermatomyositis National Registry and Repository (UK and Ireland)-clinical characteristics of children recruited within the first 5 yr. Rheumatology 2006;45(10):1255–60.
6. Rider LG, Koziol D, Giannini EH, et al. Validation of manual muscle testing and a subset of eight muscles (MMT8) for adult and juvenile idiopathic inflammatory myopathies. Arthritis Care Res (Hoboken) 2010;62(4):465–72.
7. Huber AM, Feldman BM, Rennebohm RM, et al. Validation and clinical significance of the Childhood Myositis Assessment Scale (CMAS) for assessment of muscle function in the juvenile idiopathic inflammatory myopathies. Arthritis Rheum 2004;50(5):1595–603.
8. Lovell DJ, Lindsley CB, Rennebohm RM, et al. Development of disease activity and damage indices for the juvenile idiopathic inflammatory myopathies. II. The Childhood Myositis Assessment Scale (CMAS): a quantitative tool for the evaluation of muscle function. Arthritis Rheum 1999;42(10):2213–9.
9. Rennebohm RM, Jones K, Huber AM, et al. Normal scores for nine maneuvers of the Childhood Myositis Assessment Scale (CMAS). Arthritis Rheum 2004;51(3):365–70.
10. Huber AM, Hicks JE, Lachenbruch PA, et al. Validation of the childhood health assessment questionnaire in the juvenile idiopathic inflammatory myopathies. J Rheumatol 2001;28(5):1106–11.
11. Singh G, Athreya BH, Fries JF, et al. Measurement of health status in children with juvenile rheumatoid arthritis. Arthritis Rheum 1994;37(12):1761–9.
12. Dugan EM, Huber AM, Miller FW, et al. Review of the classification and assessment of the cutaneous manifestations of the idiopathic inflammatory myopathies [review]. Dermatol Online J 2009;15(2):2.
13. Dugan EM, Huber AM, Miller FW, et al. Photoessay of the cutaneous manifestations of the idiopathic inflammatory myopathies [review]. Dermatol Online J 2009;15(2):1.
14. Dolezalova P, Young SP, Bacon PA, et al. Nailfold capillary microscopy in healthy children and in childhood rheumatic diseases: a prospective single blind observational study. Ann Rheum Dis 2003;62(5):444–9.

15. Christen-Zaech S, Seshadri R, Sundberg J, et al. Persistent association of nailfold capillaroscopy changes and skin involvement over thirty-six months with duration of untreated disease in patients with juvenile dermatomyositis. Arthritis Rheum 2008;58(2):571–6.

16. Nascif A, Terreri M, Len C, et al. Inflammatory myopathies in childhood: correlation between nailfold capillaroscopy findings and clinical and laboratory data. J Pediatr (Rio J) 2006;82(1):40–5.

17. Smith R, Sundberg J, Shamiyah E, et al. Skin involvement in juvenile dermatomyositis is associated with loss of end row nailfold capillary loops. J Rheumatol 2004;31(8):1644–9.

18. Ostrowski RA, Sullivan CL, Seshadri R, et al. Association of normal nailfold end row loop numbers with a shorter duration of untreated disease in children with juvenile dermatomyositis. Arthritis Rheum 2010;62(5):1533–8.

19. Bode RK, Klein-Gitelman MS, Miller ML, et al. Disease activity score for children with juvenile dermatomyositis: reliability and validity evidence. Arthritis Care Res 2003;49(1):7–15.

20. Huber AM, Dugan EM, Lachenbruch PA, et al. The Cutaneous Assessment Tool (CAT): development and reliability in juvenile idiopathic inflammatory myopathy. Rheumatology 2007;46(10):1606–11.

21. Huber AM, Dugan EM, Lachenbruch PA, et al. Preliminary validation and clinical meaning of the Cutaneous Assessment Tool (CAT) in juvenile dermatomyositis. Arthritis Rheum 2008;59(2):214–21.

22. Huber AM, Lachenbruch PA, Dugan EM, et al. Alternative scoring of the Cutaneous Assessment Tool (CAT) in juvenile dermatomyositis: results using an abbreviated format. Arthritis Rheum 2008;59(3):352–6.

23. Yassaee M, Fiorentino D, Okawa J, et al. Modification of the cutaneous dermatomyositis disease area and severity index, an outcome instrument. Br J Dermatol 2010;162(3):669–73.

24. Carroll CL, Lang W, Snively B, et al. Development and validation of the dermatomyositis skin severity index. Br J Dermatol 2008;158(2):345–50.

25. Klein R, Bangert C, Costner M, et al. Comparison of the reliability and validity of outcome instruments for cutaneous dermatomyositis. Br J Dermatol 2008;159(4):887–94.

26. Pachman LM, Boskey AL. Clinical manifestations and pathogenesis of hydroxyapatite crystal deposition in juvenile dermatomyositis [review]. Curr Rheumatol Rep 2006;8(3):236–43.

27. Huber AM, Lang B, LeBlanc CM, et al. Medium- and long-term functional outcomes in a multicenter cohort of children with juvenile dermatomyositis. Arthritis Rheum 2000;43(3):541–9.

28. Rider LG. Calcinosis in juvenile dermatomyositis: pathogenesis and current therapies. Pediatr Rheumatol Online J 2003;1(2):119–33.

29. Bowyer SL, Blane CE, Sullivan DB, et al. Childhood dermatomyositis: factors predicting functional outcome and development of dystrophic calcification. J Pediatr 1983;103:882–8.

30. Pachman LM, Abbott K, Sinacore JM, et al. Duration of illness is an important variable for untreated children with juvenile dermatomyositis. J Pediatr 2006;148(2):247–53.

31. Pachman LM, Veis A, Stock S, et al. Composition of calcifications in children with juvenile dermatomyositis: association with chronic cutaneous inflammation. Arthritis Rheum 2006;54(10):3345–50.

32. Bingham A, Mamyrova G, Rother K, et al. Predictors of acquired lipodystrophy in juvenile-onset dermatomyositis and a gradient of severity. Medicine 2008;87(2): 70–86.

33. Huemer C, Kitson H, Malleson P, et al. Lipodystrophy in patients with juvenile dermatomyositis—evaluation of clinical and metabolic abnormalities. J Rheumatol 2001;28:610–5.

34. Pope E, Janson A, Khambalia A, et al. Childhood acquired lipodystrophy: a retrospective study. J Am Acad Dermatol 2006;55(6):947–50.

35. Mamyrova G, Kleiner DE, James-Newton L, et al. Late-onset gastrointestinal pain in juvenile dermatomyositis as a manifestation of ischemic ulceration from chronic endarteropathy. Arthritis Rheum 2007;57(5):881–4.

36. Vega P, Ibarra M, Prestridge A, et al. Autoantibody to PL-12 (anti-alanyl-tRNA synthetase) in an African American girl with juvenile dermatomyositis and resolution of interstitial lung disease. J Rheumatol 2011;38(2):394–5.

37. Sato S, Hirakata M, Kuwana M, et al. Autoantibodies to a 140-kd polypeptide, CADM-140, in Japanese patients with clinically amyopathic dermatomyositis. Arthritis Rheum 2005;52(5):1571–6.

38. Trapani S, Camiciottoli G, Vierucci A, et al. Pulmonary involvement in juvenile dermatomyositis: a two-year longitudinal study. Rheumatology 2001;40(2):216–20.

39. Sanner H, Aalokken TM, Gran JT, et al. Pulmonary outcome in juvenile dermatomyositis: a case-control study. Ann Rheum Dis 2011;70(1):86–91.

40. Cassidy JT, Petty RE, Laxer RM, et al. Textbook of pediatric rheumatology. 6th edition. Philadelphia: Saunders Elsevier; 2011. p. 394–5.

41. Morris P, Dare J. Juvenile dermatomyositis as a paraneoplastic phenomenon: an update. J Pediatr Hematol Oncol 2010;32(3):189–91.

42. Bohan A, Peter JB. Polymyositis and dermatomyositis (first of two parts). N Engl J Med 1975;292(7):344–7.

43. Stringer E, Ota S, Bohnsack J, et al. Treatment approaches to juvenile dermatomyositis across North America: the Childhood Arthritis and Rheumatology Research Alliance (CARRA) JDM treatment survey. J Rheumatol 2009;37(9): 1953–61.

44. Wedderburn L, Varsani H, Li C, et al. International consensus on a proposed score system for muscle biopsy evaluation in patients with juvenile dermatomyositis: a tool for potential use in clinical trials. Arthritis Rheum 2007;57(7):1192–201.

45. Brown V, Pilkington C, Feldman BM, et al, on behalf of the network for juvenile dermatomyositis (PReS). An international consensus survey on the diagnostic criteria for juvenile dermatomyositis. Rheumatology 2006;45:990–3.

46. Kimball AB, Summers RM, Turner M, et al. Magnetic resonance imaging detection of occult skin and subcutaneous abnormalities in juvenile dermatomyositis. Implications for diagnosis and therapy. Arthritis Rheum 2000;43(8):1866–73.

47. Maillard SM, Jones R, Owens C, et al. Quantitative assessment of MRI T2 relaxation time of thigh muscles in juvenile dermatomyositis. Rheumatology (Oxford) 2004;43(5):603–8.

48. Gardner-Medwin JM, Irwin G, Johnson K. MRI in juvenile idiopathic arthritis and juvenile dermatomyositis [review]. Ann N Y Acad Sci 2009;1154:52–83.

49. Eisenstein D, O'Gorman M, Pachman LM. Correlations between change in disease activity and changes in peripheral blood lymphocyte subsets in patients with juvenile dermatomyositis. J Rheumatol 1997;24(9):1830–2.

50. O'Gorman M, Bianchi L, Zaas D, et al. Decreased levels of CD54 (ICAM-1)-positive lymphocytes in the peripheral blood in untreated patients with active juvenile dermatomyositis. Clin Diagn Lab Immunol 2000;7(4):693–7.

51. De Benedetti F, De Amici M, Aramini L, et al. Correlation of serum neopterin concentrations with disease activity in juvenile dermatomyositis. Arch Dis Child 1993;69(2):232–5.

52. Rider LG, Schiffenbauer A, Zito M, et al. Neopterin and quinolinic acid are surrogate measures of disease activity in the juvenile idiopathic inflammatory myopathies. Clin Chem 2002;48(10):1681–8.

53. Bloom BJ, Tucker LB, Miller LC, et al. von Willebrand factor in juvenile dermatomyositis. J Rheumatol 1995;22(2):320–5.

54. Guzman J, Petty RE, Malleson PN. Monitoring disease activity in juvenile dermatomyositis: the role of von Willebrand factor and muscle enzymes. J Rheumatol 1994;21(4):739–43.

55. Huber AM, Gaboury I, Cabral DA, et al. Prevalent vertebral fractures among children initiating glucocorticoid therapy for the treatment of rheumatic disorders. Arthritis Care Res 2010;62(4):516–26.

56. Huber AM, Giannini EH, Bowyer SL, et al. Protocols for the initial treatment of moderately severe juvenile dermatomyositis: results of a Children's Arthritis and Rheumatology Research Alliance Consensus Conference. Arthritis Care Res (Hoboken) 2010;62(2):219–25.

57. Huber AM, Robinson AB, Reed AM, et al. Consensus treatments for moderate juvenile dermatomyositis: Beyond the first two months. Arthritis Care Res (Hoboken) 2011. DOI: 10.1002/acr.20695. [Epub ahead of print].

58. Rouster-Stevens KA, Gursahaney A, Ngai KL, et al. Pharmacokinetic study of oral prednisolone compared with intravenous methylprednisolone in patients with juvenile dermatomyositis. Arthritis Rheum 2008;59(2):222–6.

59. Ramanan A, Campbell-Webster N, Ota S, et al. The effectiveness of treating juvenile dermatomyositis with methotrexate and aggressively tapered corticosteroids. Arthritis Rheum 2005;52(11):3570–8.

60. Maillard SM, Jones R, Owens CM, et al. Quantitative assessments of the effects of a single exercise session on muscles in juvenile dermatomyositis. Arthritis Rheum 2005;53(4):558–64.

61. Gualano B, Pinto AL, Perondi MB, et al. Therapeutic effects of exercise training in patients with pediatric rheumatic diseases. Rev Bras Reumatol 2011;51(5):490–6.

62. McCann L, Garay S, Ryan M, et al. Oropharyngeal dysphagia in juvenile dermatomyositis (JDM): an evaluation of videofluoroscopy swallow study (VFSS) changes in relation to clinical symptoms and objective muscle scores. Rheumatology 2007;46:1363–6.

63. Huber AM. Juvenile dermatomyositis: advances in pathogenesis, evaluation, and treatment [review]. Paediatr Drugs 2009;11(6):361–74.

64. Wedderburn LR, Rider LG. Juvenile dermatomyositis: new developments in pathogenesis, assessment and treatment [review]. Best Pract Res Clin Rheumatol 2009;23(5):665–78.

65. Bitnum S, Daeschner C Jr, Travis LB, et al. Dermatomyositis. J Pediatr 1964;64(1):101–31.

66. Hashkes PJ, Wright BM, Lauer MS, et al. Mortality outcomes in pediatric rheumatology in the US. Arthritis Rheum 2010;62(2):599–608.

67. Huber A, Feldman BM. Long-term outcomes in juvenile dermatomyositis: how did we get here and where are we going? [review]. Curr Rheumatol Rep 2005;7(6):441–6.

68. Ravelli A, Trail L, Ferrari C, et al. Long-term outcome and prognostic factors of juvenile dermatomyositis: a multinational, multicenter study of 490 patients. Arthritis Care Res 2010;62(1):63–72.

69. Rodd C, Lang BA, Ramsay T, et al. Incident vertebral fractures among children with rheumatic disorders 12 months post-glucocorticoid initiation: a national observational study. Arthritis Care Res 2012;64(1):122–31. DOI: 10.1002/acr.20589.

70. Apaz M, Saad-Magalhães C, Pistorio A, et al. Health-related quality of life of patients with juvenile dermatomyositis: results from the Pediatric Rheumatology International Trials Organisation multinational quality of life cohort study. Arthritis Rheum 2009;61(4):509–17.

71. Butbul Aviel Y, Stremler R, Benseler SM, et al. Sleep and fatigue and the relationship to pain, disease activity and quality of life in juvenile idiopathic arthritis and juvenile dermatomyositis. Rheumatology 2011;50(11):2051–60.

Pediatric Scleroderma: Systemic or Localized Forms

Kathryn S. Torok, MD

KEYWORDS

- Systemic sclerosis • Localized scleroderma • Morphea
- Pediatric rheumatology

PEDIATRIC SCLERODERMA

The term scleroderma literally means "skleros," sclerosing or hardening, of the "derma," skin. "Scleroderma" encompasses both forms of the disease: systemic sclerosis (SSc), characterized by skin, vascular, and visceral organ fibrosis, which more commonly affects adults, and localized scleroderma (LS), characterized by fibrosis of skin and underlying tissue without vascular or internal organ involvement, which more commonly affects children. Although they share a common underlying pathophysiology of excessive collagen deposition in an autoimmune setting, these two entities are clinically different, with unique morbidities and prognoses (**Fig. 1**). Both are uncommon in children, with the estimated annual incidence of LS being 1 to 3 per 100,000 children[1] and that of SSc being 1 per million children.[2] The mean age of onset for both forms of pediatric scleroderma is between 7.3 and 8.8 years of age. Although fewer than 5% of all patients with SSc have pediatric onset, most patients with LS have childhood onset.[3–6] Unfortunately there is a significant delay in diagnosis, with an average 1.9 to 2.8 years for SSc[3,4] and 1.2 to 1.6 years for LS.[5,7] For the few cases of congenital involvement of LS, the mean time to diagnosis is longer, 3.3 to 3.9 years.[7,8] The approximate female to male ratio of pediatric SSc is 4:1[3,4] and for pediatric LS 2:1.[5] There is no clear evidence for racial predilection for either form of pediatric scleroderma.

Source of support: National Institutes of Health/NIAMS K23 AR059722 and the Nancy Taylor Foundation for Chronic Diseases research grants.
The author has nothing to disclose.
Division of Rheumatology, Children's Hospital of Pittsburgh of the University of Pittsburgh Medical Center, 4401 Penn Avenue, Pittsburgh, PA 15224, USA
E-mail address: Kathryn.Torok@chp.edu

Pediatr Clin N Am 59 (2012) 381–405
doi:10.1016/j.pcl.2012.03.011
0031-3955/12/$ – see front matter © 2012 Elsevier Inc. All rights reserved.

Pediatric Scleroderma

Systemic sclerosis (SSc)
Multi-system disease

- **Diffuse cutaneous (dcSSc)**
  Cardiac, renal, pulmonary (ILD)
- **Limited cutaneous (lcSSc)**
  Gastrointestinal, pulmonary (PAH)
- **Overlap SSc**
  Cardiac, renal, pulmonary, myositis, arthritis

Localized Scleroderma (LS)
Cutaneous disease

- **Linear scleroderma**
  - Limbs/trunk
    Limitation joint ROM
  - Head
    Neurologic
- **Circumscribed morphea**
  - Superficial
  - Deep
- **Generalized morphea**
- **Mixed**
- **Pansclerotic morphea**
  Severe limitation joint ROM

Fig. 1. Pediatric scleroderma divided into systemic and localized disease, which is further differentiated into subtypes based on clinical findings of skin involvement. Clinical subsets are related, with particular morbidities as mentioned. ILD, interstitial lung disease; PAH, pulmonary arterial hypertension; ROM, range of motion.

SYSTEMIC SCLEROSIS
Categorization: Clinical and Serologic

SSc is a rare but potentially life-threatening condition. There are 3 main clinical subtypes associated with different morbidities (see **Fig. 1**): diffuse cutaneous (dc) SSc, characterized by widespread and rapidly progressive skin thickening (spreading proximal to elbows and knees) associated with early visceral disease (lung, heart, and kidney), limited cutaneous SSc (lcSSc), characterized by restricted and nonprogressive skin thickening (limited to distal extremities) associated with late visceral disease (pulmonary arterial hypertension, malabsorption), and overlap SSc, which can be dcSSc or lcSSc with features of another connective tissue disease, such as dermatomyositis or systemic lupus erythematosus (SLE).[9] Patients with CREST syndrome (calcinosis, Raynaud phenomenon (RP), esophageal dysmotility, sclerodactyly, and telangiectasia) are considered to have lcSSc. Some patients with undifferentiated or mixed connective tissue disease may have shiny or full-appearing skin of the distal fingers, but they must have the major criterion, namely skin induration or sclerosis proximal to the metacarpal phalangeal (MCP) or metatarsophalangeal (MTP) joints, to be considered to have juvenile SSc (**Fig. 2**). There are an additional 2 minor criteria required for the diagnosis of SSc in children according to international consensus agreement (**Box 1**).[10] In addition to the extent of skin thickening, particular scleroderma-related serum autoantibody profiles assist in identifying subsets of SSc and predicting their organ involvement in both adult-onset and childhood-onset SSc.[3,4,6,11,12] For example, antitopoisomerase antibody (Scl-70) would be expected in a patient with dcSSc, and would be worrisome for a rapid skin progression and the development of interstitial lung disease (ILD).[3,4,6] The 4 most common antibodies in pediatric SSc are antitopoisomerase antibody (Scl-70) (20%–34%), typically associated with dcSSc and ILD as mentioned, followed by anticentromere antibody (ACA) (2%–16%), associated with lcSSc and pulmonary arterial hypertension (PAH), and

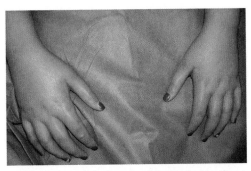

Fig. 2. Typical shiny and thick skin of the hands with skin induration traveling up the forearm (past the metacarpal phalangeal joints) in a patient with systemic sclerosis.

antiU1-RNP and Pm-Scl (polymyositis-scleroderma) antibodies (2%–16%), both of which are commonly found in those with overlap syndromes of SSc and other connective tissue diseases with more prominent arthritis and myositis features, such as dermatomyositis or SLE.[3,4,6] The U1-RNP and Pm-Scl positive proportion of patients is likely higher than reported because some investigators do not include cases of overlap SSc or mixed connective tissue disease in their pediatric SSc cohorts. Overall, the frequency of these antibodies in children reflects the clinical subset frequencies of dcSSc, lcSSc, and overlap SSc[3,4,6] Compared with adult SSc, overlap SSc is much more common in pediatric SSc (29% vs 9%), as reflected by the increased frequency of U1-RNP and Pm-Scl antibodies, and is related to the higher percentage of myositis and arthritis observed in pediatric SSc.[3] There are several other SSc-related autoantibodies that associate with different organ manifestations; however, they are much less common in childhood-onset SSc. One of these is RNA polymerase III (POL3) antibody, which relates to severe renal disease in the form of scleroderma renal crisis. POL3 is rarely observed in childhood-onset SSc, but can be found in up to 30% of adult-onset SSc patients and reflects the clinically significant higher proportion of renal disease in adult SSc.[3,6] Although many scleroderma-related autoantibodies have been identified in adult SSc, there is a high proportion of pediatric patients (20%–23%) who have a positive antinuclear antibody (ANA) test without a specific autoantibody identified.[3,6]

Clinical Manifestations

Common features at the onset of pediatric SSc are raynaud phenomenon (RP) (70%) and skin changes of hands (60%) including edema, sclerodactyly, and induration proximal to the MCPs.[4] In the largest cohort of pediatric SSc (153 patients) studied, 53% presented with both skin induration of hands and RP, and 10% of those presenting with RP also had digital infarcts (**Fig. 3**).[4] Throughout the course of the disease, almost all will have RP (97%) and skin changes of the hands (96%).[3]

RP is a vasospastic response leading to a triphasic color change of the hands (first pallor because of vasoconstriction, then blue secondary to cyanosis, and finally red because of reperfusion with subsequent swelling and pain) associated with a sensation of numbness and tingling. RP can also occur in toes and other acral areas including the ears, tip of the nose, or tongue. In SSc, arterioles are more narrow and stiff because of marked intimal hyperplasia and fibrosis from endothelial dysfunction, which leads to more pronounced RP with resultant tissue damage/ischemia.[13] These vasculopathic changes are identifiable in the nailfold capillary beds of these patients by capillary microscopy, demonstrating dilatation, tortuosity, hemorrhage, drop-off

Box 1
Provisional guidelines for the classification criteria of juvenile systemic sclerosis

Major Criterion (Required)

Skin induration/thickening proximal to the MCP or MTP joints

Minor Criteria (2 Required) (Scleroderma-Specific Organ Involvement)

Cutaneous

   Sclerodactyly

Peripheral vascular

   Raynaud phenomenon

   Nailfold capillary changes (megacapillaries and avascular areas)

   Digital-tip ulcers

Gastrointestinal

   Dysphasia

   Gastroesophageal reflux

Cardiac

   Arrhythmias

   Heart failure

Renal

   Scleroderma renal crisis

   New arterial hypertension

Respiratory

   Pulmonary fibrosis (on chest radiograph or high-resolution computed tomography)

   Decreased DLCO

   Pulmonary arterial hypertension (primary or secondary to ILD, assessed by echocardiography)

Neurologic

   Neuropathy

   Carpal tunnel syndrome

Musculoskeletal

   Tendon friction rubs

   Arthritis

   Myositis

Serologic

   Antinuclear antibody

   SSc-selective autoantibodies

      Antitopoisomerase 1 (Scl-70), anticentromere, anti–RNA polymerase I or III, anti–PM-Scl, antifibrillin

Sensitivity of 90% and specificity of 96% when the major and 2 minor criteria are present in clinical scenarios.

Age of onset of the disease must be younger than 16 years.

Abbreviations: DLCO, diffusing capacity for carbon monoxide; ILD, interstitial lung disease; MCP, metacarpal phalangeal; MTP, metatarsophalangeal.
  Data from Zulian F, Woo P, Athreya BH, et al. The Pediatric Rheumatology European Society/American College of Rheumatology/European League against Rheumatism provisional classification criteria for juvenile systemic sclerosis. Arthritis Rheum 2007;57(2):203–12.

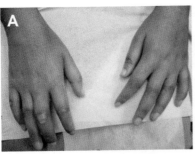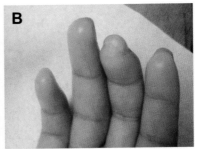

Fig. 3. A teenage girl with typical (*A*) sclerodactyly and (*B*) digital pitting and ulcers.

(avascularization), and later arborization of the capillaries.[14] The prevalence of nailfold capillary changes in pediatric SSc is reported to be 50%,[3,4] but is likely higher if standardized microscopy is performed. Poor perfusion of the fingers eventually leads to digital-tip pitting, ulceration (see **Fig. 3**B), and in more severe cases autoamputation. Healthy individuals can also experience RP without being at risk for developing an underlying connective tissue disease (primary RP). These individuals typically never develop digital-tip ulcers or have nailfold capillary changes because they do not have an underlying vasculopathy. Features that help the clinician differentiate primary RP from that secondary to a connective tissue disease in both children and adults are the following: lack of nailfold capillary changes, digital-tip pitting and/or ulceration, and a negative ANA.[15,16]

Cutaneous manifestations frequently bring children to medical attention, but because of the insidious and subtle onset of skin changes, there is often a delay in diagnosis, with a mean time of 1.9 and 2.8 years between first sign of disease and diagnosis.[3,4] Early in the clinical course, the skin is edematous with particular predilection for the distal extremities; rarely, involvement of the more proximal limb, face, and trunk is present. The induration phase, for which scleroderma is named, is characterized by loss of the natural pliability of the skin and the presence of a palpable skin thickness. The skin takes on a shiny, tense appearance with distal tapering of the fingers (see **Figs. 2** and **3**A). Over time as skin thickens and underlying structures, such as tendons, become affected and shortened, the finger joints start to lose range of motion in both extension and flexion, and in more severe cases a claw-hand deformity results, with great impact on performing activities of daily living. The typical scleroderma facies of tight skin and skin atrophy produces a pinched nose, thin pursed lips, small mouth, prominent teeth, and an expressionless appearance (**Fig. 4**). Skin thickness is measured as mild, moderate, and severe throughout the body, and a cumulative score is obtained using the modified Rodnan skin score (mRSS).[17] The mRSS is obtained over longitudinal visits, and a skin thickness progression rate (STPR) can be calculated and assist in predicting timing of internal organ involvement in those with dcSSc. A high STPR is associated with scleroderma renal crisis.[18]

Other skin findings in SSc include subcutaneous calcium deposits (calcinosis cutis), which may occur at pressure points, typically found on extensor surfaces of hand joints in SSc, and may occasionally extrude through the skin in a fashion similar to der-matomyositis. These lesions may be painful and may ulcerate. However, they are more typically associated with chronic disease and are rarely present at the time of disease onset and diagnosis. Telangiectasias are also a manifestation of SSc, most typically found in the lcSSc variant (previously known as CREST syndrome), and are commonly distributed on the face and upper extremities.

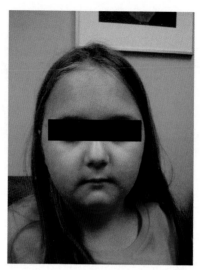

Fig. 4. Expressionless facies of scleroderma in a prepubertal girl with decreased oral aperture and pursed lips.

Other organ manifestations in SSc (in order of decreasing frequency) include gastrointestinal, pulmonary, musculoskeletal, cardiac, renal, and neurologic symptoms. Gastrointestinal symptoms occur in approximately half of the children, although more detailed investigation often indicates the presence of abnormalities in a larger percentage.[3] Esophageal dysmotility and gastroesophageal reflux often leads to dysphagia and esophagitis. Distal dysphagia, especially with solids, causing a sensation of food getting stuck mid-chest, is typical and represents dysfunction of the distal smooth muscle of the esophagus. Gastroparesis with delayed gastric emptying in addition to esophageal dysfunction can lead to increased reflux symptoms. Typically patients will complain of nighttime cough when lying prone, owing to silent aspiration, and a brackish taste in their mouth on wakening, due to silent reflux. Chronic reflux may lead to esophageal strictures. Evaluation of the gastrointestinal (GI) tract using manometry and intraesophageal 24-hour pH monitoring have been reported as sensitive indicators of lowered esophageal tone and reflux.[19] However, these modalities are used less often in pediatrics. Instead, a swallow study to evaluate for aspiration and dysmotility, followed by an upper GI study with small bowel follow-through, is typically used. If the small bowel is involved, cramps, diarrhea, and constipation may result from peristaltic dysfunction. Episodes of pseudo-obstruction with postprandial abdominal distension, pain, and nausea can occur because of a functional ileus. Bacterial overgrowth, steatorrhea, weight loss, volvulus, and even perforation can occur. Colonic disease occurs in the form of wide-mouth diverticula and a loss of the normal colonic architecture. Another complication of GI involvement with SSc is acute GI bleeding associated with gastric antral venular ectasia (GAVE) requiring photocoagulation. This condition is uncommon in children and is associated with early dcSSc, RNA polymerase III–positive patients.[20]

Pulmonary involvement in pediatric SSc ranges from 30% to 70% in the literature, and includes ILD, PAH (either primary, which results from vasculopathy, or secondary from ILD), and abnormal pulmonary function tests (PFTs). PFT abnormalities of special of concern are decreased forced vital capacity (FVC) and diffusing capacity for carbon monoxide (DLCO).[21] ILD typically begins with an inflammatory phase, alveolitis, characterized by a mixed cellular infiltrate in the lung interstitium that spills over into the alveolar spaces. Bronchoalveolar lavage (BAL) demonstrates increased neutrophils and/or eosinophils in addition to alveolar macrophages.[22] The presence of alveolitis is also suggested by ground-glass opacities on high-resolution computed tomography (HRCT) scans of the lungs. As ILD progresses, inflammation subsides, as there is a transition toward fibrosis with the thickening of alveolar walls and remodeling of the lung. Progressive pulmonary fibrosis may result in moderate to severe restrictive lung disease with significant decrease in FVC and DLCO. Clinically, ILD typically presents as slowly progressive dyspnea with exertion over years. In comparison, PAH presents with rapid progression of dyspnea on exertion over months. In the setting of PAH, PFTs demonstrate a decreased DLCO and abnormal echocardiogram findings with estimated pulmonary artery (PA) or right ventricular (RV) systolic pressure of greater than 40 mm Hg, verified by right-heart catheterization with mean PA pressure greater than 25 mm Hg. For most children with SSc or suspected SSc, initial assessment includes chest radiograph, PFTs, including DLCO, and an echocardiogram. Additional cardiopulmonary testing is pursued if abnormalities are detected or the patient is too young to appropriately complete testing (ie, PFTs). Abnormal PFTs prompt evaluation with HRCT of chest, and possibly BAL, if further evidence of inflammation (alveolitis) is required or evaluation of infection is needed before starting therapy.[21,23] Evidence of PAH on echocardiogram is more formally assessed by right-heart catheterization.

Compared with adult-onset SSc, musculoskeletal involvement is more common in pediatric SSc. Approximately 30% to 40% of those with pediatric SSc experience inflammatory arthritis (joint effusions) in addition to the typical dry synovitis of scleroderma, reflected by the fibrosis of tendons transversing the joints, which limits their range of motion. Early in the disease process, especially in those with dcSSc, tenosynovitis/bursitis causes palpable tendon friction rubs (a leathery crepitus) when the joint is extended or flexed.[24] When the patient has myopathy, typically there is a symmetric proximal weakness, especially of the shoulder girdle and humeral muscles, sometimes with pronounced atrophy. Myositis is also reflected by elevated muscle enzymes and changes on magnetic resonance imaging (MRI) of muscle groups similar to those of juvenile dermatomyositis (JDM). The muscle biopsy of SSc differs from that of JDM by having more fibrosis and the presence of thickened capillaries.[25] Children with dcSSc and myositis are particularly at risk for severe cardiac involvement, including myocardial perfusion deficits and dilated cardiomyopathy.[26]

Cardiac involvement, although infrequent, is the major cause of scleroderma-related mortality in children with SSc, and is evidenced by 10 of 15 deaths in Martini and colleagues'[4] cohort and 5 of 32 deaths in Scalapino and colleagues'[3] cohort. Cardiac manifestations result from the combination of myocardial fibrosis, vascular insufficiency, and inflammation, and include heart block, arrhythmia, congestive heart failure, cardiomyopathy, and pericarditis. In contrast to pediatric SSc, scleroderma-related mortality in adults is primarily caused by pulmonary involvement, both ILD and PAH.[27]

Mild renal dysfunction is not uncommon in SSc and is secondary to vasculopathy instead of glomerulonephritis, which is observed in SLE. This consideration is supported by pathologic findings of intimal proliferation of the interlobular arteries of the kidney and lack of active urinary sediment (ie, red blood cell casts). By contrast, a more severe and morbid form of renal disease, scleroderma renal crisis (SRC), occurs only in approximately 15% of adult patients with SSc and is even less common in children. SRC is characterized by accelerated arterial hypertension, renal insufficiency, microangiopathic hemolytic anemia, and thrombocytopenia. In adult SSc, SRC previously had a 20% survival rate at 1 year, but now has an 80% survival rate owing to the advent of angiotensin-converting enzyme inhibitors.[27] SRC is most frequently seen early in the disease course of dcSSc RNA-polymerase III–positive patients and is thought to be augmented by higher doses of corticosteroids. Renal crisis is rare in children with SSc, with fewer than 5% affected and only 5 cases reported (2 of whom died of renal disease) among the 3 large published cohorts.[3,4,28]

Outcome

Despite the potential organ involvement in pediatric SSc, it has a far more favorable prognosis at 5, 10, and 15 years compared with adult SSc, with a lower frequency of severe organ involvement. Foeldvari and colleagues[28] recently reported Kaplan-Meier survival rates at 10 years for children to be 98% versus 75% in adults. Treatment of SSc is dependent on organ involvement, but general measures such as antacid medication for GI protection, prokinetic agents for dysmotility, rotating antibiotics for malabsorption, as well as vasodilators for RP (may also help with PAH), and nonsteroidal anti-inflammatory drugs and physical therapy for arthritis or tendonitis are generally recommended. Corticosteroids for myositis, arthritis, and other inflammatory clinical features must be used with caution, as they can prompt SRC. More specific treatment recommendations for different organ manifestations have been agreed on by a consensus conference of international scleroderma experts, and were published in 2009.[29] It is notable that in the treatment of both pediatric and adult SSc early diffuse skin disease, there has been a shift from the use of D-penicillamine to mycophenolate mofetil (MMF) likely because of its potential antiproliferative effects, although it is not included in the treatment recommendations previously discussed.[30]

LOCALIZED SCLERODERMA
Classification

Localized Scleroderma (LS), also known as morphea, has a pattern of skin involvement different to that of SSc and encompasses several subtypes classified by depth and pattern of the lesion(s). The group of disorders is characterized by fibrosis that is mainly confined to the skin and subcutaneous tissue; however, deeper forms also involve the fascia, muscle, tendon, and joint capsule. The traditional classification delineated by Peterson and colleagues[31] described 5 subclassifications including plaque morphea, generalized morphea, bullous morphea, linear morphea, and deep and pansclerotic morphea (**Box 2**). However, more recently a consensus of experts made modifications to provide more clinically applicable classifications, titled the Padua criteria, which include a mixed morphea subtype, given the prevalence of this category to be 15% (**Box 3**).[32]

Disease Activity and Damage Features (Clinical and Histologic Findings)

Similar to SSc both clinically and histologically, LS exhibits an earlier more active phase of disease and a later more fibrotic phase (**Fig. 5**). Early active lesions in LS are characterized by a violaceous inflammatory border or lilac ring (**Fig. 6**) and skin induration throughout the lesion, including the border. During this active state, lesions may also expand and new lesions can accumulate.[33] Histologic findings in the early stages of disease consist of a perivascular infiltrate of predominantly lymphocytes with admixed rare plasma cells and eosinophils in the deep reticular dermis and subcutis, accompanied by thickened collagen bundles, decreased elastic fibers, and swollen endothelial cells.[34,35] Over time, disease damage accumulates and is

---

Box 2
LS subtypes: Mayo classification

Plaque morphea[a]

    Morphea en plaque[a]

    Guttate morphea

    Atrophoderma of Pasini and Pierini

Generalized morphea[a]

Bullous morphea

Linear morphea[a]

    Linear morphea (linear scleroderma)[a]

    En coup de sabre[a]

    Progressive hemifacial atrophy

Deep morphea[a]

    Subcutaneous morphea[a]

    Eosinophilic fasciitis

    Morphea profunda[a]

    Disabling pansclerotic morphea of children

[a] Most prevalent subtypes in pediatric and adult LS.
Data from Peterson LS, Nelson AM, Su WP. Classification of morphea (localized scleroderma). Mayo Clin Proc 1995;70(11):1068–76.

Box 3
Proposed subtypes for Juvenile LS: Padua preliminary classification

Circumscribed Morphea

Oval/round lesions

a. Superficial lesions (Plaque morphea): limited to epidermis and dermis

b. Deep lesions (Deep morphea): involve subcutaneous tissue

Linear Scleroderma

Linear lesions can involve dermis, subcutaneous tissue, muscle, bone

a. Trunk/limbs

b. Head: En coup de sabre or Parry-Romberg syndrome

Generalized Morphea

≥4 large plaques (>3 cm) on at least 2 of 7 anatomic areas: head/neck, right upper extremity, left upper extremity, right lower extremity, left lower extremity, anterior trunk, posterior trunk

Pansclerotic Morphea

Circumferential involvement of limb (spares fingertips/toes)

All depths of skin/subcutaneous tissue/muscle/bone

Mixed Morphea

Combination of 2 or more of above subtypes

Data from Laxer RM, Zulian F. Localized scleroderma. Curr Opin Rheumatol 2006;18(6):606–13.

Natural History of LS – Cutaneous manifestations

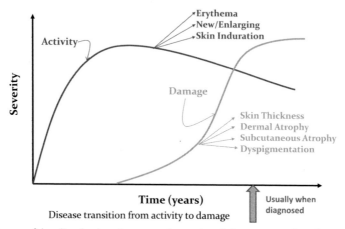

Fig. 5. Phases of localized scleroderma and associated features. Active disease features, erythema, skin induration/edema, and new or enlarging lesions occur first and give way to disease damage features, dyspigmentation, atrophy, and skin thickening.

represented by an increase in skin thickness, especially at the center of the lesion, sometimes leaving an ivory-colored sclerotic center (**Fig. 7**). Histologic evaluation of the skin reveals thickened hypocellular (homogenized) collagen that replaces the previous inflammatory infiltrate around the dermal appendages, leaving behind atrophic eccrine glands and hair follicles. In addition, capillaries are decreased in number with a fibrotic wall and narrowed lumen.[34,35] The clinical outcome of these findings is reflected in dermal and subcutaneous atrophy. On physical examination, when the dermis is atrophic there is lack of hair growth at the site of the lesion, visible veins,

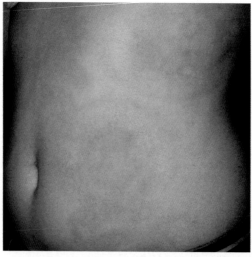

Fig. 6. Typical lilac ring observed at the border of multiple plaque lesions of the trunk, indicating active disease. (*Courtesy of* Elena Pope, Hospital for Sick Children, Toronto, ON, Canada.)

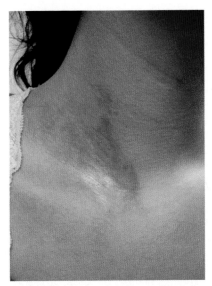

Fig. 7. Waxy yellow center of plaque lesion remaining on right side of the neck years after the onset of localized scleroderma.

and slight cliff-drop appearance to the skin (**Fig. 8**). Subcutaneous atrophy exists on a continuum and can be observed as mild as a flattening of the skin, to a more scooped-out concave appearance of the adipose tissue in more moderate lesions, and in the most severe instances, to the point one can see the muscles moving underneath the skin. Postinflammatory hyperpigmentation and hypopigmentation also are a result of previous inflammation and are often the features that bring the lesion to the attention of a medical provider. Often families will miss the early active phase

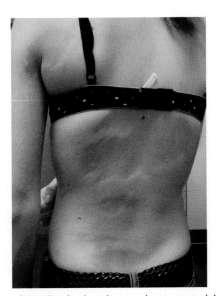

Fig. 8. Dermal atrophy of localized scleroderma, demonstrated by cliff-drop lesions in a teenage girl with generalized morphea.

and consider the erythema/violaceous color more of a bruise or injury, but in fact it is the "bruise that does not go away" (postinflammatory hyperpigmentation) that often prompts the family to seek medical attention (see **Fig. 5**).

Pathogenesis (Shared Between LS and SSc)

The shared histologic findings between the skin of those with SSc and LS exemplify their common pathophysiology despite different clinical disease features. Both are autoimmune diseases with an inflammatory, fibrotic, and vascular component. Mononuclear cell populations identified in both SSc and LS skin specimens are predominately T cells, both CD8- and CD4-positive, with a higher percentage of CD4 cells (T-helper).[36,37] T-helper cell–associated cytokines and chemokines such as interleukin (IL)-2, IL-4, IL-6, IL-8, IL-13, and tumor necrosis factor α (TNF-α), have been identified in the circulating sera and stimulated peripheral blood mononuclear cells from LS and SSc patients.[38–43] Of note, some serum cytokines have been found in higher concentrations in LS subjects than in SSc subjects, which is interesting because LS is termed a localized disease; however, this may support the high frequency of extracutaneous manifestations (approximately 25%) demonstrated in LS.[44] There have been several correlations between clinical variables of disease severity in LS and cytokines and their soluble receptors, such as number of plaque and linear lesions (IL-13, TNF-α, sIL-2r, sIL-6r), generalized morphea and linear scleroderma subsets (IL-2, -4, -6, -8, -13, TNF-α, sIL-2r, sIL-6r), and antibody correlation, antihistone, and/or anti-single-stranded DNA antibodies (IL-4, -6, TNF-α, sIL-2r, sIL-6r).[38–40,45–47] These T-cell–associated cytokines, in turn, further stimulate fibroblasts and endothelial cells to produce transforming growth factor β and connective tissue growth factor, which are thought to be the main stimulators of tissue fibrosis (via increased collagen production) and endothelial cell damage (via influence of intercellular adhesion molecule 1 and vascular cell adhesion molecule 1).[48–51]

Microchimerism is another area of interest being investigated regarding a shared pathogenesis between LS and SSc. Clinically and histologically, LS and SSc share characteristics with chronic graft-versus-host disease (**Fig. 9**), a type of microchimerism that plays a role in pathogenesis. Chimeric cells have been identified in patients with LS and SSc using real-time polymerase chain reaction techniques.[52,53]

Autoimmunity, as one of the components propagating LS, is supported by the autoantibody profile, concurrent associated autoimmune diseases, and family history of

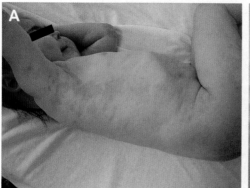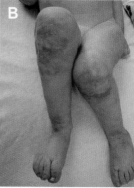

Fig. 9. Linear lesion down trunk (*A*) and legs (*B*) of a toddler with sclerodermatous chronic graft-versus-host disease.

autoimmune disease observed in patients with LS. Autoantibodies are commonly positive in LS, including ANA, antihistone antibody (AHA), and anti–single-stranded DNA antibody (ss-DNA Ab).[54] ANA is a classic serologic marker of autoimmune disease and is found in a high frequency of LS patients, with a reported range between 42% and 73%.[5,55] It is thought that higher titers are associated with early disease[55] and increased risk for extracutaneous manifestations.[44,56] The prevalence of ss-DNA in LS is approximately 50%[57] and is associated with linear scleroderma (especially those with joint contractures), deep muscle involvement, and increased number of anatomic sites, all reflecting an increase in disease severity.[56,58] In a subgroup of LS patients, ss-DNA Ab has been shown to reflect disease-activity status, with titers decreasing as the skin lesions improve clinically.[54,56] AHA is found in a similar frequency in LS (47%)[59] and is also correlated with indicators of disease severity; including total surface area of body involved, number of lesions, linear disease, and the presence of joint contractures.[54,56] In a study focusing on linear scleroderma, the combination of positive ss-DNA and AHA was found in 23% of patients (adult and pediatric LS) and was significantly correlated with the presence of joint contractures.[56] The aforementioned antibodies indicate disease severity and may help in stratifying patients with early diagnosed disease, suggesting the possible initiation of more aggressive therapy and increased surveillance.

Concomitant and familial rheumatic and autoimmune disease is more prevalent in LS (pediatric and adult) than in the general population.[60] Concomitant disease was reported in 5% to 10% of children[7,44,60] and in 30% of adults with LS.[60] The most common disorders present were dermatologic autoimmune disease (psoriasis, vitiligo, alopecia areata), followed by rheumatic conditions (juvenile idiopathic arthritis, rheumatoid arthritis [RA], SLE. and Sjögren syndrome).[7,60] When evaluated by LS subtype, the frequency of concomitant autoimmune disease was significantly higher in patients with generalized morphea.[60] Familial rheumatic diseases and other autoimmune disorders were reported in 12% to 25% of all patients (both pediatric and adult), with the most common being psoriasis, followed by RA, SLE, SSc, LS, multiple sclerosis, and thyroiditis.[5,7,60] Again, an association between generalized morphea and increased frequency of these diseases was demonstrated.[5]

Clinical Manifestations

Although the term LS or morphea encompasses all of the subtypes into a single category, their cutaneous/subcutaneous findings and extra cutaneous associations are quite unique. Linear scleroderma (LiScl) is the most common subtype occurring in 50% to 60% of children with LS, and is characterized by a linear streak or band involving the dermis, subcutis, and often, the underlying muscle, tendons and bone. LiScl typically occurs as a single, linear unilateral band on the extremities, trunk or head (**Fig. 10**).[5,7] Legs are the most commonly involved sites, followed by arms, frontal head and trunk. Lesions of LiScl affecting the extremities are most worrisome when they transverse a joint, because there is the potential for sclerosis and tightening of the underlying muscle, tendon and joint capsule, resulting in joint contracture and associated limb dysfunction. Of particular concern in pediatric patients with LiScl is involvement of the epiphyseal growth plate, which can lead to permanent shortening or atrophy of the limb. Orthopedic complications are reported in approximately 30% to 50% of patients with LiScl of the limb(s).[7,58,61] Peterson and colleagues[1] reported mild to moderate disability at follow-up in those with LiScl of the extremity in their cohort (mean follow-up time of 9.2 years).

Approximately 25% of those with LiScl have scalp/head involvement.[5] Linear lesions involving the scalp and forehead are termed en coup de sabre (ECDS) because

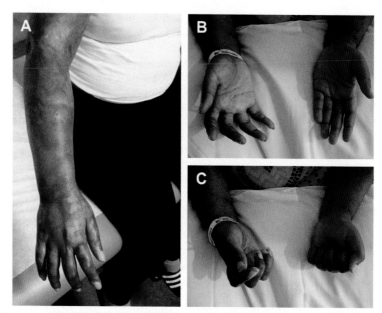

Fig. 10. Linear scleroderma lesion affecting unilateral right upper extremity (*A*). This young woman has associated joint contractures of the wrist and metacarpal and phalangeal joints. Joint contractures of the hand are grossly apparent in comparison with the contralateral side during active extension (*B*) and flexion (*C*).

the linear depression resembles a saber-wound scar (**Fig. 11**). Progressive hemifacial atrophy, also known as Parry-Romberg syndrome (PRS), is another linear variant of LS causing hemiatrophy of the face, including mandible, maxilla, and tongue, and subcutaneous and muscle tissue (**Fig. 12**). Typically, ECDS is associated with cutaneous

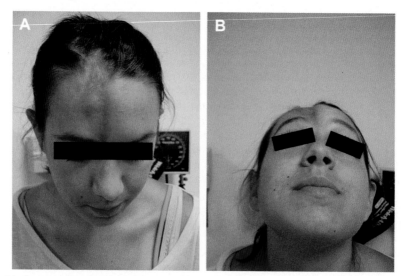

Fig. 11. En coup de sabre (ECDS) lesion affecting the scalp and head in a unilateral fashion (*A*), causing moderate amount of subcutaneous tissue loss and skeletal deformity (*B*).

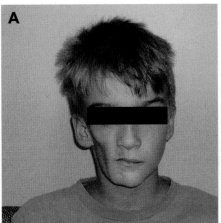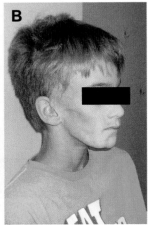

Fig. 12. A severe example of Parry-Romberg syndrome/hemifacial atrophy of the right face.

findings of dyspigmentation and skin thickness, whereas PRS is not and usually has more pronounced subcutaneous atrophy. These disorders can occur together, either at the same location (side of face) or opposing sides.[62] Although controversial, ECDS and PRS are likely different spectra of the same condition, supported by similar manifestations and prevalence of neurologic symptoms[62,63] and cellular infiltrates (lymphocytic infiltrate of neurovascular bundles) of the skin[64] and brain tissue.[65] PRS and ECDS carry the same risks for neurologic involvement, with 8% to 20% of the patients with these conditions demonstrating central nervous involvement expressed as seizures, chronic headaches, optic neuritis and, less frequently, neuropsychiatric changes or ischemic stroke.[62,63] Orthodontic and ophthalmologic abnormalities also have been reported in similar prevalence in both conditions.[63] If the onset of the disease (ECDS or PRS) occurs before 10 years of age, there is a particular risk for skeletal hypoplasia of the affected side of the face, due to the immaturity of the skeleton, resulting in significant dental and cosmetic abnormalities.[66]

Superficial circumscribed morphea, previously termed plaque morphea in the Peterson classification, is the most common presentation of LS in adults (60%) and accounts for approximately one-quarter of LS in children.[5,60] It is characterized by one or few oval or rounded areas of induration with an ivory waxy center and peripheral violaceous halo, ranging from 1 to 30 cm in diameter. These lesions typically arise on the trunk or proximal extremities (**Fig. 13**). The superficial variant is limited to the epidermis and dermis. Deep circumscribed morphea, previously referred to as subcutaneous morphea, morphea profunda, or deep morphea, presents as a round/oval lesion deeper in the tissue. These lesions affect the dermis and subcutis with variable penetration into the fascia and muscle. Typically there are only subtle cutaneous changes (such as slight erythema and thinning of the dermis) but a great deal of inflammatory infiltrate in deep subcutaneous tissue and fascia is present, causing a depression in the adipose tissue (scooped-out appearance) and thickened, bound-down skin.

Generalized morphea (GM) is defined by more than 3 plaque lesions that are each greater than 3 cm wide. Typically the plaques become confluent and affect several anatomic areas, the trunk being most common. GM is an uncommon subtype, occurring in less than 10% of LS patients.[5,7] As mentioned previously, this subtype is often associated with several autoimmune phenomena, including ss-DNA and AHA

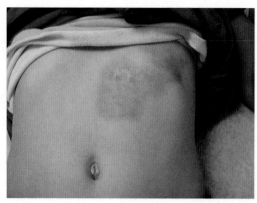

Fig. 13. Typical isolated oval lesion on the trunk consistent with superficial circumscribed morphea.

antibodies, and concomitant and family history of autoimmune disorders. Systemic symptoms, such as myalgia, arthralgia, and fatigue, are more common in GM.[7,60]

Pansclerotic morphea is a rare subset of LS that affects only 1% to 2% of patients and is typically disabling. It initially involves the extremities, but later may migrate to the trunk, only sparing the face and distal areas of fingers and toes (**Fig. 14**). There is a rapidly progressive fibrosis of the deep dermis, subcutis, fascia, and muscles, with occasional bone involvement. This process leads to significant contracture of joints, muscle atrophy, cutaneous ulcerations, and sometimes restrictive pattern respiratory insufficiency if the trunk is involved. The development of squamous cell carcinoma is an additional complication in pansclerotic morphea, especially in areas of chronic wounds.[67]

Mixed morphea is the final subtype considered from the Padua consensus, and is defined by the presence of more than one clinical subtype in a single LS patient. Mixed morphea is rather common and is seen in approximately 15% of the pediatric LS population. The most frequent presentation of mixed morphea is a combination of linear and plaque morphea.[5]

Bullous morphea is sometimes considered a rare subtype of LS. However, many experts agree that the bullous lesions are secondary to aggressive linear or deep LS disease and likely reflect disruption of the lymphatic drainage. Eosinophilic fasciitis

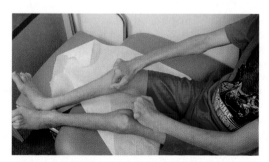

Fig. 14. Pansclerotic morphea affecting limbs circumferentially and sparing the distal toes and fingers.

(EF), once considered a type of deep morphea by Peterson criteria, is not considered a subtype of LS by Padua criteria. EF often behaves as a mixture of deep morphea and linear scleroderma, resulting in deep infiltration and joint contractures.[31]

Extracutaneous Manifestations

Extracutaneous manifestations (ECM) are not uncommon in LS and occur in approximately one-quarter of patients throughout the course of disease.[44] According to a large international study of 750 children with LS, ECM are more frequent in patients with LiScl and consist essentially of orthopedic complications (19% of the entire group, 50% in those with LiScl of the extremity), neurologic or ocular findings (5% of the entire group, 40% in those with LiScl of the head), RP (2.1% of the entire group) and other autoimmune conditions such as thyroiditis (2% all subtypes).[44] Less common ECM are gastrointestinal, respiratory, and renal, all of which occurred in fewer than 2% of the 750 patients examined.[44] These estimates may be lower than the true percentage of ECM, because only symptomatic patients were included in the analysis. Another limitation of the study was a lack of a control population to evaluate the prevalence of these manifestations in a comparable pediatric population. In another series, which screened for GI manifestations in LS patients (such as gastroesophageal reflux) and neurologic imaging changes in ECDS/PRS patients, investigators found a higher occurrence of ECM (20% and 60%, respectively).[63,68] In the study by Zulian and colleagues[44] of 750 children with LS, of the 168 patients with ECM 25% had articular, neurologic, and ocular manifestations unrelated to the site of skin lesions, that is, arthritis of a peripheral joint with uninvolved overlying skin and subcutaneous tissue, further supporting the hypothesis that localized scleroderma is more of a systemic process. Twenty-four of the 750 children (3.2%) had significant ocular involvement, most of whom had linear scleroderma of the head (67%).[69] These findings support routine screening of LS patients by ophthalmology for inflammatory eye findings, especially for those with linear scleroderma of the head. This benign screening tool can detect clinically silent disease, and treatment can prevent long-term visual sequela.

Evaluation

No laboratory test is diagnostic of LS. Although a localized disease, there have been several autoantibodies associated with LS that can be supportive of diagnosis and indicate more severe/involved disease (see the section on autoimmunity). Specifically, ANA, AHA, and ss-DNA positivity have been detected at a relatively high frequency (40%–50%). In addition, rheumatoid factor is present in one-third of patients, particularly those who have GM, and is also correlated to disease severity (number of lesions).[5] General markers of inflammation, including erythrocyte sedimentation rate and serum immunoglobulin levels, may be useful markers of disease activity in select patients with LS, particularly those with deep or eosinophilic-like variants. However, most patients presenting with active LS lesions do not have elevation of these markers. Diagnosis of LS is usually made by clinical examination, and if there is uncertainty, a skin and subcutaneous biopsy can aid in the diagnosis. Differential diagnosis is limited and includes 2 skin conditions with well-defined plaque lesions: lichen sclerosus et atrophicus and atrophoderma of Pasini and Pierini. Both are superficial dermal and epidermal inflammatory conditions thought by some to be on the milder spectrum of LS. Cutaneous T-cell lymphoma, especially if there is a deeper purple skin discoloration, and collagenoma, usually presenting with induration of the skin and subcutis without pigmentary changes from birth or early childhood, are included in the differential. Other possible conditions are associated with certain exposures and generally have more widespread lesions, such as graft-versus-host disease (status post transplant), nephrogenic fibrosing dermatopathy (gadolinium administered in renal compromised state), and porphyria cutanea tarda (sun exposure).

Several tools have been used for the assessment of skin and subcutaneous involvement in LS, such as clinical skin scores, measurement tools, and imaging. Clinical skin scores are commonly used by physicians and include the modified Rodnan Skin Score[17] and the Localized Scleroderma Cutaneous Assessment Tool (LoSCAT), which combines disease activity and damage parameters.[33,70] A computerized skin score (CSS) can be used to determine the size of lesion in an objective manner.[71] Measurement tools, including a durometer, which measures the degree of skin hardness,[72] and a cutometer, which measures skin elasticity,[73] have also been proposed as useful. In addition, several types of imaging can be used for diagnostic or assessment purposes, such as thermography,[74,75] laser Doppler flowmetry,[76] ultrasonography,[77,78] and MRI.[79] Some of these techniques have been validated in LS, including the LoSCAT, the CSS, ultrasonography using higher frequencies (10–25 MHz), and MRI. However, currently standard measures are not widely used and assessment depends on center-specific modalities that rely on the investigator's experience.

Recent efforts through the Childhood Arthritis and Rheumatology Research Alliance (CARRA) have focused on collaborative projects among pediatric rheumatology and dermatology investigators in North America. Their goal is to establish specific clinical measures to assess activity and damage, which will assist in monitoring progression and disease state in LS. These projects are in the process of assessing clinical measures such as the LoSCAT and identifying others through multicentered studies with the Localized Scleroderma Clinical and Ultrasound Study group (LOCUS). The LOCUS group is composed of experts in LS, both pediatric rheumatologists and pediatric dermatologists, who were asked to rank clinical variables that most strongly reflect disease activity and damage in LS. There was greater than 75% consensus agreement and high content validity (modified kappa statistic 0.88–1.00) regarding 4 activity parameters; the appearance of new lesions, expansion of current lesions, erythematous/violaceous hue at the border, and skin induration at the border of a lesion.[33] Cutaneous disease damage parameters ranked highest amongst the group were postinflammatory hyperpigmentation and hypopigmentation, dermal atrophy, and subcutaneous atrophy (88% agreement and Inter-Item Content Validity Index of 0.88–1.0).[70]

Once systemic immunosuppressive therapy is initiated in patients with moderate to severe LS, the signs of disease activity typically resolve within months and some of the damage features improve mildly to moderately.[80–86] It is after this initial improvement that the detection of subclinical disease is important, so as to not wean off of immunosuppression too early, potentially resulting in relapse.[80,83,84] A recent study in pediatric LS found a 28% relapse rate after a mean duration of treatment with Methotrexate (MTX) of 2.4 years. Linear extremity subtype and older age at disease onset were found to be significant predictors of relapse, and although not significant, there was a noticeable difference in duration of MTX treatment between relapsers and nonrelapsers.[86] However, it remains difficult to detect subclinical disease, which is why multiple imaging and thermal modalities are being pursued.

Treatment

The approach to the treatment of LS initially depends on the severity of the disease, which is characterized by the subtype of LS, potential involvement of deeper tissue and structures (such as joints), location of LS, and disease-activity state. The length of disease duration does have an impact on disease-activity state, with most superficial circumscribed or plaque lesions "burning out" in 3 to 5 years. Any remaining central sclerosis may soften over time without intervention. If only disease-damage parameters remain and there is no expansion, erythema, or other clinical disease-activity parameters present, simply monitoring the lesion is acceptable. However, if there is any sign of active disease, pediatric rheumatologists and dermatologists agree that a single superficial circumscribed lesion in a noncosmetically concerning location can be treated either topically with corticosteroids, calcineurin inhibitors, imiquimod, or vitamin D, or via recurrent phototherapy with ultraviolet (UV) light. All modalities have had clinical success in case series or uncontrolled trials, shown by lightening of hyperpigmentation and decreased skin thickness. Many dermatologists prescribe these medications in combination, and recommend using occlusive dressing to increase absorption of topical therapies.[87] UV treatment has several modalities; broad-band UVA, narrow-band UVB, and UVA-1. UVA-1 was successful in 2 randomized control trials, especially regarding early inflammatory and superficial dermal lesions.[88,89] However, access to UV therapy is limited and treatment is time consuming (often requiring three 30–60-minute sessions per week), making this a difficult option for many. In addition, the risk for potential long-term effects such as skin aging and carcinogenesis are unknown in children.

There is growing consensus among both rheumatologists and dermatologists that systemic therapy is warranted for more moderate to severe LS. Features that might indicate moderate to severe disease include deeply involved subcutis, fascia, and muscle that can transverse a joint and potentially cause functional impairment, linear or atrophic lesions affecting the face/scalp, rapidly progressive or widespread active disease, and failed topical or UV therapy.[87,90] The most commonly used systemic therapy is MTX in conjunction with corticosteroids, confirmed by a recent survey of 158 North American pediatric rheumatologists by Li and colleagues.[90] Clinical vignettes describing patients with moderate to severe LS were distributed to clinicians, who were asked to respond with their treatment recommendations. The clinicians' response as to initial therapy was overwhelmingly MTX combined with corticosteroids (more than 80% would use both). Although there was excellent agreement as to the choice of medications, treatment regimens varied broadly regarding administration (oral vs subcutaneous vs intravenous) as well as corticosteroid taper and length of therapy.[90]

A subcommittee of CARRA is deriving consensus best-treatment protocols for those with moderate to severe LS to help address this issue and narrow down spectrum of regimens to a handful that would be useful to the clinician. These protocols have 4 treatment plans for induction of therapy. Three protocols involve subcutaneous MTX (1 mg/kg, with a maximum dose of 25 mg/wk) and the fourth was derived for those who either fail MTX or are intolerant to MTX. The protocols are divided into MTX alone, MTX with oral corticosteroids and taper, MTX with intravenous corticosteroids, and MMF in addition to either oral or intravenous corticosteroids. These protocols are currently being submitted for publication and are not in their final state. MMF has been shown to be effective in severe MTX-resistant pediatric LS, as exemplified by a case series of 10 patients (2 with pansclerotic morphea, 3 with GM, 2 with LiScl extremities, and 3 with LiScl head). All cases improved with MMF, with weaning of corticosteroid dose.[91]

The first double-blind randomized, controlled trial using objective measures in children with LS was performed by Zulian and colleagues,[84] who compared MTX and oral corticosteroids with placebo and oral corticosteroids. MTX was found to be effective and safe, confirming the community's support for the use of MTX in LS. In addition,

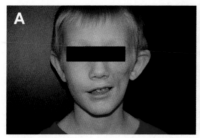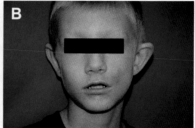

Fig. 15. Parry-Romberg syndrome affecting left face before (*A*) and after (*B*) subcutaneous fat grafting. (*Courtesy of* Joseph Losee, Children's Hospital of Pittsburgh, Pittsburgh, PA.)

those treated with MTX significantly improved and had significantly less relapse compared with those on corticosteroids alone.

Other Therapies

Intensive physical and occupational therapy in conjunction with systemic immunosuppressive therapy is recommended for those with linear or deep scleroderma of the extremity, to help avoid and/or minimize joint contractures. Also, for those with ECDS and/or PRS, plastic-surgery intervention is considered reasonable after the disease has been in remission without any signs of clinical activity. Augmentation includes fat grating with microdroplets from the patient's abdominal subcutis, to assist in filling in some of the subcutaneous atrophy in order to yield a more symmetric facial contour (**Fig. 15**). For more severe disease, fasciocutaneous flaps and facial bone reconstruction are also options, although they are typically reserved for the late teenage years, after the skeleton has matured.[92] One center reports that of 10 teenagers with ECDS and/or PRS who underwent surgical intervention to correct facial deformity, 9 reported satisfaction with the results of the procedure(s) and all would recommend surgical intervention to others with this condition, signifying a potentially great impact on quality of life for these patients.[93]

REFERENCES

1. Peterson LS, Nelson AM, Su WP, et al. The epidemiology of morphea (localized scleroderma) in Olmsted County 1960-1993. J Rheumatol 1997;24(1):73–80.
2. Pelkonen PM, Jalanko HJ, Lantto RK, et al. Incidence of systemic connective tissue diseases in children: a nationwide prospective study in Finland. J Rheumatol 1994;21(11):2143–6.
3. Scalapino K, Arkachaisri T, Lucas M, et al. Childhood onset systemic sclerosis: classification, clinical and serologic features, and survival in comparison with adult onset disease. J Rheumatol 2006;33(5):1004–13.
4. Martini G, Foeldvari I, Russo R, et al. Systemic sclerosis in childhood: clinical and immunologic features of 153 patients in an international database. Arthritis Rheum 2006;54(12):3971–8.
5. Zulian F, Athreya BH, Laxer R, et al. Juvenile localized scleroderma: clinical and epidemiological features in 750 children. An international study. Rheumatology (Oxford) 2006;45(5):614–20.
6. Foeldvari I, Zhavania M, Birdi N, et al. Favourable outcome in 135 children with juvenile systemic sclerosis: results of a multi-national survey. Rheumatology (Oxford) 2000;39(5):556–9.

7. Christen-Zaech S, Hakim MD, Afsar FS, et al. Pediatric morphea (localized scleroderma): review of 136 patients. J Am Acad Dermatol 2008;59(3):385–96.

8. Zulian F, Vallongo C, de Oliveira SK, et al. Congenital localized scleroderma. J Pediatr 2006;149(2):248–51.

9. Medsger TA Jr. Natural history of systemic sclerosis and the assessment of disease activity, severity, functional status, and psychologic well-being. Rheum Dis Clin North Am 2003;29(2):255–73, vi.

10. Zulian F, Woo P, Athreya BH, et al. The Pediatric Rheumatology European Society/ American College of Rheumatology/European League against Rheumatism provisional classification criteria for juvenile systemic sclerosis. Arthritis Rheum 2007;57(2):203–12.

11. LeRoy EC, Black C, Fleischmajer R, et al. Scleroderma (systemic sclerosis): classification, subsets and pathogenesis. J Rheumatol 1988;15(2):202–5.

12. Steen VD. The many faces of scleroderma. Rheum Dis Clin North Am 2008;34(1): 1–15, v.

13. Rodnan GP, Myerowitz RL, Justh GO. Morphologic changes in the digital arteries of patients with progressive systemic sclerosis (scleroderma) and Raynaud phenomenon. Medicine (Baltimore) 1980;59(6):393–408.

14. Maricq HR. Wide-field capillary microscopy. Arthritis Rheum 1981;24(9):1159–65.

15. LeRoy EC, Medsger TA Jr. Raynaud's phenomenon: a proposal for classification. Clin Exp Rheumatol 1992;10(5):485–8.

16. Duffy CM, Laxer RM, Lee P, et al. Raynaud syndrome in childhood. J Pediatr 1989;114(1):73–8.

17. Clements P, Lachenbruch P, Siebold J, et al. Inter and intraobserver variability of total skin thickness score (modified Rodnan TSS) in systemic sclerosis. J Rheumatol 1995;22(7):1281–5.

18. Domsic RT, Rodriguez-Reyna T, Lucas M, et al. Skin thickness progression rate: a predictor of mortality and early internal organ involvement in diffuse scleroderma. Ann Rheum Dis 2011;70(1):104–9.

19. Weber P, Ganser G, Frosch M, et al. Twenty-four hour intraesophageal pH monitoring in children and adolescents with scleroderma and mixed connective tissue disease. J Rheumatol 2000;27(11):2692–5.

20. Ingraham KM, O'Brien MS, Shenin M, et al. Gastric antral vascular ectasia in systemic sclerosis: demographics and disease predictors. J Rheumatol 2010; 37(3):603–7.

21. Panigada S, Ravelli A, Silvestri M, et al. HRCT and pulmonary function tests in monitoring of lung involvement in juvenile systemic sclerosis. Pediatr Pulmonol 2009;44(12):1226–34.

22. Silver RM, Miller KS, Kinsella MB, et al. Evaluation and management of scleroderma lung disease using bronchoalveolar lavage. Am J Med 1990;88(5): 470–6.

23. Rabinovich CE. Challenges in the diagnosis and treatment of juvenile systemic sclerosis. Nat Rev Rheumatol 2011;7(11):676–80.

24. Rodnan GP, Medsger TA. The rheumatic manifestations of progressive systemic sclerosis (scleroderma). Clin Orthop Relat Res 1968;57:81–93.

25. Ringel RA, Brick JE, Brick JF, et al. Muscle involvement in the scleroderma syndromes. Arch Intern Med 1990;150(12):2550–2.

26. Quartier P, Bonnet D, Fournet JC, et al. Severe cardiac involvement in children with systemic sclerosis and myositis. J Rheumatol 2002;29(8):1767–73.

27. Steen VD, Medsger TA. Changes in causes of death in systemic sclerosis, 1972-2002. Ann Rheum Dis 2007;66(7):940–4.

28. Foeldvari I, Nihtyanova SI, Wierk A, et al. Characteristics of patients with juvenile onset systemic sclerosis in an adult single-center cohort. J Rheumatol 2010; 37(11):2422–6.

29. Kowal-Bielecka O, Landewe R, Avouac J, et al. EULAR recommendations for the treatment of systemic sclerosis: a report from the EULAR Scleroderma Trials and Research group (EUSTAR). Ann Rheum Dis 2009;68(5):620–8.

30. Nihtyanova SI, Denton CP. Current approaches to the management of early active diffuse scleroderma skin disease. Rheum Dis Clin North Am 2008;34(1):161–79, viii.

31. Peterson LS, Nelson AM, Su WP. Classification of morphea (localized sclero-derma). Mayo Clin Proc 1995;70(11):1068–76.

32. Laxer RM, Zulian F. Localized scleroderma. Curr Opin Rheumatol 2006;18(6): 606–13.

33. Arkachaisri T, Vilaiyuk S, Li S, et al. The localized scleroderma skin severity index and physician global assessment of disease activity: a work in progress toward development of localized scleroderma outcome measures. J Rheumatol 2009; 36(12):2819–29.

34. Lever WF, Elder DE, Elenitsas R, et al. Lever's histopathology of the skin. 8th edition. Philadelphia: Lippincott-Raven; 1997.

35. McKee PH. Pathology of the skin: with clinical correlations. 2nd edition. London: Mosby-Wolfe; 1996.

36. Roumm AD, Whiteside TL, Medsger TA Jr, et al. Lymphocytes in the skin of patients with progressive systemic sclerosis. Quantification, subtyping, and clin-ical correlations. Arthritis Rheum 1984;27(6):645–53.

37. Torres JE, Sanchez JL. Histopathologic differentiation between localized and systemic scleroderma. Am J Dermatopathol 1998;20(3):242–5.

38. Ihn H, Sato S, Fujimoto M, et al. Demonstration of interleukin-2, interleukin-4 and interleukin-6 in sera from patients with localized scleroderma. Arch Dermatol Res 1995;287(2):193–7.

39. Hasegawa M, Sato S, Nagaoka T, et al. Serum levels of tumor necrosis factor and interleukin-13 are elevated in patients with localized scleroderma. Dermatology 2003;207(2):141–7.

40. Ihn H, Sato S, Fujimoto M, et al. Demonstration of interleukin 8 in serum samples of patients with localized scleroderma. Arch Dermatol 1994;130(10):1327–8.

41. Hasegawa M, Fujimoto M, Kikuchi K, et al. Elevated serum levels of interleukin 4 (IL-4), IL-10, and IL-13 in patients with systemic sclerosis. J Rheumatol 1997; 24(2):328–32.

42. Needleman BW, Wigley FM, Stair RW. Interleukin-1, interleukin-2, interleukin-4, interleukin-6, tumor necrosis factor alpha, and interferon-gamma levels in sera from patients with scleroderma. Arthritis Rheum 1992;35(1):67–72.

43. Hasegawa M, Sato S, Ihn H, et al. Enhanced production of interleukin-6 (IL-6), on-costatin M and soluble IL-6 receptor by cultured peripheral blood mononuclear cells from patients with systemic sclerosis. Rheumatology (Oxford) 1999;38(7): 612–7.

44. Zulian F, Vallongo C, Woo P, et al. Localized scleroderma in childhood is not just a skin disease. Arthritis Rheum 2005;52(9):2873–81.

45. Ihn H, Sato S, Fujimoto M, et al. Clinical significance of serum levels of soluble interleukin-2 receptor in patients with localized scleroderma. Br J Dermatol 1996;134(5):843–7.

46. Uziel Y, Krafchik BR, Feldman B, et al. Serum levels of soluble interleukin-2 receptor. A marker of disease activity in localized scleroderma. Arthritis Rheum 1994;37(6):898–901.

47. Nagaoka T, Sato S, Hasegawa M, et al. Serum levels of soluble interleukin 6 receptor and soluble gp130 are elevated in patients with localized scleroderma. J Rheumatol 2000;27(8):1917–21.

48. Varga J, Rosenbloom J, Jimenez SA. Transforming growth factor beta (TGF beta) causes a persistent increase in steady-state amounts of type I and type III collagen and fibronectin mRNAs in normal human dermal fibroblasts. Biochem J 1987;247(3):597–604.

49. Gore-Hyer E, Pannu J, Smith EA, et al. Selective stimulation of collagen synthesis in the presence of costimulatory insulin signaling by connective tissue growth factor in scleroderma fibroblasts. Arthritis Rheum 2003;48(3):798–806.

50. Uziel Y, Feldman BM, Krafchik BR, et al. Increased serum levels of TGFbeta1 in children with localized scleroderma. Pediatr Rheumatol Online J 2007;5:22.

51. Higley H, Persichitte K, Chu S, et al. Immunocytochemical localization and serologic detection of transforming growth factor beta 1. Association with type I procollagen and inflammatory cell markers in diffuse and limited systemic sclerosis, morphea, and Raynaud's phenomenon. Arthritis Rheum 1994;37(2):278–88.

52. Lambert NC, Pang JM, Yan Z, et al. Male microchimerism in women with systemic sclerosis and healthy women who have never given birth to a son. Ann Rheum Dis 2005;64(6):845–8.

53. Rak JM, Pagni PP, Tiev K, et al. Male microchimerism and HLA compatibility in French women with scleroderma: a different profile in limited and diffuse subset. Rheumatology (Oxford) 2009;48(4):363–6.

54. Takehara K, Sato S. Localized scleroderma is an autoimmune disorder. Rheumatology (Oxford) 2005;44(3):274–9.

55. Takehara K, Moroi Y, Nakabayashi Y, et al. Antinuclear antibodies in localized scleroderma. Arthritis Rheum 1983;26(5):612–6.

56. Arkachaisri T, Fertig N, Pino S, et al. Serum autoantibodies and their clinical associations in patients with childhood- and adult-onset linear scleroderma. A single-center study. J Rheumatol 2008;35(12):2439–44.

57. Falanga V, Medsger TA Jr, Reichlin M. Antinuclear and anti-single-stranded DNA antibodies in morphea and generalized morphea. Arch Dermatol 1987;123(3):350–3.

58. Falanga V, Medsger TA Jr, Reichlin M, et al. Linear scleroderma. Clinical spectrum, prognosis, and laboratory abnormalities. Ann Intern Med 1986;104(6):849–57.

59. Sato S, Fujimoto M, Ihn H, et al. Clinical characteristics associated with antihistone antibodies in patients with localized scleroderma. J Am Acad Dermatol 1994;31(4):567–71.

60. Leitenberger JJ, Cayce RL, Haley RW, et al. Distinct autoimmune syndromes in morphea: a review of 245 adult and pediatric cases. Arch Dermatol 2009;145(5):545–50.

61. Marzano AV, Menni S, Parodi A, et al. Localized scleroderma in adults and children. Clinical and laboratory investigations on 239 cases. Eur J Dermatol 2003;13(2):171–6.

62. Tollefson MM, Witman PM. En coup de sabre morphea and Parry-Romberg syndrome: a retrospective review of 54 patients. J Am Acad Dermatol 2007;56(2):257–63.

63. Kister I, Inglese M, Laxer RM, et al. Neurologic manifestations of localized scleroderma: a case report and literature review. Neurology 2008;71(19):1538–45.

64. Pensler JM, Murphy GF, Mulliken JB. Clinical and ultrastructural studies of Romberg's hemifacial atrophy. Plast Reconstr Surg 1990;85(5):669–74 [discussion: 675–6].

65. Holland KE, Steffes B, Nocton JJ, et al. Linear scleroderma en coup de sabre with associated neurologic abnormalities. Pediatrics 2006;117(1):e132–6.

66. Thorne C, Grabb WC, Smith JW. Grabb and Smith's plastic surgery. 6th edition. Philadelphia: Lippincott Williams & Wilkins; 2007.

67. Wollina U, Buslau M, Heinig B, et al. Disabling pansclerotic morphea of childhood poses a high risk of chronic ulceration of the skin and squamous cell carcinoma. Int J Low Extrem Wounds 2007;6(4):291–8.

68. Dehen L, Roujeau JC, Cosnes A, et al. Internal involvement in localized scleroderma. Medicine (Baltimore) 1994;73(5):241–5.

69. Zannin ME, Martini G, Athreya BH, et al. Ocular involvement in children with localised scleroderma: a multi-centre study. Br J Ophthalmol 2007;91(10):1311–4.

70. Arkachaisri T, Vilaiyuk S, Torok KS, et al. Development and initial validation of the localized scleroderma skin damage index and physician global assessment of disease damage: a proof-of-concept study. Rheumatology (Oxford) 2010;49(2):373–81.

71. Zulian F, Meneghesso D, Grisan E, et al. A new computerized method for the assessment of skin lesions in localized scleroderma. Rheumatology (Oxford) 2007;46(5):856–60.

72. Seyger MM, van den Hoogen FH, de Boo T, et al. Reliability of two methods to assess morphea: skin scoring and the use of a durometer. J Am Acad Dermatol 1997;37(5 Pt 1):793–6.

73. de Rie MA, Enomoto DN, de Vries HJ, et al. Evaluation of medium-dose UVA1 phototherapy in localized scleroderma with the cutometer and fast Fourier transform method. Dermatology 2003;207(3):298–301.

74. Birdi N, Shore A, Rush P, et al. Childhood linear scleroderma: a possible role of thermography for evaluation. J Rheumatol 1992;19(6):968–73.

75. Martini G, Murray KJ, Howell KJ, et al. Juvenile-onset localized scleroderma activity detection by infrared thermography. Rheumatology (Oxford) 2002;41(10):1178–82.

76. Weibel L, Howell KJ, Visentin MT, et al. Laser Doppler flowmetry for assessing localized scleroderma in children. Arthritis Rheum 2007;56(10):3489–95.

77. Hoffmann K, Gerbaulet U, el-Gammal S, et al. 20-MHz B-mode ultrasound in monitoring the course of localized scleroderma (morphea). Acta Derm Venereol Suppl (Stockh) 1991;164:3–16.

78. Li SC, Liebling MS, Haines KA, et al. Initial evaluation of an ultrasound measure for assessing the activity of skin lesions in juvenile localized scleroderma. Arthritis Care Res (Hoboken) 2011;63(5):735–42.

79. Horger M, Fierlbeck G, Kuemmerle-Deschner J, et al. MRI findings in deep and generalized morphea (localized scleroderma). AJR Am J Roentgenol 2008;190(1):32–9.

80. Cox D, O' Regan G, Collins S, et al. Juvenile localised scleroderma: a retrospective review of response to systemic treatment. Ir J Med Sci 2008;177(4):343–6.

81. Uziel Y, Feldman BM, Krafchik BR, et al. Methotrexate and corticosteroid therapy for pediatric localized scleroderma. J Pediatr 2000;136(1):91–5.

82. Fitch PG, Rettig P, Burnham JM, et al. Treatment of pediatric localized scleroderma with methotrexate. J Rheumatol 2006;33(3):609–14.

83. Weibel L, Sampaio MC, Visentin MT, et al. Evaluation of methotrexate and corticosteroids for the treatment of localized scleroderma (morphoea) in children. Br J Dermatol 2006;155(5):1013–20.

84. Zulian F, Martini G, Vallongo C, et al. Methotrexate treatment in juvenile localized scleroderma: a randomized, double-blind, placebo-controlled trial. Arthritis Rheum 2011;63(7):1998–2006.

85. Torok KS, Arkachaisri T. Methotrexate and corticosteroids in the treatment of localized scleroderma: a standardized prospective longitudinal single-center study. J Rheumatol 2012;39(2):286–94.

86. Mirsky L, Chakkittakandiyil A, Laxer RM, et al. Relapse after systemic treatment in paediatric morphoea. Br J Dermatol 2012;166(2):443–5.

87. Zwischenberger BA, Jacobe HT. A systematic review of morphea treatments and therapeutic algorithm. J Am Acad Dermatol 2011;65(5):925–41.

88. Kreuter A, Hyun J, Stucker M, et al. A randomized controlled study of low-dose UVA1, medium-dose UVA1, and narrowband UVB phototherapy in the treatment of localized scleroderma. J Am Acad Dermatol 2006;54(3):440–7.

89. Sator PG, Radakovic S, Schulmeister K, et al. Medium-dose is more effective than low-dose ultraviolet A1 phototherapy for localized scleroderma as shown by 20-MHz ultrasound assessment. J Am Acad Dermatol 2009;60(5):786–91.

90. Li SC, Feldman BM, Higgins GC, et al. Treatment of pediatric localized scleroderma: results of a survey of North American pediatric rheumatologists. J Rheumatol 2010;37(1):175–81.

91. Martini G, Ramanan AV, Falcini F, et al. Successful treatment of severe or methotrexate-resistant juvenile localized scleroderma with mycophenolate mofetil. Rheumatology (Oxford) 2009;48(11):1410–3.

92. Asai S, Kamei Y, Nishibori K, et al. Reconstruction of Romberg disease defects by omental flap. Ann Plast Surg 2006;57(2):154–8.

93. Palmero ML, Uziel Y, Laxer RM, et al. En coup de sabre scleroderma and Parry-Romberg syndrome in adolescents: surgical options and patient-related outcomes. J Rheumatol 2010;37(10):2174–9.

Pediatric Vasculitis

Pamela F. Weiss, MD, MSCE[a,b,*]

KEYWORDS

- Vasculitis - Pediatrics - Review

Childhood vasculitis is a challenging and complex group of conditions that are multi-system in nature and often require integrated care from multiple subspecialties, including rheumatology, dermatology, cardiology, nephrology, neurology, and gastro-enterology. Vasculitis is defined as the presence of inflammation in the blood vessel wall. The site of vessel involvement, size of the affected vessels, extent of vascular injury, and underlying pathology determine the disease phenotype and severity. Vasculitis can be secondary to infection, malignancy, drug exposure, and other rheumatic conditions, such as systemic lupus erythematosus and juvenile dermatomyositis. This article explores the classification and general features of vasculitis, as well as the clinical presentation, diagnostic evaluation, and therapeutic options for the most common primary systemic vasculitides.

DIAGNOSIS

Making the diagnosis of vasculitis is often challenging, as presenting symptoms may be subacute, nonspecific, and nondiagnostic. Fever, malaise, diffuse pain, and laboratory evidence of elevated acute-phase reactants may be the only early symptoms to suggest systemic inflammation. As vessel damage evolves, more specific clinical features, such as a purpuric rash, evidence of organ involvement, such as glomerulonephritis, or detection of certain antibodies, such as antineutrophil cytoplasmic antibodies (ANCA), may heighten the suspicion of vasculitis. The presenting symptoms can vary widely depending on the size and location of involved vasculature.

If vasculitis is suspected, then a thorough history and physical examination are paramount. The history should include recent infections, drug exposure, and a detailed family history. The physical examination should include a 4-extremity blood pressure evaluation. Takayasu arteritis (TA) may present with a blood pressure difference of greater than 10 mm Hg between arms, and hypertension is common with many of the vasculitides. In addition, careful auscultation for bruits (carotid, axillary, aortic,

Disclosures: None.
[a] Division of Rheumatology and Center for Pediatric Clinical Effectiveness, Children's Hospital of Philadelphia, 3401 Civic Center Boulevard, Colkett Translational Research Building, Philadelphia, PA 19104; [b] Center for Clinical Epidemiology and Biostatistics, University of Pennsylvania, Philadelphia, PA, USA
* Division of Rheumatology, The Children's Hospital of Philadelphia, Room 1526, North Campus, 3535 Market Street, Philadelphia, PA 19104.
E-mail address: weisspa@email.chop.edu

Pediatr Clin N Am 59 (2012) 407–423
doi:10.1016/j.pcl.2012.03.013
0031-3955/12/$ – see front matter © 2012 Elsevier Inc. All rights reserved.

renal, and iliac vessels) and palpation of peripheral pulses is essential. Absent peripheral pulses may help identify areas of vessel involvement. A thorough skin examination is also important; the presence of painful nodules, purpura, ulcerations, microinfarctions, or livedo reticularis is common. A neurologic examination should evaluate for peripheral neuropathy; polyarteritis nodosa (PAN) is associated with mononeuritis multiplex. A fundoscopic examination and nailfold capillaroscopy are also helpful to visualize small vessel abnormalities.

The laboratory evaluation for vasculitis should include a complete blood count and acute phase reactants, such as the erythrocyte sedimentation rate and C-reactive protein, which can be markedly elevated. Liver enzymes, blood urea nitrogen and creatinine, and urinalysis will evaluate for hepatic and renal involvement. Specific antibody testing, such as antinuclear antibodies and ANCA, and complements should be sent depending on the vasculitis being considered. When clinical suspicion is high, imaging, such as computed tomography (CT) angiography, magnetic resonance (MR) angiography, or conventional angiography may help detect blood vessel abnormalities. Imaging may demonstrate prototypical patterns of vessel involvement, such as beading and aneurysms in PAN and TA, respectively. Typically, imaging is most useful when there is suspicion for medium-vessel or large-vessel disease. The diagnostic gold standard for diagnosis, however, is tissue biopsy.

CLASSIFICATION

Primary vasculitis can be classified according to clinical manifestations, size of the affected vessels, or histopathology, including the presence or absence of granuloma. In 2005, the European League Against Rheumatism (EULAR) and the Pediatric Rheumatology European Society (PReS) developed the first pediatric-specific classification of vasculitis (**Box 1**).[1] This classification system is primarily based on size of affected vessels and the presence or absence of granuloma.

EPIDEMIOLOGY AND PATHOGENESIS

The annual incidence of primary vasculitis in children and adolescents younger than 17 years is approximately 23 per 100,000.[2] Primary vasculitis accounts for approximately 2% to 10% of all pediatric conditions evaluated in pediatric rheumatology clinics.[3–6] Of the primary vasculitides, Henoch Schönlein purpura (HSP) and Kawasaki disease (KD) are the most common, accounting for 49% and 23% of all childhood vasculitis, respectively.[6] The prevalence of diseases may be different based on the population studied. For example, the incidence of KD and Behçet's disease is higher in Asian and Turkish children, respectively, than in other ethnicities.

These ethnic differences in prevalence suggest that genetics and environment may play an important role in disease susceptibility and pathogenesis. Other theories of pathogenesis include humoral factors, as manifest by ANCA-associated vasculitides. Abnormal regulation of immune complex formation may be contributory, as in HSP. Impaired lymphocyte regulation, specifically T-regulatory cell dysfunction, may also be involved. Antecedent infections, particularly streptococcal infections, have been implicated in many of the vasculitides including HSP, granulomatosis with polyangiitis (GPA), and PAN.

Henoch Schönlein Purpura

Etiology and epidemiology
HSP is a leukocytoclastic vasculitis that predominantly affects the small blood vessels. It is also known as anaphylactoid purpura or purpura rheumatica. The EULAR/PReS

Box 1
EULAR/PReS classification of pediatric vasculitis

Vasculitis category

Predominately large vessel

    Takayasu arteritis

Predominately medium vessel

    Childhood polyarteritis nodosa

    Cutaneous polyarteritis

    Kawasaki disease

Predominately small vessel

    Granulomatous

        Wegener granulomatosis[a]

        Churg-Strauss syndrome

    Nongranulomatous

        Microscopic polyangiitis

        Henoch-Schönlein purpura

        Isolated cutaneous leucocytoclastic vasculitis

        Hypocomplementemic urticarial vasculitis

Other

    Behçet disease

    Vasculitis secondary to infection, malignancy, drugs

    Vasculitis associated with connective tissue disease

    Isolated vasculitis of the central nervous system

    Cogan syndrome

    Unclassified

[a] Granulomatosis with polyangiitis.
Adapted from Ozen S, Ruperto N, Dillon MJ, et al. EULAR/PReS endorsed consensus criteria for the classification of childhood vasculitides. Ann Rheum Dis 2006;65:936–41.

classification criteria are listed in **Box 2**.[7] Among children younger than 17 years, the annual incidence of HSP is approximately 20 per 100,000 and the peak age of onset is between 4 and 6 years.[2] Caucasians have the highest incidence and African Americans have the lowest incidence. Unlike most vasculitides, males are affected more commonly than females, with a ratio of approximately 2 to 1. Certain autoimmune risk factors, such as complement deficiencies,[8] and hereditary fever syndromes,[9] such as Familial Mediterranean Fever syndrome, may predispose a child to HSP. HSP is most prevalent during the winter and spring. This seasonal distribution supports the hypothesis that an infectious agent triggers this condition.[10] Group A β–hemolytic streptococcus, *Staphylococcus aureus,* influenza, parainfluenza, Epstein-Barr virus, adenovirus, parvovirus, and mycoplasma have all been reported as triggers for HSP.

Clinical presentation
The classic presentation of HSP includes lower-extremity purpura, arthritis, abdominal pain, and renal disease. The purpuric rash is usually on dependent areas but may be

Box 2
EULAR/PReS classification criteria for HSP

Purpura or petechiae with lower limb predominance and at least 1 of the following:

1. Arthritis or arthralgias

2. Abdominal pain

3. Histopathology demonstrating immunoglobulin A deposition

4. Renal involvement (hematuria or proteinuria)

Data from Ozen S, Pistorio A, Iusan SM, et al. EULAR/PRINTO/PRES criteria for Henoch-Schönlein purpura, childhood polyarteritis nodosa, childhood Wegener granulomatosis and childhood Takayasu arteritis: Ankara 2008. Part II: final classification criteria. Ann Rheum Dis 2010; 69:798–806.

seen on the arms, face, and ears (**Fig. 1**A). The purpura may be preceded by a maculopapular or urticarial rash that usually disappears within 24 hours.[11] The rash may appear as bullae, necrotic lesions (see **Fig. 1**B), or deep bruising (see **Fig. 1**C).

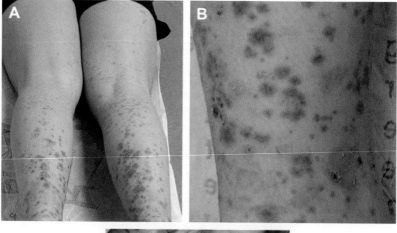

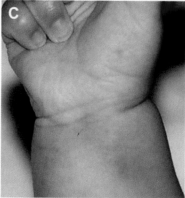

Fig. 1. Skin lesions of HSP: (*A*) classic lower extremity purpura, (*B*) necrotic lesions, (*C*) deep bruising. (*Courtesy of* David D. Sherry, MD, Philadelphia, PA.)

Arthritis affects three-quarters of children, and the most commonly affected joints are the knees and ankles. The arthritis is usually oligoarticular, self-limited, and nondestructive. It is the presenting symptom in 15% of patients.[12]

The gastrointestinal (GI) manifestations of HSP affect 50% to 75% of children and may include bleeding, intussusception, and abdominal pain. GI manifestations may precede the purpura by up to 2 weeks in as many as 20% of children.[11] Intestinal bleeding, manifested as gross or occult blood per rectum, occurs in approximately one-third of children. Intussusception occurs in 1% to 5% of children and is mostly ileo-ileal in location.[13]

Renal disease affects 20% to 60% of children, and the most common manifestation is microscopic hematuria with or without proteinuria. Renal disease rarely precedes the onset of rash. Children may present with nephritic or nephrotic syndrome, or rarely renal failure. Most children who develop renal disease do so within the first 6 weeks and 97% within 6 months.[14] In longitudinal studies of unselected patients, the risk of chronic renal impairment and end-stage renal disease is 2% to 15% and less than 1%, respectively.[14,15]

Unusual clinical manifestations of HSP may include edema of scrotum, eyes, or hands; pulmonary hemorrhage; seizures; stroke; and mental status changes. The mean duration of symptoms is 3 to 4 weeks and up to one-third of children have at least 1 recurrence.[16]

HSP must be distinguished from other causes of purpura in childhood, including acute hemorrhagic edema of infancy, immune thrombocytopenic purpura, acute poststreptococcal glomerulonephritis, hemolytic-uremic syndrome, disseminated intravascular coagulation, infections, and hypersensitivity vasculitis. Hypersensitivity vasculitis is also known as cutaneous leukocytoclastic vasculitis and microscopic polyarteritis. It typically affects the small vessels and is idiopathic or triggered by infection or drug exposure. Clinical manifestations include urticaria, purpura, or a maculopapular rash, arthralgias, hypocomplementemia, and elevated inflammatory markers (**Fig. 2**).

Treatment

Therapy for mild HSP cases is primarily supportive, with analgesics and nonsteroidal anti-inflammatory drugs. Current literature, however, supports the notion that in the

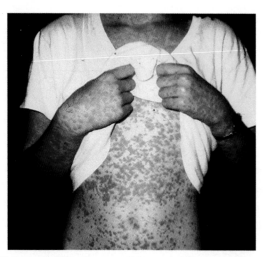

Fig. 2. Hypersensitivity vasculitis. Hypersentivity vasculitis secondary to propylthiouracil exposure. (*Courtesy of* David D. Sherry, MD, Philadelphia, PA.)

hospital setting, early use of corticosteroids for HSP is associated with improved outcomes, particularly GI comorbidities.[17] In more severe hospitalized cases, pulse methylprednisolone (30 mg/kg up to 1 g) may be warranted. The optimal dose and duration of corticosteroids has not been well studied. In some cases, oral corticosteroid doses of 2 mg/kg per day may be adequate; however, too short a course of corticosteroids or a rapid tapering of corticosteroids may precipitate a flare of symptoms. Corticosteroid treatment for mild cases of HSP remains controversial. A meta-analysis of 15 studies of patients with HSP treated at diagnosis with corticosteroids versus supportive care revealed that corticosteroid treatment significantly reduced the mean resolution time of abdominal pain and reduced the odds of developing persistent renal disease.[18] In a 6-month prospective clinical trial of 223 children, prednisone was effective in reducing the severity of abdominal and joint pain and in treating renal disease[19]; however, in that same study, prophylaxis with prednisone did not prevent the development of nephritis.[19] In life-threatening cases or acute renal failure, plasmapheresis followed by a more potent immunosuppressive agent, such as cyclophosphamide, azathioprine, or cyclosporine, should be considered.

Kawasaki Disease

Etiology and epidemiology

KD is the second most common childhood vasculitis, accounting for 23% of all vasculitides.[6] It affects primarily medium-sized blood vessels and is also known as mucocutaneous lymph node syndrome. The EULAR/PReS classification criteria for KD are listed in **Box 3**. Fewer than 4 criteria are required if there are characteristic coronary artery changes and fever[7]; 90% of cases occur in children younger than 5 years. In the United States, the annual incidence in children younger than 5 years is 20 per 100,000.[20] The incidence is higher among children who live in eastern Asia, at 100 per 100,000 in Japan[21] and 69 per 100,000 in Taiwan.[22] Similar to HSP, KD is more common in boys. Children younger than 6 months are more likely to have atypical features and to develop coronary aneurysms. The cause of KD remains unknown, although bacterial and viral infections, superantigens, genetics, and humoral factors, such as antiendothelial cell antibodies, ANCA, and circulating immune complexes may be involved.

Clinical presentation

KD is a triphasic disease consisting of an acute febrile period that lasts up to 14 days, a subacute phase of 2 to 4 weeks, and a convalescent phase that can last months to

---

Box 3
EULAR/PReS classification criteria for KD

Fever that persists for at least 5 days plus at least 4 of the following:

1. Bilateral conjunctival injection

2. Changes of the lips and oral cavity

3. Cervical lymphadenopathy

4. Polymorphous exanthem

5. Changes in the peripheral extremities or perineal area

Data from Ozen S, Pistorio A, Iusan SM, et al. EULAR/PRINTO/PRES criteria for Henoch-Schönlein purpura, childhood polyarteritis nodosa, childhood Wegener granulomatosis and childhood Takayasu arteritis: Ankara 2008. Part II: final classification criteria. Ann Rheum Dis 2010; 69:798–806.

years. The acute period is characterized by a persistent and high (>38.5° C) fever. The fever is typically minimally responsive to antipyretics. The fever is likely related to elevated concentrations of proinflammatory cytokines, particularly interleukin-6 and tumor necrosis factor alpha (TNF-α).[23] Conjunctivitis affects 85% of children and is bilateral, nonexudative, and limbic sparing. Other ocular symptoms include anterior uveitis, keratitis, papilledema, vitreous opacities, and subconjunctival hemorrhages (**Fig. 3**A).[24] Oral mucosal changes may include dry and cracked lips and strawberry tongue. Cervical adenopathy is the least common of the diagnostic criteria, detectable in 25% of children.[25] The adenopathy is usually unilateral and limited to the anterior cervical chain (see **Fig. 3**B). Diffuse lymphadenopathy is unusual. The rash associated with KD is typically nonpruritic, macular, or target lesions on the trunk and extremities. A perineal rash that desquamates by the end of the first week is common. Early extremity changes include diffuse erythema of the palms and soles and swelling of the dorsum of the hands and feet (see **Fig. 3**C); these changes usually last for fewer than 3 days. Sheetlike desquamation on the fingers and toes occurs toward the end of the acute phase.

There are also many symptoms of KD that are not part of diagnostic criteria. GI symptoms include diarrhea, vomiting, abdominal pain, and hydrops of the gallbladder. Genitourinary symptoms include scrotal pain and swelling, dysuria, and sterile pyuria. Arthritis affects up to 25% of children[26] and the most commonly affected joints are the knees, ankles, and hips. The arthritis can be oligoarticular or polyarticular and is usually self-limited and nondestructive. Most children with KD are very irritable, likely secondary to aseptic meningitis and headache.[27]

Cardiovascular disease during the acute phase may include valvulitis, myocarditis, and pericarditis. Coronary dilation and aneurysms may be detected during the acute phase, but most develop during the convalescent phase. Up to 10% of children who

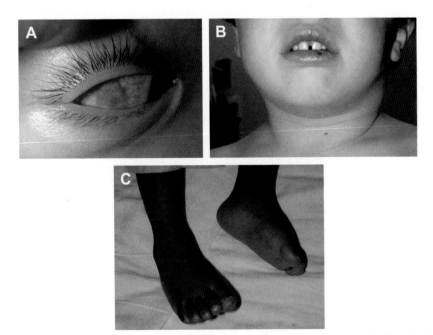

Fig. 3. Kawasaki disease: (*A*) subconjunctival hemorrhage; (*B*) unilateral cervical lymphadenopathy; (*C*) pedal edema. (*Courtesy of* Jon M. Burnham, MD, MSCE, Philadelphia, PA.)

develop coronary changes do not meet full criteria for KD.[28] As many as 20% of untreated children develop aneurysms. Treatment with intravenous immunoglobulin (IVIG) reduces the incidence of aneurysms by approximately 80%.[29] Children younger than 12 months are at the highest risk for coronary aneurysms.

Several conditions can mimic KD, including infections (Epstein-Barr virus, adenovirus, echovirus, measles), toxin-mediated illnesses (toxic shock syndrome, scarlet fever), inflammatory conditions (systemic juvenile idiopathic arthritis, polyarteritis nodosa), hypersensitivity reactions (mercury), and drug reactions (Stevens-Johnson syndrome).

Treatment

The goal of treatment in KD is to reduce inflammation and prevent the formation of coronary aneurysms. The American Heart Association (AHA) recommends treatment with high-dose aspirin (80–100 mg/kg per day) and IVIG (2 g/kg) within the first 10 days of disease.[30] Once afebrile for 48 hours, the aspirin should be adjusted to an anti-platelet dosage of 3 to 5 mg/kg per day. Although corticosteroids are the cornerstone of therapy for most vasculitides, their use in KD for the primary treatment of KD is controversial.[31,32] Approximately 10% to 15% of patients fail to respond to initial IVIG therapy; failure is defined as persistent fever or recurrence of fever within 36 hours of IVIG therapy. Persistent or recurring fever is concerning because it likely indicates ongoing inflammation and is associated with an increased risk of developing coronary aneurysms.[33] In a small multicenter randomized prospective trial of a second IVIG infusion versus infliximab, an anti–TNF-α agent (5 mg/kg), for refractory KD, there were no statistically significant differences between the 2 treatment groups in recurrence of fever, coronary artery outcomes, or laboratory markers of inflammation.[34] Current AHA guidelines, however, recommend re-dosing IVIG at least once in the event of IVIG failure.[30] If 2 or more doses of IVIG are ineffective, then corticosteroid pulse therapy (30 mg/kg for 1–3 doses) or treatment with infliximab (5 mg/kg) should be considered.[30] For uncomplicated KD, an echocardiogram should be performed at diagnosis, at 2 weeks, and then again at 6 to 8 weeks to assess treatment efficacy for the prevention of aneurysm formation.[30]

Polyarteritis Nodosa

PAN is the third most common childhood vasculitis. PAN is predominantly a medium-sized vasculitis and accounts for 3% of all childhood vasculitides in the United States.[6] Classification of childhood-onset PAN is listed in **Box 4**. Similar to HSP, several

---

Box 4
EULAR/PReS classification criteria for childhood PAN

Systemic inflammation with evidence of necrotizing vasculitis or angiographic abnormalities of medium-sized or small-sized arteries plus 1 of the following:

1. Skin involvement (livedo reticularis, nodules, infarcts)

2. Myalgias

3. Hypertension

4. Peripheral neuropathy

5. Renal involvement (proteinuria, hematuria, or impaired function)

Data from Ozen S, Pistorio A, Iusan SM, et al. EULAR/PRINTO/PRES criteria for Henoch-Schönlein purpura, childhood polyarteritis nodosa, childhood Wegener granulomatosis and childhood Takayasu arteritis: Ankara 2008. Part II: final classification criteria. Ann Rheum Dis 2010; 69:798–806.

reports suggest an association with familial mediterranean fever. Peak age of onset in children is 9 years.[35] In adults, PAN is classically associated with hepatitis B; however, this association is less common in childhood. Childhood PAN is associated with fewer relapses and improved survival compared with adult-onset disease.[35]

PAN can affect the vascular supply to any organ, although the lungs are typically spared. Vascular insufficiency is most common to the skin, muscles, kidneys, and GI tract. Involvement of the heart, and peripheral and central nervous systems are less common. Children may have fever, malaise, weight loss, myalgias, and arthralgias at presentation. Depending on the distribution of involved vessels, children may have hypertension, ischemic heart disease, testicular pain, abdominal pain, hematuria, or proteinuria. Neurologic involvement may include mononeuritis multiplex with both sensory and motor deficits. Inflammation of the small arteries leads to vasculitic skin rashes, including livedo reticularis, purpura, necrosis, and possibly digital gangrene (see **Fig. 4**A and B). Painful subcutaneous nodules along affected vessels are also a characteristic feature. Laboratory markers of systemic inflammation are usually elevated.

There have not been any randomized clinical trials to compare different induction or maintenance therapies for childhood systemic PAN. Therefore, treatment is primarily based on clinical experience and adult studies. Corticosteroids (1–2 mg/kg per day with or without initial corticosteroid pulses of 30 mg/kg) are the cornerstone of therapy. Additional therapy with cyclophosphamide (oral: 2 mg/kg per day, or IV: 750 mg/m^2 monthly) may be warranted during the induction phase. In life-threatening or organ-threatening situations, plasmapheresis is indicated. Maintenance agents include azathioprine, methotrexate, IVIG, and mycophenolate mofetil. More recently, the efficacies of biologic agents and rituximab have been explored.[36]

Cutaneous PAN is limited to the skin and musculoskeletal system. Characteristic features include fever, painful subcutaneous nodules, purpura, livedo reticularis, myalgias, arthralgias, and nondestructive arthritis. The skin manifestations are usually limited to the lower extremities. Cutaneous PAN is often associated with antecedent streptococcal infection.[37] Nonsteroidal anti-inflammatory drugs and corticosteroids are the mainstay of therapy. In cases of persistent or relapsing disease, steroid-sparing agents, such as methotrexate, colchicine, and IVIG have been used. Cutaneous PAN rarely evolves into systemic PAN.

Takayasu Arteritis

TA is a granulomatous vasculitis that predominantly affects the aorta and its major branches. The EULAR/PReS consensus criteria for childhood TA are listed in

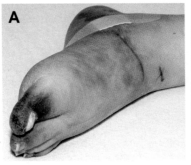 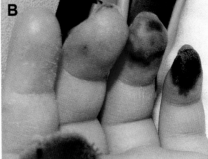

Fig. 4. Polyarteritis nodosa. Digital necrosis of toes (*A*) and fingers (*B*) from PAN. (*Courtesy of* David D. Sherry, MD, Philadelphia, PA.)

Box 5.[7] Most children are diagnosed during adolescence, with a mean age of 13 years.[38] It is more common in females than males (3:1).[38] The most commonly involved vessels in children are the aorta and renal, subclavian, and carotid arteries.[38]

Early diagnosis of TA in children is challenging, because the presenting symptoms are usually nonspecific. The most common complaints at diagnosis are headache (84%), dizziness (37%), abdominal pain (37%), claudication of the extremities (32%), fever (26%), and weight loss (10%).[38] Other early indicators of disease are night sweats, back pain, myalgias, and arthralgias. Hypertension is present in approximately 90% of children at diagnosis.[38] If left untreated, more specific disease manifestations develop and are determined by the distribution of vessel involvement. Involvement of the aortic arch or its major branches is associated with central nervous system (CNS) symptoms, claudication, absent peripheral pulses, and cardiac manifestations. CNS involvement may include headache, ischemic strokes, cerebral aneurysms, and seizures. Cardiac manifestations may include cardiomyopathy, congestive heart disease, and valvular disease. Involvement of the mid-aorta is associated with hypertension, abdominal pain, and lower extremity claudication.

Once TA is suspected, imaging often helps to confirm the diagnosis. The gold standard for TA imaging is angiography; however, it is invasive and cannot detect thickened vessel walls, an early sign of inflammation. CT and MR angiograms are less invasive than conventional angiography and can detect luminal diameter changes (**Fig. 5**A) and vessel wall thickening (see **Fig. 5**B).[39]

Treatment of TA is challenging. Corticosteroids may induce remission in up to 60% of patients; however, half of these patients flare with tapering.[40] There are anecdotal reports of treatment with methotrexate, azathioprine, and biologics, such as infliximab. Cyclophosphamide should be considered for life-threatening or organ-threatening cases.

Childhood Primary Central Nervous System Vasculitis

Previously healthy children with childhood primary central nervous system vasculitis (cPACNS) may present with devastating subacute-onset or acute-onset neurologic changes and psychiatric symptoms. If the disease is diagnosed early, the inflammation and neurologic damage may be reversible. The Calabrese criteria, designed for adults, requires a new neurologic deficit plus angiographic or histologic evidence of

---

Box 5
EULAR/PReS classification criteria for childhood-onset TA

Characteristic angiographic abnormalities of the aorta or its main branches and pulmonary arteries plus 1 of the following:

1. Absent peripheral pulses or claudication

2. Blood pressure discrepancy in any limb

3. Bruits

4. Hypertension

5. Elevated acute phase reactants

Data from Ozen S, Pistorio A, Iusan SM, et al. EULAR/PRINTO/PRES criteria for Henoch-Schönlein purpura, childhood polyarteritis nodosa, childhood Wegener granulomatosis and childhood Takayasu arteritis: Ankara 2008. Part II: final classification criteria. Ann Rheum Dis 2010; 69:798–806.

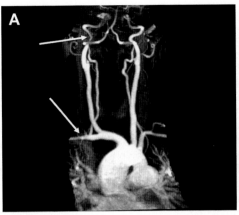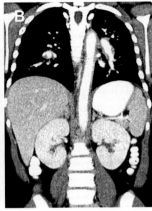

Fig. 5. Takayasu arteritis. (*A*) Contrast-enhanced MR angiography demonstrating narrowed right internal carotid and subclavian arteries. (*B*) Thoracoabdominal CT angiography demonstrating thickening of the aortic wall.

CNS vasculitis.[41] Two subtypes of cPACNS are recognized: (1) angiography-positive cPACNS, which affects the medium and large vessels, and (2) angiography-negative cPACNS, which primarily affects the small vessels. Children with angiography-positive cPACNS typically present with focal neurologic symptoms, such as unilateral sensory or motor deficits. Systemic inflammatory markers and cerebrospinal fluid (CSF) analysis may be normal.[42] The classic MR imaging (MRI) finding is a focal area of acute ischemia in a vascular distribution. Diagnosis is confirmed by conventional angiography or MR angiography, which demonstrates large-sized or medium-sized vessel stenosis, tortuosity, beading, or occlusion.

Angiography-positive cPACNS is further defined as progressive or nonprogressive, based on the appearance of new lesions 3 months after diagnosis. Diffuse neurologic symptoms, such as headaches, cognitive dysfunction, and behavioral issues, are more common in progressive disease.[43] Progressive disease also tends to be multifocal. The treatment of nonprogressive cPACNS is controversial but may include anticoagulation and corticosteroids. Corticosteroids may help prevent recurrence and improve neurologic recovery.[44] Treatment of progressive cPACNS includes 6 months of induction therapy with cyclophosphamide (500–750 mg/m^2 per month) and corticosteroids (2 mg/kg per day initially) followed by maintenance therapy with mycophenolate mofetil or azathioprine for 18 months.[45]

Angiography-negative cPACNS may present with systemic features, including fever and malaise in addition to diffuse or focal neurologic symptoms.[43] Systemic inflammatory markers may be normal but CSF analysis typically reveals pleocytosis, elevated protein, or increased opening pressure. MRI findings are usually multifocal and may can be unilateral or bilateral and involve the gray or white matter.[43] Leptomeningeal enhancement on imaging can help to distinguish this disease from demyelinating conditions. Conventional angiography, by definition, is negative. If cPACNS is suspected, then a brain biopsy must be performed to confirm the diagnosis. Typical histologic findings are a lymphocytic and nongranulomatous vasculitis.[46,47] Treatment of angiography-negative cPACNS includes 6 months of induction therapy with cyclophosphamide (500–750 mg/m^2) and corticosteroids (2 mg/kg per day initially) followed by maintenance therapy with mycophenolate mofetil or azathioprine for 18 months.[45,46]

ANCA-vasculitis

The ANCA-associated vasculitides (AAV) are a group of pediatric conditions classified by small-vessel and medium-vessel inflammation, multiorgan system involvement, and potentially life-threatening disease. They are associated with a high frequency of disease-related and treatment-related morbidities. The 3 classic vasculitides in the AAV group are GPA (formerly known as Wegener's granulomatosis), microscopic polyangiitis (MPA), and Churg-Strauss syndrome (CSS). In the acute phase of disease, the major comorbid conditions may include pulmonary hemorrhage, respiratory failure, rapidly progressive glomerular nephritis, and acute renal failure. Untreated AAV follows a severe course, with near 100% mortality[48] and a mean survival of 5 months.[49] In addition, renal failure at presentation confers a high risk of end-stage renal disease and death despite potent immunosuppressive therapy.[50] Relapses are very common and occur in up to 60% of patients.[51,52] In comparison with adults, children are more likely to have multiple organ involvement, renal involvement, and subglottic stenosis.[53,54]

GPA primarily affects the upper and lower respiratory tracts and the kidneys. The pediatric GPA classification criteria are listed in **Box 6**.[7] The median age of diagnosis in childhood-onset disease is 14 years.[53] Constitutional symptoms, such as fever, malaise, and weight loss are present in 90% of children at diagnosis.[53] Eighty percent have pulmonary manifestations that may include pulmonary hemorrhage, nodules, infiltrates, pleurisy, oxygen dependency, and respiratory failure (**Fig. 6**A).[53] Eighty percent have upper respiratory disease that may include oral or nasal ulcerations, nasal septum perforation (with subsequent saddle nose deformity), recurrent epistaxis, sinusitis, mastoiditis, hearing loss, and subglottic stenosis (see **Fig. 6**B).[53] Seventy-five percent have renal involvement that may include hematuria, proteinuria, glomerulonephritis, and kidney failure.[53] The renal disease is classically necrotizing and pauci-immune on biopsy. Ninety percent of patients with GPA are ANCA positive, and 80% to 90% of those patients are cytoplasmic-ANCA (c-ANCA)/pr3-positive.[55] Biopsy of inflamed tissue is helpful to confirm the diagnosis.

MPA is a necrotizing, nongranulomatous, pauci-immune disease that affects the small vessels. The most common features of MPA include pulmonary capillaritis and necrotizing glomerulonephritis. Almost all children have constitutional symptoms,

---

Box 6
EULAR/PReS classification criteria for childhood-onset GPA

Diagnosis requires 3 of the following 6 criteria:

1. Histopathological evidence of granulomatous inflammation

2. Upper airway involvement

3. Laryngo-tracheo-bronchial involvement

4. Pulmonary involvement (by radiograph or CT)

5. ANCA positivity

6. Renal involvement (proteinuria, hematuria, red blood cell casts, necrotizing pauci-immune glomerulonephritis)

Data from Ozen S, Pistorio A, Iusan SM, et al. EULAR/PRINTO/PRES criteria for Henoch-Schönlein purpura, childhood polyarteritis nodosa, childhood Wegener granulomatosis and childhood Takayasu arteritis: Ankara 2008. Part II: final classification criteria. Ann Rheum Dis 2010; 69:798–806.

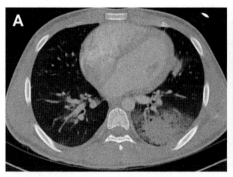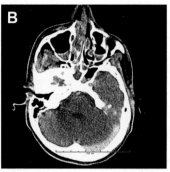

Fig. 6. Granulomatosis with polyangiitis. (*A*) Contrast-enhanced CT of the chest demonstrating pulmonary nodules and infiltrates. (*B*) Contrast-enhanced CT of head showing diffuse sinus disease.

such as fever, malaise, arthralgias, myalgias, and weight loss.[56] One-third of children present with renal failure, and nearly 100% have renal disease that may include hypertension, hematuria, or proteinuria.[56] Ischemic cerebral insults (30%) and necrotizing vasculitic lesions of the skin (30%) are common.[56] MPA is associated with a high titer of c-ANCA or peri-nuclear ANCA.

CSS is a granulomatous vasculitis of small-sized and medium-sized vessels that primarily affects individuals with severe asthma or allergies. Pediatric-specific criteria for CSS do not exist. The American College of Rheumatology (ACR) disease criteria for adult-onset disease are listed in **Box 7**. CSS usually has an insidious onset over years. The most common features in children at diagnosis are asthma (91%), pulmonary infiltrates (85%), sinusitis (77%), skin involvement (66%), cardiac disease (55%), GI symptoms (40%), peripheral neuropathy (39%), and kidney disease (16%).[57] Vasculitic skin rashes are also common. The renal disease is usually mild and rarely progresses.[58] Twenty-five percent of children are ANCA-positive.

Treatment regimens for AAV depend on the specific type of vasculitis and the end-organ manifestations. Almost all knowledge about the optimal treatment and outcomes of children with AAV have been adapted from adult studies or come from a small collection of case series. Standard induction therapy for adults with severe systemic AAV includes corticosteroids and cyclophosphamide (oral or IV).[59] This regimen, however, is suboptimal, as there are not only significant treatment-related toxicities, including serious infection, hemorrhagic cystitis, infertility, and malignancy,

---

Box 7
ACR classification criteria for adult-onset CSS

Diagnosis requires 4 of the following:

1. History of asthma

2. History of allergies (seasonal, foods, contact)

3. Peripheral eosinophilia greater than 10%

4. Mononeuropathy or polyneuropathy

5. Migratory pulmonary infiltrates

6. Paranasal sinus pain or radiographic opacification

7. Biopsy demonstrating extravascular eosinophils

but, in addition, a high risk of relapse.[51,52] Recent studies in adults, therefore, have examined the role of biologic medications and plasmapheresis as adjunct therapy in an effort to find strategies with comparable efficacy, lower toxicity, and fewer relapses. Methotrexate and corticosteroids are used for induction in milder cases. Maintenance therapy is typically with mycophenolate mofetil or azathioprine for 18 to 24 months. Infliximab (5 mg/kg twice a month), rituximab (375 mg/m^2 per week for 4 weeks), and IVIG (2 g/kg per month) are options for refractory disease.

SUMMARY

Pediatric vasculitis is a challenging and complex group of conditions. The site of vessel involvement, size of the affected vessels, extent of vascular injury, and underlying pathology determine the disease phenotype and severity. The most common vasculitides are HSP and KD. Almost all knowledge about the optimal treatment and outcomes of children with vasculitis, with the exception of HSP and KD, have been adapted from adult studies or come from a small collection of case series. Early diagnosis, which requires a high level of clinical suspicion, may help to improve outcomes. Pediatricians should consider vasculitis as part of the differential diagnosis in children with evidence of systemic inflammation and multisystem disease that cannot be otherwise explained.

REFERENCES

1. Ozen S, Ruperto N, Dillon MJ, et al. EULAR/PReS endorsed consensus criteria for the classification of childhood vasculitides. Ann Rheum Dis 2006;65:936–41.
2. Gardner-Medwin JM, Dolezalova P, Cummins C, et al. Incidence of Henoch-Schönlein purpura, Kawasaki disease, and rare vasculitides in children of different ethnic origins. Lancet 2002;360:1197–202.
3. Natter M, Winsor J, Fox K, et al. The childhood arthritis & rheumatology research alliance network registry: demographics and characteristics of the initial 6-month cohort. In: Pediatric rheumatology symposium (PRSYM). Miami (FL): Rheumatology ACo; 2011. p. 43–4.
4. Denardo BA, Tucker LB, Miller LC, et al. Demography of a regional pediatric rheumatology patient population. Affiliated Children's Arthritis Centers of New England. J Rheumatol 1994;21:1553–61.
5. Malleson PN, Fung MY, Rosenberg AM. The incidence of pediatric rheumatic diseases: results from the Canadian Pediatric Rheumatology Association Disease Registry. J Rheumatol 1996;23:1981–7.
6. Bowyer S, Roettcher P. Pediatric rheumatology clinic populations in the United States: results of a 3 year survey. Pediatric Rheumatology Database Research Group. J Rheumatol 1996;23:1968.
7. Ozen S, Pistorio A, Iusan SM, et al. EULAR/PRINTO/PRES criteria for Henoch-Schönlein purpura, childhood polyarteritis nodosa, childhood Wegener granulomatosis and childhood Takayasu arteritis: Ankara 2008. Part II: final classification criteria. Ann Rheum Dis 2010;69:798–806.
8. Stefansson Thors V, Kolka R, Sigurdardottir SL, et al. Increased frequency of C4B*Q0 alleles in patients with Henoch-Schönlein purpura. Scand J Immunol 2005;61:274–8.
9. Gershoni-Baruch R, Broza Y, Brik R. Prevalence and significance of mutations in the familial Mediterranean fever gene in Henoch-Schönlein purpura. J Pediatr 2003;143:658–61.

10. Weiss PF, Klink AJ, Luan X, et al. Temporal association of *Streptococcus, Staphylococcus,* and parainfluenza pediatric hospitalizations and hospitalized cases of Henoch-Schönlein purpura. J Rheumatol 2010;37:2587–94.
11. Saulsbury FT. Henoch-Schönlein purpura in children. Report of 100 patients and review of the literature. Medicine (Baltimore) 1999;78:395–409.
12. Trapani S, Micheli A, Grisolia F, et al. Henoch Schönlein purpura in childhood: epidemiological and clinical analysis of 150 cases over a 5-year period and review of literature. Semin Arthritis Rheum 2005;35:143–53.
13. Saulsbury FT. Henoch-Schönlein purpura. Curr Opin Rheumatol 2010;22: 598–602.
14. Narchi H. Risk of long term renal impairment and duration of follow up recommended for Henoch-Schönlein purpura with normal or minimal urinary findings: a systematic review. Arch Dis Child 2005;90:916–20.
15. Stewart M, Savage JM, Bell B, et al. Long-term renal prognosis of Henoch-Schönlein purpura in an unselected childhood population. Eur J Pediatr 1988;147: 113–5.
16. Saulsbury FT. Epidemiology of Henoch-Schönlein purpura. Cleve Clin J Med 2002;69(Suppl 2):SII87–9.
17. Weiss PF, Klink AJ, Localio R, et al. Corticosteroids may improve clinical outcomes during hospitalization for Henoch-Schönlein purpura. Pediatrics 2010;126:674–81.
18. Weiss PF, Feinstein JA, Luan X, et al. Effects of corticosteroid on Henoch-Schönlein purpura: a systematic review. Pediatrics 2007;120:1079–87.
19. Jauhola O, Ronkainen J, Koskimies O, et al. Renal manifestations of Henoch-Schönlein purpura in a 6-month prospective study of 223 children. Arch Dis Child 2010;95:877–82.
20. Holman RC, Belay ED, Christensen KY, et al. Hospitalizations for Kawasaki syndrome among children in the United States, 1997–2007. Pediatr Infect Dis J 2010;29:483–8.
21. Yanagawa H, Nakamura Y, Yashiro M, et al. Results of the nationwide epidemiologic survey of Kawasaki disease in 1995 and 1996 in Japan. Pediatrics 1998; 102:E65.
22. Huang WC, Huang LM, Chang IS, et al. Epidemiologic features of Kawasaki disease in Taiwan, 2003–2006. Pediatrics 2009;123:e401–5.
23. Leung DY. The potential role of cytokine-mediated vascular endothelial activation in the pathogenesis of Kawasaki disease. Acta Paediatr Jpn 1991;33:739–44.
24. Kumagai N, Ohno S. Kawasaki disease. In: Holland G, Wilhelmus K, editors. Ocular immunity and infection. St Louis (MO): Mosby; 1996.
25. Sung RY, Ng YM, Choi KC, et al. Lack of association of cervical lymphadenopathy and coronary artery complications in Kawasaki disease. Pediatr Infect Dis J 2006; 25:521–5.
26. Melish ME. Kawasaki syndrome: a 1986 perspective. Rheum Dis Clin North Am 1987;13:7–17.
27. Dengler LD, Capparelli EV, Bastian JF, et al. Cerebrospinal fluid profile in patients with acute Kawasaki disease. Pediatr Infect Dis J 1998;17:478–81.
28. Sundel RP. Update on the treatment of Kawasaki disease in childhood. Curr Rheumatol Rep 2002;4:474–82.
29. Newburger JW, Takahashi M, Burns JC, et al. The treatment of Kawasaki syndrome with intravenous gamma globulin. N Engl J Med 1986;315:341–7.
30. Newburger JW, Takahashi M, Gerber MA, et al. Diagnosis, treatment, and long-term management of Kawasaki disease: a statement for health professionals

from the Committee on Rheumatic Fever, Endocarditis, and Kawasaki Disease, Council on Cardiovascular Disease in the Young, American Heart Association. Pediatrics 2004;114:1708–33.

31. Newburger JW, Sleeper LA, McCrindle BW, et al. Randomized trial of pulsed corticosteroid therapy for primary treatment of Kawasaki disease. N Engl J Med 2007;356:663–75.

32. Sundel RP, Baker AL, Fulton DR, et al. Corticosteroids in the initial treatment of Kawasaki disease: report of a randomized trial. J Pediatr 2003;142:611–6.

33. Beiser AS, Takahashi M, Baker AL, et al. A predictive instrument for coronary artery aneurysms in Kawasaki disease. US Multicenter Kawasaki Disease Study Group. Am J Cardiol 1998;81:1116–20.

34. Burns JC, Best BM, Mejias A, et al. Infliximab treatment of intravenous immunoglobulin-resistant Kawasaki disease. J Pediatr 2008;153:833–8.

35. Ozen S, Anton J, Arisoy N, et al. Juvenile polyarteritis: results of a multicenter survey of 110 children. J Pediatr 2004;145:517–22.

36. Eleftheriou D, Melo M, Marks SD, et al. Biologic therapy in primary systemic vasculitis of the young. Rheumatology 2009;48:978–86.

37. David J, Ansell BM, Woo P. Polyarteritis nodosa associated with streptococcus. Arch Dis Child 1993;69:685–8.

38. Cakar N, Yalcinkaya F, Duzova A, et al. Takayasu arteritis in children. J Rheumatol 2008;35:913–9.

39. Kissin EY, Merkel PA. Diagnostic imaging in Takayasu arteritis. Curr Opin Rheumatol 2004;16:31–7.

40. Kerr GS, Hallahan CW, Giordano J, et al. Takayasu arteritis. Ann Intern Med 1994; 120:919–29.

41. Calabrese LH, Furlan AJ, Gragg LA, et al. Primary angiitis of the central nervous system: diagnostic criteria and clinical approach. Cleve Clin J Med 1992;59:293–306.

42. Benseler SM, Silverman E, Aviv RI, et al. Primary central nervous system vasculitis in children. Arthritis Rheum 2006;54:1291–7.

43. Cellucci T, Benseler SM. Central nervous system vasculitis in children. Curr Opin Rheumatol 2010;22:590–7.

44. Soon G, Yau I, Branson H, et al. Nonprogressive primary CNS vasculitis in children: immunosuppression reduces recurrent ischemic event risk. Arthritis & Rheumatism 2008;58(S9):s942.

45. Sen ES, Leone V, Abinun M, et al. Treatment of primary angiitis of the central nervous system in childhood with mycophenolate mofetil. Rheumatology 2010;49:806–11.

46. Benseler SM, deVeber G, Hawkins C, et al. Angiography-negative primary central nervous system vasculitis in children: a newly recognized inflammatory central nervous system disease. Arthritis Rheum 2005;52:2159–67.

47. Elbers J, Halliday W, Hawkins C, et al. Brain biopsy in children with primary small-vessel central nervous system vasculitis. Ann Neurol 2010;68(5):602–10.

48. Cassidy JT, Petty RE, Laxer RM, et al. Textbook of pediatric rheumatology. 6th ed. Philadelphia: Saunders Elsevier; 2011.

49. Walton EW. Giant-cell granuloma of the respiratory tract (Wegener's granulomatosis). Br Med J 1958;2:265–70.

50. Jayne DR, Gaskin G, Rasmussen N, et al. Randomized trial of plasma exchange or high-dosage methylprednisolone as adjunctive therapy for severe renal vasculitis. J Am Soc Nephrol 2007;18:2180–8.

51. Nachman PH, Hogan SL, Jennette JC, et al. Treatment response and relapse in antineutrophil cytoplasmic autoantibody-associated microscopic polyangiitis and glomerulonephritis. J Am Soc Nephrol 1996;7:33–9.

52. Wegener's Granulomatosis Etanercept Trial (WGET) Research Group. Etanercept plus standard therapy for Wegener's granulomatosis. N Engl J Med 2005;352: 351–61.
53. Cabral DA, Uribe AG, Benseler S, et al. Classification, presentation, and initial treatment of Wegener's granulomatosis in childhood. Arthritis Rheum 2009;60: 3413–24.
54. Akikusa JD, Schneider R, Harvey EA, et al. Clinical features and outcome of pediatric Wegener's granulomatosis. Arthritis Rheum 2007;57:837–44.
55. Hoffman GS, Specks U. Antineutrophil cytoplasmic antibodies. Arthritis Rheum 1998;41:1521–37.
56. Peco-Antic A, Bonaci-Nikolic B, Basta-Jovanovic G, et al. Childhood microscopic polyangiitis associated with MPO-ANCA. Pediatr Nephrol 2006;21:46–53.
57. Zwerina J, Eger G, Englbrecht M, et al. Churg-Strauss syndrome in childhood: a systematic literature review and clinical comparison with adult patients. Semin Arthritis Rheum 2009;39:108–15.
58. Lanham JG, Elkon KB, Pusey CD, et al. Systemic vasculitis with asthma and eosinophilia: a clinical approach to the Churg-Strauss syndrome. Medicine 1984;63:65–81.
59. Molloy ES, Langford CA. Advances in the treatment of small vessel vasculitis. Rheum Dis Clin North Am 2006;32:157–72, x.

Kawasaki Disease

Rosie Scuccimarri, MD, FRCPC

KEYWORDS

- Kawasaki disease • Coronary artery • Aneurysm
- Intravenous immunoglobulin • Vasculitis
- Mucocutaneous lymph node syndrome

HISTORICAL PERSPECTIVES

Kawasaki disease (KD) is a systemic vasculitis of unknown cause and the leading cause of acquired heart disease in North American and Japanese children.[1,2] This disease was first reported in 1967 by Dr Tomisaku Kawasaki.[3] His original case series of pediatric acute mucocutaneous lymph node syndrome described 50 Japanese patients with the clinical signs and symptoms that we now refer to as KD.[3] In 1965, Dr Noboru Tanaka was the first pathologist to recognize the potentially serious and fatal complications of this disease when he discovered coronary artery thrombosis in a child who died unexpectedly.[4] Dr Takajiro Yamamoto was the first physician to note cardiac complications in nonfatal cases.[4,5] He described electrocardiogram abnormalities in these patients and published this finding in a report in 1968.[4,5]

In 1970, the first Japanese nationwide epidemiologic survey of KD was undertaken.[6] This study clearly established the link between KD and coronary vasculitis.[4,6] Although KD was first described in Japan, similar cases were being seen around the world in the 1960s and 1970s.[4] The first North American description was published in 1976 from Hawaii.[7]

EPIDEMIOLOGY

There have been 20 nationwide epidemiologic surveys of KD in Japan. The average annual incidence in 2005 and 2006 was 184.6 per 100 000 children less than 5 years of age.[8] In 2008, in the latest survey, the incidence increased to 218.6 per 100 000 children less than 5 years of age.[9] The latest incidence is even higher than the rates seen in the epidemic years of 1979, 1982, and 1986.[9] As in previous surveys, the incidence was highest in children aged 6 to 11 months.[9] Patients with affected siblings were seen in 1.4%; and 0.7% of patients had at least 1 parent with a previous history of KD.[9] Recurrence of the disease was seen in 3.5% of patients.[9]

KD has been described in more than 60 countries.[10] The annual incidence of KD is highest in Asian countries.[11] After Japan, Korea (105/100 000)[12] and Taiwan

Division of Pediatric Rheumatology, Department of Pediatrics, Montreal Children's Hospital, McGill University, 2300 Tupper, Room C-505, Montreal, Quebec H3H 1P3, Canada
E-mail address: rosie.scuccimarri@muhc.mcgill.ca

Pediatr Clin N Am 59 (2012) 425–445
doi:10.1016/j.pcl.2012.03.009
0031-3955/12/$ – see front matter

(68/100 000)[13] have the next highest incidences. It is presumed that the incidence is high in other Asian countries but cases may not be as well documented as in Japan.[11]

In the United States, the incidence in the year 2006 was estimated to be 20.8/100,000 in children less than 5 years of age.[14] Race-specific incidence rates showed that the disease was most common among Americans of Asian and Pacific Island descent.[14] In Ontario, the most populous province in Canada, the incidence increased over time from 14.4/100 000 in children less than 5 years of age in 1995 to 1997 to 26.2/100 000 in 2004 to 2006.[11] This is most likely because of better disease recognition over the years, particularly for incomplete cases.[11] In this study, a seasonal pattern was observed, with an increase in cases in the late fall and winter, similar to Japan.[11] The male/female ratio was 1.62:1.[11] Children less than 5 years of age made up 73% of cases seen.[11] Although race was not evaluated, Ontario has a large Asian population and it was suggested that the incidence of KD in Ontario, and possibly of Canada, may be one of the highest outside Asia.[11] Other reported incidences include Ireland (15.2/100 000),[15] England (8.1/100 000),[16] New Zealand (8.0/100 000),[17] and Australia (3.7/100 000).[18]

CAUSE

The cause of KD remains unknown. It is suspected that there is activation of the immune system by an infectious trigger in a genetically susceptible host.[19] An infectious cause is suspected for several reasons. First, the clinical characteristics of KD resemble an infection and the illness is self-limited.[20] Second, the epidemiologic features, such as age of affected children, seasonality of cases, and occurrence of community outbreaks and epidemics, are all consistent with an infectious trigger.[20] However, no known infectious agent has been consistently found. Genetics may explain why certain ethnicities are at increased risk.[20] This risk persists despite a move from 1 country to another.[21] As well, the risk of disease in a child born to a parent with a history of KD, or in siblings of affected children, is higher than in the general population.[22]

There is still significant controversy about the mechanism of immune system activation in patients with KD. Some investigators believe that a bacterial superantigen leads to massive stimulation of T lymphocytes.[23] Others suggest that an oligoclonal IgA immune response is occurring rather than a polyclonal one.[24] This theory is supported by the discovery of IgA plasma cells infiltrating the coronary artery aneurysms in patients who died in the acute phase of KD,[24,25] as well as the detection of viral-like cytoplasmic inclusion bodies in ciliated bronchial epithelial cells of patients with KD.[24,26]

Recent data have suggested that T-cell activation is important in determining the susceptibility and severity of KD.[19] A genetic association study identified a polymorphism in the inositol 1,4,5-triphosphate 3-kinase C (ITPKC) gene on chromosome 19q13.2, which acts as a negative regulator of T-cell activation and may contribute to immune hyperreactivity in KD.[27] This polymorphism was significantly associated with KD susceptibility, and with an increased risk of coronary artery abnormalities (CAA), in both Japanese and American children.[27] An animal mouse model of KD has also identified regulation of T-cell activation as a critical determinant of coronary disease.[19]

Multiple studies are under way to identify genetic markers that influence disease susceptibility, disease severity, and treatment resistance in KD. Genetic studies to date have made significant contributions to this field,[27–31] and it is hoped that with further studies, the cause of KD will also be elucidated.

CLINICAL, LABORATORY, AND CARDIAC FEATURES
Diagnostic Criteria

The diagnosis of KD is made clinically. There is currently no diagnostic test for this disease. Clinical criteria were established to help clinicians make the diagnosis of KD (**Box 1**).[20] The diagnostic criteria can be applied once other diseases with similar findings have been excluded (**Box 2**).[20,32] However, it is not uncommon to document a concomitant infection in patients with KD[33,34]; in 1 study, 33% of children diagnosed with typical KD had a confirmed concomitant infection.[33] Therefore, suspicion for KD needs to remain high, especially if the documented infection cannot explain all the clinical features.

The fever of KD is usually high and unresponsive to antibiotics, and often to antipyretics as well.[32] The clinical features may not all be present at 1 time and therefore, it is important to inquire about these features on history. At times, the diagnosis may become clear as one notes the evolution of symptoms over time. Therefore, it is important to reevaluate a child with a persistent fever or a fever without a focus or a child whose fever is not responding to antibiotics, because the diagnosis may become clear on reevaluation. If untreated, the febrile illness typically lasts 10 to 14 days.[32]

Conjunctivitis, oropharyngeal changes, and rash are the most common clinical features. The conjunctivitis is nonexudative and primarily involves the bulbar rather than the palpebral conjunctivae (**Fig. 1**A). Oropharyngeal changes may include erythema, cracking, fissuring, or bleeding of the lips (see **Fig. 1**B), strawberry tongue (see **Fig. 1**C), and diffuse erythema of the oropharynx without exudate. The rash is polymorphous. The most common rash is a nonspecific, diffuse maculopapular eruption.[20] Many different rashes have been described with KD, except for bullous or vesicular eruptions.[20] Accentuation of the rash in the perineal region with

---

Box 1
Diagnostic criteria and definitions

Classic/Complete KD:

- Fever for ≥5 days and ≥4 of the 5 following clinical criteria:
  - ○ Bilateral, nonexudative, bulbar conjunctivitis
  - ○ Oropharyngeal changes with any of the following:
    - ■ Strawberry tongue
    - ■ Diffuse erythema of the oropharyngeal mucosa
    - ■ Erythema or cracking of the lips
  - ○ Cervical lymphadenopathy (>1.5 cm diameter, usually unilateral)
  - ○ Polymorphous rash
  - ○ Peripheral extremity changes with any of the following:
    - ■ Erythema or edema of the palms or soles
    - ■ Periungal desquamation in the subacute phase

Incomplete KD:

- Fever ≥5 days with 2 or 3 of the above clinical criteria

Atypical KD:

- This term is used for patients who fulfill criteria for KD but who have a clinical feature that is not usually seen with KD (eg, a patient with KD with renal impairment)

Box 2
Differential diagnosis

Infectious:

Viruses: measles, adenovirus, Epstein-Barr virus, enterovirus, influenza, roseola infantum

Bacterial illnesses: cervical adenitis, scarlet fever, staphylococcal scalded skin syndrome, toxic shock syndrome, leptospirosis

Rickettsial illness: Rocky Mountain spotted fever

Immune-mediated:

Stevens-Johnson syndrome, serum sickness, rheumatic fever, systemic onset juvenile idiopathic arthritis, other systemic vasculitis (eg, polyarteritis nodosa), connective tissue diseases (eg, systemic lupus erythematosus)

Hereditary autoinflammatory syndromes:

Tumor necrosis factor (TNF) receptor associated periodic syndrome, hyper-IgD syndrome, cryopyrin-associated periodic syndrome

Poisoning:

Mercury

---

desquamation occurs frequently.[35] Unlike the periungual desquamation that occurs in the subacute phase (see later discussion), the perineal desquamation occurs during the acute phase.

Peripheral extremity changes can include erythema or edema of the palms or soles in the acute phase (**Fig. 2**A) and periungual desquamation in the subacute phase (see **Fig. 2**B). In 1 North American series, 68% had desquamation on follow-up and this correlated with having had peripheral extremity changes in the acute phase.[36] It is important to evaluate the periungual region even in the acute phase, because periungual lifting, or detachment of the skin beneath the nail plate (hyponychium) without frank desquamation, can occur within the febrile period and may help when evaluating a child with prolonged fever. Within 1 to 2 months after the onset of fever, a variety of

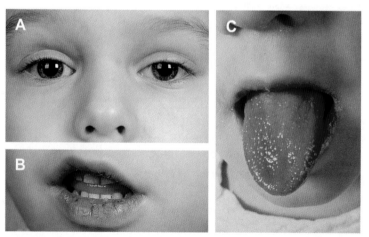

Fig. 1. (*A*) Bilateral, nonexudative, bulbar conjunctivitis. (*B*) Red, cracked lips. (*C*) Strawberry tongue. ([*C*] *From* Yoskovitch A, Tewfik TL, Duffy CM, et al. Head and neck manifestations of Kawasaki disease. Int J Pediatr Otorhinolaryngol 2000;52(2):125; with permission.)

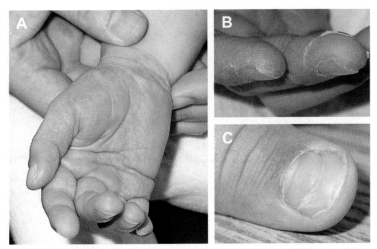

Fig. 2. Peripheral extremity changes. (*A*) Erythema and edema of the palm. (*B*) Peringual desquamation. (*C*) Beau's line. (*Courtesy of* Dr Gaëlle Chédeville.)

nail abnormalities have been described in these patients[37] of which Beau's lines (deep transverse grooves across the nails) are the most characteristic (see **Fig. 2**C).[20,32]

Cervical adenopathy is the least common clinical manifestation of KD.[20] It is usually unilateral, with a diameter greater than 1.5 cm, and the node is usually firm but non-fluctuant (**Fig. 3**). It can be confused with bacterial cervical adenitis and the diagnosis of KD needs to be considered in children with this diagnosis who are not responding to antibiotics. In 1 study, approximately 12% of patients had fever and cervical adenopathy as the initial presenting features of KD.[38]

Other Clinical Features

Other clinical features may be seen besides those included in the diagnostic criteria. These features may help support the diagnosis of KD. Severe irritability occurs commonly. Aseptic meningitis may also be seen.[20,32] Mild acute iridocyclitis or anterior uveitis may be noted on slit lamp examination.[39,40] Obtaining an ophthalmologic evaluation may be warranted in those who do not fulfill criteria. Arthritis and arthralgias can occur, and in 1 study, the reported prevalence of arthritis was 7.5%.[41] Oligoarticular and polyarticular involvement were almost equally observed.[41] In another study, gastrointestinal complaints including diarrhea, vomiting, and abdominal pain were seen in 61% of patients, and respiratory symptoms including rhinorrhea or cough were seen in 35%.[42] Otitis media or tympanitis can also be seen in KD[32,38] and may represent inflammation rather than infection. Urethritis or meatitis is common and may result in sterile pyuria.[32] Hydrops of the gallbladder occurs in approximately 15% of patients in the acute phase and can be seen on abdominal ultrasonography.[20,43] In those who do not fulfill diagnostic criteria, abdominal ultrasonography may also be useful in supporting the diagnosis of KD. Facial nerve palsies have been described.[44] Transient sensorineural hearing loss can also occur.[45–47] In countries where the BCG vaccine is administered, erythema and induration are commonly seen at the previous site of this vaccine.[48,49] Psoriatic skin eruptions can occur in both the acute and conva-lescent phases of KD.[50] Two of the potentially rare but devastating features of KD are peripheral gangrene[51] and macrophage activation syndrome.[52,53]

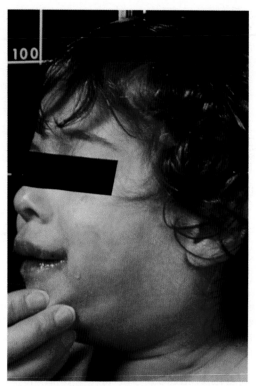

Fig. 3. Unilateral, cervical adenopathy. (*From* Yoskovitch A, Tewfik TL, Duffy CM, et al. Head and neck manifestations of Kawasaki disease. Int J Pediatr Otorhinolaryngol 2000;52(2): 126; with permission.)

Laboratory Findings

Results of laboratory investigations in the acute phase of KD are nonspecific; however, in children who do not fulfill diagnostic criteria, these may also help support the diagnosis. Acute phase reactants are almost always increased and include erythrocyte sedimentation rate (ESR) and C-reactive protein (CRP). In a child suspected of KD, if the acute phase reactants are not increased in the early febrile period, repeat testing usually shows this finding. Increased white blood cell count with a predominance of neutrophils is frequently seen. It is also not uncommon to see toxic granulations within the neutrophils.[54,55] Anemia may be seen especially with prolonged inflammation. A characteristic feature of KD is thrombocytosis; however, this finding usually occurs in the second week of the illness (subacute phase, see later discussion). Hypoalbuminemia is common, as are increased serum transaminase levels. Sterile pyuria can also be seen.

Leukopenia and thrombocytopenia are both rare in KD.[20] When seen, particularly in association with a lymphocytosis, a viral infection should be suspected.[20] Leukopenia and thrombocytopenia can be present in KD in association with macrophage activation syndrome.[52,53] Index of suspicion for this entity needs to be high given that this is a potentially fatal complication.[52,53] Although thrombocytopenia is uncommon at presentation in KD, it is considered a risk factor for the development of CAA.[56]

Cardiovascular biomarkers are being evaluated in KD. One such biomarker is *N*-terminal pro-B-type natriuretic peptide (NT-proBNP).[57,58] This biomarker is associated with cardiomyocyte stress.[58] It correlates with markers of inflammation, oxidative stress, and echocardiographic measurements, suggesting diastolic dysfunction.[58] Some investigators suggest that subclinical myocardial inflammation occurs to some degree in all patients with KD and therefore, NT-proBNP may be an excellent biomarker to help support the diagnosis of KD.[57] These investigators showed that NT-proBNP was increased in both patients with KD who fulfilled criteria and those who did not, compared with febrile controls.[57] They suggested that NT-proBNP may be a valid adjunctive diagnostic test in patients with KD particularly in those with incomplete diagnostic criteria.[57] Another study showed that NT-proBNP was increased in patients with KD who were developing CAA and therefore suggested that this could be a valuable tool for disease prognosis.[59]

Clinical Phases

KD has 3 clinical phases: acute, subacute, and convalescent. The acute phase begins with the onset of fever and ends with its resolution.[32] It usually lasts for a mean of 11 days (or shorter if therapy is instituted).[20] The subacute phase begins with the resolution of fever and ends when all clinical features resolve.[32] It typically begins 10 days into the illness and lasts for 2 weeks.[32] Thrombocytosis and periungual desquamation of the fingers or toes occur at this stage. The convalescent phase begins at the end of the subacute phase and continues until the sedimentation rate and platelet count return to normal, which is usually 4 to 8 weeks after the onset of illness.[32] This stage is when the nail abnormalities can be seen.

Cardiac Manifestations

Children suspected of having KD should be admitted to hospital and treated. During admission, all children with KD should undergo a two-dimensional echocardiogram and electrocardiogram. In the acute phase, the myocardium, pericardium, endocardium, valves, conduction system, and coronary arteries may all be involved.[20] Myocarditis, when present, occurs during the acute phase.[60] Myocarditis may present with tachycardia, gallop rhythm, electrocardiographic changes, or wall motion abnormalities on echocardiogram.[32,60] Other cardiovascular abnormalities include pericarditis,[60] valvulitis,[60,61] and involvement of the conduction system.[62]

KD shock syndrome is another cardiovascular manifestation that, when present, occurs in the acute phase.[63] Patients present with hypotension and a shocklike state.[63] They more often have left ventricular systolic dysfunction, mitral regurgitation, CAA, and resistance to treatment compared with hemodynamically normal patients with KD.[63]

CAA can occur in the acute phase and have been detected as early as 3 days from onset of illness.[64] However, CAA develop more commonly in the subacute phase.[64] They develop in approximately 20% of untreated children and are the most common cause of morbidity and mortality in this disease.[64] Two-dimensional echocardiography has been shown to be sensitive and specific in detecting aneurysms in the proximal portions of the right and left coronary arteries; isolated distal coronary artery aneurysms are uncommon.[65] Children with uncomplicated KD should undergo an echocardiogram at diagnosis, at 2 weeks, and 6 to 8 weeks after the onset of disease.[20] Repeat echocardiography should be considered optional beyond 8 weeks in those patients with previously normal studies.[20] More frequent echocardiograms are required in those with CAA.[20] These patients may eventually also require other investigations such as an angiogram (**Fig. 4**). Although KD has a predilection for the

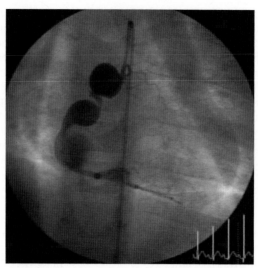

Fig. 4. Angiogram in a 2-year-old with 3 giant aneurysms of the right coronary artery. (*Courtesy of* Dr Nagib Dahdah.)

coronary arteries, other arteries may be involved, including the axillary, iliac, and renal arteries.[60,66]

Risk Factors for the Development of CAA

Many scoring systems have been developed to try to identify those who are at highest risk for the development of CAA, with the goal of using these to target treatment.[20] The scoring systems are imperfect and it is recommended that all children diagnosed with KD receive treatment.[20] Nonetheless, there are both clinical and laboratory findings that are associated with an increase risk of CAA in KD. The clinical features include male gender, extremes of age, prolonged fever, delay in diagnosis, and persistent fever after treatment.[32] The laboratory features include low hemoglobin, increased white blood cell count, high absolute band count, very increased or persistently increased ESR or CRP, low platelet count, and low albumin.[67]

Incomplete KD

KD is a diagnostic challenge. The signs and symptoms are nonspecific and are often found in viral illnesses. Adding to this challenge are the patients with KD who do not fulfill diagnostic criteria. These patients are considered as having incomplete KD, with at least 5 days of fever but only 2 or 3 of the other clinical criteria (see **Box 1**).[20] The diagnostic criteria serve as a guideline to prevent overdiagnosis; however, they fail to identify children with incomplete forms of the disease.[20] Incomplete KD needs to be considered in children with some of the clinical features and supportive laboratory findings seen in classic KD, especially in children at the extremes of age at which incomplete KD occurs more frequently. Incomplete KD should not be considered as mild KD because the risk of CAA in these patients is comparable with, if not higher than, classic KD.[68]

Children less than 1 year of age, and those older than 9 years, are more likely to present with incomplete KD.[69] Infants less than 6 months of age are more likely to have an incomplete presentation, late intravenous immunoglobulin (IVIG) treatment,

CAA, and poor outcome.[70] A high index of suspicion is required for infants younger than 6 months who present with fever for 5 or more days, despite not fulfilling criteria for KD. One study found that although children less than 6 months old and those greater than 9 years old were at an increased risk for CAA, there seemed to be different associated factors.[69] Those less than 6 months of age had the coexistence of 2 associated risk factors: poor laboratory profile and delay in diagnosis.[69] The poor laboratory profile included lower albumin levels, lower hemoglobin levels, and higher platelet counts.[69] Children in the older age group had a delay in diagnosis and a lower rate of receiving appropriate treatment but a more benign laboratory profile.[69] There may be an inherent risk for worse disease in the group less than 6 months of age but it is often coupled with a delay in diagnosis, leading to a worse outcome. This study also found that those more than 9 years of age were more likely to have resistant disease, with longer duration of fever despite treatment.[69] Another study similarly showed that older children more often had a delay in diagnosis, took longer to defervesce, and had a more complicated course compared with younger children.[71] Failing to consider the diagnosis of KD at the extremes of age puts children at risk for CAA.

In the 2004 American Heart Association (AHA) scientific statement, an algorithm was proposed to assist in evaluating children with suspected incomplete KD.[20] This algorithm had not been tested prospectively before publication. The goal of this algorithm was to allow for earlier diagnosis and treatment of incomplete KD. As part of the algorithm, the authors suggested that an infant 6 months of age or younger, who is on the seventh day of fever or greater, without a focus, should have laboratory test looking for signs of inflammation.[20] If systemic inflammation is found, with an increased CRP of 3 mg/dL or greater or ESR 40 mm/h or greater, then the authors suggest that the child undergo an echocardiogram even if no clinical criteria are present.[20] If abnormal findings are seen on echocardiogram, treatment of KD is suggested.[20] The definition of an abnormal echocardiogram includes a Z score of left anterior descending (LAD) or right coronary artery (RCA) 2.5 or greater; aneurysm as per the Japanese Ministry of Health Criteria; or at least 3 of the following: perivascular brightness, lack of tapering, decreased left ventricular function, mitral regurgitation, pericardial effusion, or Z score between 2 and 2.5 of LAD or RCA.[20] In children more than 6 months of age with incomplete criteria, if their clinical characteristics are consistent with KD, an ESR and CRP are also advised.[20] If no signs of inflammation are found, these authors suggest that the patient be reevaluated within 48 hours and that the algorithm be repeated at that time.[20] If there is evidence of inflammation, it is suggested that supplemental laboratory testing be carried out to see if there are findings that would support this diagnosis.[20] These findings include low albumin level, anemia, increased alanine aminotransferase level, increased platelet count after the seventh day, increased white blood cell count, and pyuria.[20] If the patient fulfills at least 3 supplemental laboratory criteria, it is suggested that they be treated for KD.[20] If the child has fewer than 3 supplemental laboratory criteria, an echocardiogram is advised.[20] If the echocardiogram is abnormal, treatment is suggested.[20] If negative but fever persists, these authors suggest repeating an echocardiogram and consulting a KD expert.[20] The algorithm helps to use the knowledge of the clinical, laboratory, and echocardiographic features to assist in making the diagnosis of KD in children with incomplete disease.

The 2004 AHA scientific statement also helped to clarify the terms incomplete and atypical KD. Previously, atypical KD referred to a patient who did not fulfill criteria but who had echocardiographic findings of CAA consistent with KD.[20] It has since been suggested that the term incomplete be used for all patients who do not fulfill criteria and that atypical be reserved for patients who fulfill criteria but who have a clinical feature that is not usually seen with KD, such as renal impairment (see **Box 1**).[20]

TREATMENT
AHA Recommendations

The AHA recommends that all children suspected of having the diagnosis of KD be treated with a single dose of 2 g/kg of IVIG infused over 12 hours plus high-dose (or antiinflammatory dose) aspirin (ASA) at a dose of 80 to 100 mg/kg per day in 4 divided doses (**Box 3**).[20,64] Treatment should be started within the first 10 days of illness and ideally within the first 7 days.[20] IVIG should also be given to children who present after the 10th day of illness if fever is still present, or aneurysms are seen with evidence of persistent inflammation.[20] Some centers switch the child to low-dose (or antiplatelet dose) ASA (3–5 mg/kg/d) once the child is afebrile for 48 to 72 hours; others only do so at the 14th day of illness if the child has been afebrile for at least 48 to 72 hours (see **Box 3**).[20] Low-dose ASA is discontinued if there is a normal echocardiogram 6 to 8 weeks after the onset of illness.[20] If the coronary arteries at that time are not normal, then low-dose ASA is continued.[20]

IVIG

In the era before IVIG, children were treated with ASA alone, and CAA were seen in up to 20%[64] of patients, with a mortality as high as 2%.[72] Studies using IVIG to treat KD were first reported in 1984 in Japan.[73] North American studies showed that treating KD with 400 mg/kg/d of IVIG for 4 consecutive days decreased the incidence of CAA to 8%.[74] In 1991, the same group showed that a single infusion of 2 g/kg of IVIG was better than the 4-day infusion regimen, because CAA were detected in

---

Box 3
Treatment

Initial Treatment:

IVIG 2 g/kg as a single infusion over 12 h plus

ASA (orally) 80–100 mg/kg per day in 4 divided doses (keep until afebrile for at least 48–72 h)

Once afebrile for 48–72 h decrease ASA dose to 3–5 mg/kg/d (maintain until 6-wk to 8-wk echo is normal; if abnormal, continue ASA)

Treatment of IVIG Resistance:

Re-treat with second dose of IVIG if fever persists beyond 48 h from completion of IVIG

Give IVIG 2 g/kg as a single infusion over 12 h

If no response to second IVIG:

- Most give methylprednisolone intravenously pulse 30 mg/kg over 3 h, once daily for 1–3 days
- Some give infliximab 5 mg/kg intravenously

If no response to the above:

- If methylprednisolone was given, then try infliximab
- If infliximab was given, then try methylprednisolone; or another dose of infliximab
- Another option: give oral prednisone 1–2 mg/kg/d; continue until CRP has normalized; once normal taper over 2 wk
- Other options: cyclosporin A, methotrexate, cyclophosphamide

4.6% compared with 9.1%.[75] Recent reports have suggested that mortality is now as low as 0.026%.[9]

IVIG is a blood product that consists of concentrated IgG manufactured from pooled human plasma.[76] A standard preparation of IVIG, for intravenous use, comes from more than 5000 individual donors.[76] Its mechanism of action is not completely understood; however, it seems to have antiinflammatory effects.[76] IVIG works by interfering with the idiotype network; it downregulates inflammatory cytokines and increases production and release of interleukin 1 receptor antagonist; it downregulates T-cell activation by neutralizing bacterial toxins and other agents[76]; it increases T-cell suppressor activity and decreases antibody synthesis.[20]

IVIG is considered to be a safe product.[77] To decrease the infectious risk, in addition to donor and plasma screening and testing, current preparations have protocols to purify the product.[78] Side effects are rare but can include infusion reactions, anaphylaxis, urticaria, aseptic meningitis, autoimmune hemolytic anemia, thromboembolic events, and acute renal failure.[77] In the last few years, there seems to have been an increase in cases of hemolytic anemia associated with IVIG in KD.[79,80] It seems to occur more frequently after retreatment with IVIG.[80] If signs of hemolysis are seen, and retreatment is required, corticosteroids should be given rather than another dose of IVIG. Hemoglobin should be closely monitored after IVIG therapy,[79,80] particularly after IVIG retreatment.[80] Measles and varicella vaccinations should be deferred for 11 months after the patient has received high-dose IVIG for KD[20]; the IVIG may render these vaccinations ineffective.

Treatment Controversies

No controversy exists in regards to treating KD with IVIG. Evidence shows that IVIG (2 g/kg) has made a significant impact on the morbidity and mortality of this disease. A Cochrane review[81] confirmed that children with KD should receive IVIG. Controversy persists on the appropriate dose of ASA to be used with IVIG in the treatment of the acute phase of KD.[82] High-dose ASA was used in all the large IVIG trials conducted in the United States, and the current AHA recommendations incorporate data from these studies. The use of high-dose ASA is not the practice in Japan, where moderate-dose (30–50 mg/kg/d) ASA is used in the acute phase.[83–85] No prospective study has shown that ASA, at any dose, reduces the incidence of CAA.[82]

ASA has been used for both its antithrombotic and antiinflammatory effects in KD.[86] Even when high doses are used, therapeutic salicylate levels are difficult to achieve.[87] High-dose ASA, unlike lower doses of ASA, can decrease prostacyclin, which has an important role in interfering with thrombus formation.[85,88] As well, high-dose ASA can have potential toxicity, including Reye syndrome,[89] raised liver enzymes,[85] gastrointestinal bleeding,[90] and sensorineural hearing loss.[46]

Although high-dose ASA has been shown to shorten the duration of fever compared with moderate-dose[85] or low-dose ASA,[91] it is unclear if it has any effect on CAA. The incidence of CAA, within 3 months of diagnosis, in a cohort of 221 children treated from 1985 to 1999, with low-dose ASA and IVIG in the acute phase of disease, showed that 9.1% developed CAA.[92] The incidence decreased to 7.2% when only those who were treated with the 2-g/kg regimen of KD were included.[92] This finding is similar to the incidence of CAA using high-dose ASA with the same IVIG regimen. Another study comparing high-dose ASA with low-dose ASA showed no difference in the incidence of CAA.[91] Hsieh and colleagues[93] used IVIG alone, without ASA, during the febrile period and initiated low-dose ASA only once the fever subsided. The investigators concluded that ASA had no effect on the response rate of IVIG, duration of fever, or incidence of CAA.[93] In 2 meta-analyses, the prevalence of CAA was shown to be dependent on the total dose of IVIG but independent of the ASA dose.[94,95] A Cochrane review[96] stated that until good-quality randomized controlled trials are performed, there is insufficient evidence to indicate whether children with KD need ASA as part of their treatment regimen. In a murine model of KD, at therapeutic concentrations, IVIG but not salicylate was able to reduce the immune responses that were examined.[97] This finding implies that the usefulness of ASA is limited to its anticoagulant and antipyretic actions.[97] These actions can be achieved at lower doses than presently recommended by the AHA.[97] Many question the need for high-dose ASA in KD.[98] Some believe that an argument can be made to use low-dose ASA instead of high-dose in the acute phase of KD.[86]

Treatment Resistance

After initial treatment with 2 g/kg of IVIG, between 11.6%[99] and 38.3%[100] have persistent or recrudescent fever beyond 48 hours after completion of IVIG. This is a risk factor for the development of CAA.[101] Treatment of KD before the fifth day of illness is associated with persistent and recrudescent fever that required retreatment; however, in this scenario, an increase in CAA was not seen.[102,103] From these studies, it is suggested that there may be no benefit in treating patients on day 4 or earlier because this may result in IVIG retreatment.[102,103]

If children persist with fever or redevelop fever beyond 48 hours after completion of IVIG, the recommendation is to administer a second dose of 2 g/kg of IVIG.[20] It is unclear why some patients require retreatment and others do not; this may be determined by individual patient genotype.[31] As well, the optimal dose of IVIG is unknown and may vary among patients.[104] Response to IVIG may be related to postinfusion IgG levels because improved outcomes have been associated with higher levels.[75] There is also a suggestion of a dose-response effect with IVIG.[75] This dose-response relationship forms the theoretic basis for IVIG retreatment.[104,105]

It is known that refractory disease, and thus prolonged fever, are risk factors for the development of CAA. Predicting who will be IVIG resistant has not been successful. When risk-scoring systems for IVIG resistance, developed in Japan, are applied to North American children, they are not found to be accurate enough to be clinically useful.[106] Some laboratory factors have been shown to be associated with IVIG resistance and these include low hemoglobin level,[99] high neutrophil count,[99] high band count,[99] low albumin level,[99] increased aspartate aminotransferase level,[107] increased CRP,[107] increased total bilirubin,[107,108] and increased lactate dehydrogenase level.[108] In the future, better scoring systems or genetic markers may permit the clinician to select who should receive more aggressive therapy at the onset of disease or they may allow for more individualized treatment regimens.

Despite retreatment with IVIG, there are still approximately 3% to 4% who do not respond.[109,110] For these patients, corticosteroids may be considered.[20] Because KD is a systemic vasculitis and corticosteroids are the treatment of choice in most vasculitides, it is reasonable to consider corticosteroids in KD. Before the use of IVIG, 1 study described the high incidence of CAA in a group treated with oral prednisolone.[111] In the same study, none of the children treated with oral prednisolone plus ASA had CAA,[111] but despite this, concern was raised about the use of corticosteroids in KD.[112] After this publication, several studies showed the beneficial effects of corticosteroids in KD; however, in North America, it was not used until 1996 as rescue therapy in IVIG nonresponders.[113] Many publications have described its use.[114–116] Patients treated with corticosteroids seem to have a rapid and sustained resolution of fever with no serious adverse events.[115,116] There are conflicting studies as to whether corticosteroids are associated with better or worse regression rates of coronary artery aneurysms.[117,118] A meta-analysis of corticosteroid therapy plus ASA showed positive results for its use.[119] Overall, it does not appear that corticosteroids have a negative effect and therefore should be considered in children for rescue therapy.

Infliximab has also been used instead of corticosteroids as rescue therapy in IVIG nonresponders.[120] Infliximab is a chimeric mouse/human monoclonal antibody that binds TNF-α.[120] It has been shown that TNF-α is markedly increased in the acute phase of KD and that this correlates with the development of CAA.[121] In a trial, patients who did not respond to the first infusion of IVIG were randomized to receive a second dose of IVIG or infliximab.[120] This study was small and did not observe any differences between treatment groups; both treatment regimens were safe and well tolerated.[120] Another study used cyclosporine A in the treatment of IVIG-resistant patients; it was considered safe, was well tolerated, and provides another option for patients with resistant KD.[122] A study is examining the efficacy of etanercept, a soluble TNF receptor, in reducing the rate of IVIG resistance.[123]

In those studies in which corticosteroids were used for rescue therapy in KD, not all patients responded. Corticosteroid resistance also occurs. In this scenario, there have been several case reports and case series in the literature that have suggested beneficial effects from infliximab,[124–126] cyclosporine A,[127] methotrexate,[128] and cyclophosphamide.[129]

Corticosteroids as First-line Treatment

Despite significant success with IVIG in decreasing the incidence of CAA, there are still approximately 5% of the population with KD who continue to have CAA.[75] This concern has led clinicians to consider more aggressive treatment at diagnosis. For this reason, the role of corticosteroids as first-line treatment has been revisited. A Japanese trial combining IVIG with prednisolone at treatment onset was compared with IVIG alone and showed fewer CAA in the group with combination therapy.[130] A similar trial was conducted in North America combining intravenous methylprednisolone pulse with IVIG.[131] No differences were seen in regards to coronary dimensions, days of fever or hospitalization, and rates of retreatment.[131] However, in a subgroup analysis, there was a suggestion of better coronary outcomes with combination therapy in those who required retreatment.[131] The data in this study did not support the addition of corticosteroids to standard therapy for routine primary treatment of KD.[131] For a summary of treatment recommendations see **Box 3**.

LONG-TERM

Children with KD who have not had any CAA, or who have transient abnormalities that disappear within the first 8 weeks, generally do well. The current AHA recommendations do not advise any pharmacologic therapy beyond the first 8 weeks of illness in these patients.[20] As well, no physical activity restrictions or invasive cardiologic testing are required.[20] However, cardiovascular risk assessment and counseling are recommended at 5-year intervals for those without any abnormalities, and 3 to 5 years for those with transient CAA,[20] which may be performed by the primary care provider.[132] The reason for follow-up is that some studies have shown endothelial dysfunction in patients with KD, years after the diagnosis, which may put them at risk for early atherosclerosis.[133] The AHA suggests counseling and surveying for atherosclerotic risk factors such as smoking, obesity, diabetes, hypertension, and lipid abnormalities in all children with KD.[134]

In children with aneurysms, more than 50% of these lesions regress within the first 2 years of onset.[135] At the site of the CAA, regression is associated with marked thickening of the intima[136] and increased stiffness of the coronary artery.[137] These sites may later stimulate atherosclerosis with a risk for ischemic heart disease.[135] Also, some aneurysms may become stenotic over time, which is an important risk factor for ischemic heart disease.[138] Children with small to medium coronary artery aneurysms should be maintained on low-dose ASA at least until regression of the CAA.[20] Those with large, giant, or multiple aneurysms require long-term antiplatelet therapy as well as anticoagulation.[20] Some have physical activity restrictions and all have regular follow-up with a cardiologist for noninvasive and invasive imaging as required.[20]

Abnormalities in the coronary arteries and other structures of the heart are being identified in long-term follow-up in survivors of KD. These abnormalities include valvular abnormalities,[139] increase in aortic root size, decrease in high-density lipoprotein, presence of endothelial dysfunction, increase in carotid intima-media thickness, decrease in arterial compliance, increase in myocardial fibrosis, and alterations in coronary artery microvasculature.[132] This information suggests that long-term follow-up is necessary for all patients with KD.

SUMMARY

KD is a systemic vasculitis that is complicated by the development of CAA. Its epidemiology and cause are suggestive of an infectious trigger in a genetically susceptible host. Because the diagnosis of KD is made clinically, it is important to use the knowledge of all the clinical and laboratory features together to help establish the diagnosis. Biomarker and genetic studies seem promising and may one day help clinicians make an earlier diagnosis, particularly in incomplete cases, as well as help identify high-risk patients. Early recognition and prompt treatment are critical for this disease because a delay in diagnosis is an important risk factor for CAA. IVIG resistance is a significant problem that is associated with a higher incidence of CAA. Further research is required to help predict IVIG nonresponders, and those at highest risk for CAA, so that these patients can be identified and treated more aggressively at the outset. Although the mortality of KD has decreased throughout the years, long-term follow-up is important to assure that atherosclerotic risk factors and symptoms of cardiac disease are identified and managed early.

REFERENCES

1. Taubert KA, Rowley AH, Shulman ST. A nationwide survey of Kawasaki disease and acute rheumatic fever. J Pediatr 1991;119:279–82.
2. Yanagawa H, Nakamura Y, Ojima T, et al. Changes in epidemic patterns of Kawasaki disease in Japan. Pediatr Infect Dis J 1999;18:64–6.
3. Kawasaki T. [Pediatric acute mucocutaneous lymph node syndrome: clinical observation of 50 cases]. Arerugi (Jpn J Allergy) 1967;16:178–222 [in Japanese].
4. Burns JC, Kushner HI, Bastian JF, et al. Kawasaki disease: a brief history. Pediatrics 2000;106(2):e27.
5. Yamamoto T, Kimura J. [Acute febrile mucocutaneous lymph node syndrome (Kawasaki): subtype of mucocutaneous ocular syndrome of erythema multiforme complicated with carditis]. Shonika Rinsho (Jpn J Pediatr) 1968;21: 336–9 [in Japanese].
6. Shigematsu I. [Epidemiology of mucocutaneous lymph node syndrome]. Nippon Shonika Gakkai Zasshi (J Jpn Pediatr Soc) 1972;76:695–6 [in Japanese].

7. Melish ME, Hicks RM, Larson EJ. Mucocutaneous lymph node syndrome in the United States. Am J Dis Child 1976;130:599–607.
8. Nakamura Y, Yashiro M, Uehara R, et al. Epidemiologic features of Kawasaki disease in Japan: results from the nationwide survey in 2005-2006. J Epidemiol 2008;18(4):167–72.
9. Nakamura Y, Yashiro M, Uehara R, et al. Epidemiologic features of Kawasaki disease in Japan: results of the 2007-2008 nationwide survey. J Epidemiol 2010;20(4):302–7.
10. Nakamura Y, Yanagawa H. The worldwide epidemiology of Kawasaki disease. Prog Pediatr Cardiol 2004;19:99–108.
11. Lin YT, Manlhiot C, Ching JC, et al. Repeated systematic surveillance of Kawasaki disease in Ontario from 1995 to 2006. Pediatr Int 2010;52:699–706.
12. Park YW, Han JW, Park IS, et al. Kawasaki disease in Korea, 2003-2005. Pediatr Infect Dis J 2007;26:821–3.
13. Huang WC, Huang LM, Chang IS, et al. Epidemiologic features of Kawasaki disease in Taiwan, 2003-2006. Pediatrics 2009;123:e401–5.
14. Holman RC, Belay ED, Christensen KY, et al. Hospitalizations for Kawasaki syndrome among children in the United States, 1997-2007. Pediatr Infect Dis J 2010;29:483–8.
15. Lynch M, Holman RC, Mulligan A, et al. Kawasaki syndrome hospitalizations in Ireland, 1996 through 2000. Pediatr Infect Dis J 2003;22:959–63.
16. Harnden A, Alves B, Sheikh A. Rising incidence of Kawasaki disease in England: analysis of hospital admission data. BMJ 2002;324:1424–5.
17. Heaton P, Wilson N, Nicholson R, et al. Kawasaki disease in New Zealand. J Paediatr Child Health 2006;42:184–90.
18. Royle JA, Williams K, Elliott E, et al. Kawasaki disease in Australia, 1993-95. Arch Dis Child 1998;78:33–9.
19. Yeung RS. Kawasaki disease: update on pathogenesis. Curr Opin Rheumatol 2010;22:551–60.
20. Newburger JW, Takahashi M, Gerber MA, et al. Diagnosis, treatment, and long-term management of Kawasaki disease. Circulation 2004;110:2747–71.
21. Holman RC, Curns AT, Belay ED, et al. Kawasaki syndrome in Hawaii. Pediatr Infect Dis J 2005;24:429–33.
22. Uehara R, Yashiro M, Nakamura Y, et al. Kawasaki disease in parents and children. Acta Paediatr 2003;92:694–7.
23. Leung DY, Giorno RC, Kazemi LV, et al. Evidence for superantigen involvement in cardiovascular injury due to Kawasaki syndrome. J Immunol 1995;155(10):5018–21.
24. Rowley AH, Shulman ST. Recent advances in the understanding and management of Kawasaki disease. Curr Infect Dis Rep 2010;12(2):96–102.
25. Rowley AH, Eckerley CA, Jack HM, et al. IgA plasma cells in vascular tissue of patients with Kawasaki syndrome. J Immunol 1997;159(12):5946–55.
26. Rowley AH, Baker SC, Orenstein JM, et al. Searching for the cause of Kawasaki disease—cytoplasmic inclusion bodies provide new insight. Nat Rev Microbiol 2008;6(5):394–401.
27. Onouchi Y, Gunji T, Burns JC, et al. ITPKC functional polymorphism associated with Kawasaki disease susceptibility and formation of coronary artery aneurysms. Nat Genet 2008;40(1):35–42.
28. Burgner D, Davila S, Breunis WB, et al. A genome-wide association study identifies novel and functionally related susceptibility loci for Kawasaki disease. PLoS Genet 2009;5(1):e1000319.

29. Khor CC, Davila S, Shimizu C, et al. Genome-wide linkage and association mapping identify susceptibility alleles in ABCC4 for Kawasaki disease. J Med Genet 2011;48(7):467–72.
30. Kim JJ, Hong YM, Sohn S, et al. A genome-wide association analysis reveals 1p31 and 2p13.3 as susceptibility loci for Kawasaki disease. Hum Genet 2011;129(5):487–95.
31. Shrestha S, Wiener HW, Olson AK, et al. Functional FCGR2B gene variants influence intravenous immunoglobulin response in patients with Kawasaki disease. J Allergy Clin Immunol 2011;128(3):677–80.
32. Lang B. Recognizing Kawasaki disease. Paediatr Child Health 2001;6(9): 638–43.
33. Benseler SM, McCrindle BW, Silverman ED, et al. Infections and Kawasaki disease: implications for coronary artery outcome. Pediatrics 2005;116(6): e760–6.
34. Jordan-Villegas A, Chang ML, Ramilo O, et al. Concomitant respiratory viral infections in children with Kawasaki disease. Pediatr Infect Dis J 2010;29(8): 770–2.
35. Friter BS, Lucky AW. The perineal eruption of Kawasaki syndrome. Arch Dermatol 1988;124(12):1805–10.
36. Wang S, Best BM, Burns JC. Periungual desquamation in patients with Kawasaki disease. Pediatr Infect Dis J 2009;28(6):538–9.
37. Berard R, Scuccimarri R, Chédeville G. Leukonychia striata in Kawasaki disease. J Pediatr 2008;152(6):889.
38. Yoskovitch A, Tewfik TL, Duffy CM, et al. Head and neck manifestations of Kawasaki disease. Int J Pediatr Otorhinolaryngol 2000;52(2):123–9.
39. Ohno S, Miyajima T, Higuchi M, et al. Ocular manifestations of Kawasaki's disease (mucocutaneous lymph node syndrome). Am J Ophthalmol 1982;93: 713–7.
40. Burns JC, Joffe L, Sargent RA, et al. Anterior uveitis associated with Kawasaki syndrome. Pediatr Infect Dis 1985;4(3):258–61.
41. Gong GW, McCrindle BW, Ching JC, et al. Arthritis presenting during the acute phase of Kawasaki disease. J Pediatr 2006;148(6):800–5.
42. Baker AL, Lu M, Minich LL, et al. Associated symptoms in the ten days prior to diagnosis of Kawasaki disease. J Pediatr 2009;154(4):592–5.
43. Suddleson EA, Reid B, Woolley MM, et al. Hydrops of the gallbladder associated with Kawasaki syndrome. J Pediatr Surg 1987;22(10):956–9.
44. Wright H, Waddington C, Geddes J, et al. Facial nerve palsy complicating Kawasaki disease. Pediatrics 2008;122(3):e783–5.
45. Sundel RP, Cleveland SS, Beiser AS, et al. Audiologic profiles of children with Kawasaki disease. Am J Otol 1992;13(6):512–5.
46. Knott PD, Orloff LA, Harris JP, et al. Sensorineural hearing loss and Kawasaki disease: a prospective study. Am J Otolaryngol 2001;22(5):343–8.
47. Magalhães CM, Mãgalhaes Alves NR, Oliveira KM, et al. Sensorineural hearing loss: an underdiagnosed complication of Kawasaki disease. J Clin Rheumatol 2010;16(7):322–5.
48. Kuniyuki S, Asada M. An ulcerated lesion at the BCG vaccination site during the course of Kawasaki disease. J Am Acad Dermatol 1997;37(2 Pt 2):303–4.
49. Bertotto A, Spinozzi F, Vagliasindi C, et al. Tuberculin skin test reactivity in Kawasaki disease. Pediatr Res 1997;41(4 Pt 1):560–2.
50. Eberhard BA, Sundel RP, Newburger JW, et al. Psoriatic eruption in Kawasaki disease. J Pediatr 2000;137(4):578–80.

51. Tomita S, Chung K, Mas M, et al. Peripheral gangrene associated with Kawasaki disease. Clin Infect Dis 1992;14(1):121–6.
52. Muise A, Tallett SE, Silverman ED. Are children with Kawasaki disease and prolonged fever at risk for macrophage activation syndrome? Pediatrics 2003;112: e495–7.
53. Latino GA, Manlhiot C, Yeung RS, et al. Macrophage activation syndrome in the acute phase of Kawasaki disease. J Pediatr Hematol Oncol 2010;32(7): 527–31.
54. Rowe PC, Quinlan A, Luke BK. Value of degenerative change in neutrophils as a diagnostic test for Kawasaki syndrome. J Pediatr 1991;119:370–4.
55. Birdi N, Klassen TP, Quinlan A, et al. Role of the toxic neutrophil count in the early diagnosis of Kawasaki disease. J Rheumatol 1999;26:904–8.
56. Harada K. Intravenous gamma-globulin treatment in Kawasaki disease. Acta Paediatr Jpn 1991;33(6):805–10.
57. Dahdah N, Siles A, Fournier A, et al. Natriuretic peptide as an adjunctive diagnostic test in the acute phase of Kawasaki disease. Pediatr Cardiol 2009;30(6): 810–7.
58. Sato YZ, Molkara DP, Daniels LB, et al. Cardiovascular biomarkers in acute Kawasaki disease. Int J Cardiol 2011. [Epub ahead of print].
59. Kaneko K, Yoshimura K, Ohashi A, et al. Prediction of the risk of coronary arterial lesions in Kawasaki disease by brain natriuretic peptide. Pediatr Cardiol 2011; 32(8):1106–9.
60. Kato H. Cardiovascular involvement in Kawasaki disease: evaluation and natural history. Prog Clin Biol Res 1987;250:277–86.
61. Akagi T, Kato H, Inoue HK, et al. Valvular heart disease in Kawasaki syndrome– incidence and natural history. Kurume Med J 1989;36(3):137–49.
62. Fujiwara H, Hamashima Y. Pathology of the heart in Kawasaki disease. Pediatrics 1978;61:100–7.
63. Kanegaye JT, Wilder MS, Molkara D, et al. Recognition of a Kawasaki disease shock syndrome. Pediatrics 2009;123(5):e783–9.
64. Dajani AS, Taubert KA, Gerber MA, et al. Diagnosis and therapy of Kawasaki disease in children. Circulation 1993;87(5):1776–80.
65. Capannari TE, Daniels SR, Meyer RA, et al. Sensitivity, specificity and predictive value of two-dimensional echocardiography in detecting coronary artery aneurysms in patients with Kawasaki disease. J Am Coll Cardiol 1986;7(2):355–60.
66. Foster BJ, Bernard C, Drummond KN. Kawasaki disease complicated by renal artery stenosis. Arch Dis Child 2000;83(3):253–5.
67. Newburger JW. Kawasaki disease: who is at risk? J Pediatr 2000;137(2):149–52.
68. Sonobe T, Kiyosawa N, Tsuchiya K, et al. Prevalence of coronary artery abnormality in incomplete Kawasaki disease. Pediatr Int 2007;49(4):421–6.
69. Manlhiot C, Yeung RS, Clarizia NA, et al. Kawasaki disease at the extremes of the age spectrum. Pediatrics 2009;124(3):e410–5.
70. Chang FY, Hwang B, Chen SJ, et al. Characteristics of Kawasaki disease in infants younger than 6 months of age. Pediatr Infect Dis J 2006;25(3):241–4.
71. Momenah T, Sanatani S, Potts J, et al. Kawasaki disease in the older child. Pediatrics 1998;102(1):e7.
72. Kawasaki T, Kosaki F, Okawa S, et al. A new infantile acute febrile mucocutaneous lymph node syndrome (MCLS) prevailing in Japan. Pediatrics 1974;54: 271–6.
73. Furusho K, Nakano H, Shinomiya K, et al. High-dose intravenous gammaglobulin for Kawasaki disease. Lancet 1984;2:1055–8.

74. Newburger JW, Takahashi M, Burns JC, et al. The treatment of Kawasaki syndrome with intravenous gamma globulin. N Engl J Med 1986;315:341–7.
75. Newburger JW, Takahashi M, Beiser AS, et al. A single intravenous infusion of gamma globulin as compared with four infusions in the treatment of acute Kawasaki syndrome. N Engl J Med 1991;324:1633–9.
76. Wolf HM, Eibl MM. Immunomodulatory effect of immunoglobulins. Clin Exp Rheumatol 1996;14(Suppl 15):S17–25.
77. Orbach H, Katz U, Sherer Y, et al. Intravenous immunoglobulins: adverse effects and safe administration. Clin Rev Allergy Immunol 2005;29(3):173–84.
78. Ballow M. Safety of IGIV therapy and infusion-related adverse events. Immunol Res 2007;38(1–3):122–32.
79. Gordon DJ, Sloan SR, de Jong JL. A pediatric case series of acute hemolysis after administration of intravenous immunoglobulin. Am J Hematol 2009;84:771–2.
80. Berard R, Scuccimarri R. Hemolytic anemia following intravenous immunoglobulin therapy in patients treated for Kawasaki disease: a report of 4 cases [abstract p182]. Programs and abstracts of the ninth international Kawasaki disease symposium. Taipei (Taiwan); 2008. p. 92. Available at: http://www.tspc.org.tw/IX_IKDS_Abstracts/Abstracts.pdf. Accessed March 6, 2012.
81. Oates-Whitehead RM, Baumer JH, Haines L, et al. Intravenous immunoglobulin for the treatment of Kawasaki disease in children. Cochrane Database Syst Rev 2003;4:CD004000.
82. Lang B, Duffy CM. Controversies in the management of Kawasaki disease. Best Pract Res Clin Rheumatol 2002;16(3):427–42.
83. Akagi T, Kato H, Inoue O, et al. A study on the optimal dose of aspirin therapy in Kawasaki disease–clinical evaluation and arachidonic acid metabolism. Kurume Med J 1989;37:203–8.
84. Kato H, Koike S, Tanaka C, et al. Coronary heart disease in children with Kawasaki disease. Jpn Circ J 1979;43:469–75.
85. Akagi T, Kato H, Inoue O, et al. Salicylate treatment in Kawasaki disease: high dose or low dose? Eur J Pediatr 1991;150(9):642–6.
86. Newburger JW. Treatment of Kawasaki disease. Lancet 1996;347:1128.
87. Koren G, MacLeod SM. Difficulty in achieving therapeutic serum concentrations of salicylate in Kawasaki disease. J Pediatr 1984;105(6):991–5.
88. Hanley SP, Bevan J, Cockbill SR, et al. Differential inhibition by low-dose aspirin of human venous prostacyclin synthesis and platelet thromboxane synthesis. Lancet 1981;1:969–71.
89. Wei CM, Chen HL, Lee PI, et al. Reye's syndrome developing in an infant on treatment of Kawasaki syndrome. J Paediatr Child Health 2005;41:303–4.
90. Matsubara T, Mason W, Kashani IA, et al. Gastrointestinal hemorrhage complicating aspirin therapy in acute Kawasaki disease. J Pediatr 1996;128(5 Pt 1):701–3.
91. Melish ME, Takahashi M, Shulman ST, et al. Comparison of low dose aspirin (LDA) vs high dose aspirin (HDA) as an adjunct to intravenous gamma globulin (IVIG) in the treatment of Kawasaki syndrome (KS). Pediatr Res 1992;31:170A.
92. Scuccimarri R, Rohlicek C, Watanabe Duffy KN, et al. Incidence of early cardiac abnormalities in children with Kawasaki disease treated with low dose aspirin and intravenous immunoglobulin in the acute phase [abstract 700]. Arthritis Rheum 2001;44(9):S169.
93. Hsieh KS, Weng KP, Lin CC, et al. Treatment of acute Kawasaki disease: aspirin's role in the febrile stage revisited. Pediatrics 2004;114(6):e689–93.

94. Terai M, Shulman ST. Prevalence of coronary artery abnormalities in Kawasaki disease is highly dependent on gamma globulin dose but independent of salicylate dose. J Pediatr 1997;131(6):888–93.

95. Durongpisitkul K, Gururaj VJ, Park JM, et al. The prevention of coronary artery aneurysm in Kawasaki disease: a meta-analysis on the efficacy of aspirin and immunoglobulin treatment. Pediatrics 1995;96(6):1057–61.

96. Baumer JH, Love SJL, Gupta A, et al. Salicylate for the treatment of Kawasaki disease in children. Cochrane Database Syst Rev 2006;4:CD004175.

97. Lau AC, Duong TT, Ito S, et al. Intravenous immunoglobulin and salicylate differentially modulate pathogenic processes leading to vascular damage in a model of Kawasaki disease. Arthritis Rheum 2009;60(7):2131–41.

98. Saphyakhajon P, Greene GR. Do we need high-dose acetylsalicylic acid (ASA) in Kawasaki disease? J Pediatr 1998;133(1):167.

99. Durongpisitkul K, Soongswang J, Laohaprasitiporn D, et al. Immunoglobulin failure and retreatment in Kawasaki disease. Pediatr Cardiol 2003;24(2):145–8.

100. Tremoulet AH, Best BM, Song S, et al. Resistance to intravenous immunoglobulin in children with Kawasaki disease. J Pediatr 2008;153(1):117–21.

101. Burns JC, Capparelli EV, Brown JA, et al. Intravenous gamma-globulin treatment and retreatment in Kawasaki disease. Pediatr Infect Dis J 1998;17(12):1144–8.

102. Fong NC, Hui YW, Li CK, et al. Evaluation of the efficacy of treatment of Kawasaki disease before day 5 of illness. Pediatr Cardiol 2004;25(1):31–4.

103. Muta H, Ishii M, Egami K, et al. Early intravenous gamma-globulin treatment for Kawasaki disease: the nationwide surveys in Japan. J Pediatr 2004;144(4):496–9.

104. Sundel RP, Burns JC, Baker A, et al. Gamma globulin re-treatment in Kawasaki disease. J Pediatr 1993;123(4):657–9.

105. Newburger JW. Treatment of Kawasaki disease: corticosteroids revisited. J Pediatr 1999;135(4):411–3.

106. Sleeper LA, Minich LL, McCrindle BM, et al. Evaluation of Kawasaki disease risk-scoring systems for intravenous immunoglobulin resistance. J Pediatr 2011;158:831–5.

107. Sano T, Kurotobi S, Matsuzaki K, et al. Prediction of non-responsiveness to standard high-dose gamma-globulin therapy in patients with acute Kawasaki disease before starting initial treatment. Eur J Pediatr 2007;166(2):131–7.

108. Fukunishi M, Kikkawa M, Hamana K, et al. Prediction of non-responsiveness to intravenous high-dose γ-globulin therapy in patients with Kawasaki disease at onset. J Pediatr 2000;137(2):172–6.

109. Freeman AF, Shulman ST. Refractory Kawasaki disease. Pediatr Infect Dis J 2004;23(5):463–4.

110. Han RK, Silverman ED, Newman A, et al. Management and outcome of persistent or recurrent fever after initial intravenous gamma globulin therapy in acute Kawasaki disease. Arch Pediatr Adolesc Med 2000;154(7):694–9.

111. Kato H, Koike S, Yokoyama T. Kawasaki disease: effect of treatment on coronary artery involvement. Pediatrics 1979;63(2):175–9.

112. Shulman ST. Is there a role for corticosteroids in Kawasaki disease? J Pediatr 2003;142(6):601–3.

113. Wright DA, Newburger JW, Baker A, et al. Treatment of immune globulin-resistant Kawasaki disease with pulsed doses of corticosteroids. J Pediatr 1996;128(1):146–9.

114. Hashino K, Ishii M, Iemura M, et al. Re-treatment for immune globulin-resistant Kawasaki disease: a comparative study of additional immune globulin and steroid pulse therapy. Pediatr Int 2001;43(3):211–7.

115. Lang BA, Yeung RS, Oen KG, et al. Corticosteroid treatment of refractory Kawasaki disease. J Rheumatol 2006;33(4):803–9.

116. Ogata S, Bando Y, Kimura S, et al. The strategy of immune globulin resistant Kawasaki disease: a comparative study of additional immune globulin and steroid pulse therapy. J Cardiol 2009;53(1):15–9.

117. Adachi S, Sakaguchi H, Kuwahara T, et al. High regression rate of coronary aneurysms developed in patients with immune globulin-resistant Kawasaki disease treated with steroid pulse therapy. Tohoku J Exp Med 2010;220(4): 285–90.

118. Millar K, Manlhiot C, Yeung RS, et al. Corticosteroid administration for patients with coronary artery aneurysms after Kawasaki disease may be associated with impaired regression. Int J Cardiol 2012;154(1):9–13.

119. Wooditch AC, Aronoff SC. Effect of initial corticosteroid therapy on coronary artery aneurysm formation in Kawasaki disease: a meta-analysis of 862 children. Pediatrics 2005;116(4):989–95.

120. Burns JC, Best BM, Mejias A, et al. Infliximab treatment of intravenous immunoglobulin-resistant Kawasaki disease. J Pediatr 2008;153(6):833–8.

121. Matsubara T, Furukawa S, Yabuta K, et al. Serum levels of tumor necrosis factor, interleukin 2 receptor, and interferon-gamma in Kawasaki disease involved coronary-artery lesions. Clin Immunol Immunopathol 1990;56(1):29–36.

122. Suzuki H, Terai M, Hamada H, et al. Cyclosporin A treatment for Kawasaki disease refractory to initial and additional intravenous immunoglobulin. Pediatr Infect Dis J 2011;30(10):871–6.

123. Portman MA, Olson A, Soriano B, et al. Etanercept as adjunctive treatment for acute Kawasaki disease: study design and rationale. Am Heart J 2011;161(3): 494–9.

124. Weiss JE, Eberhard BA, Chowdhury D, et al. Infliximab as a novel therapy for refractory Kawasaki disease. J Rheumatol 2004;31(4):808–10.

125. Stenbøg EV, Windelborg B, Hørlyck A, et al. The effect of TNFα blockade in complicated, refractory Kawasaki disease. Scand J Rheumatol 2006;35(4): 318–21.

126. Burns JC, Mason WH, Hauger SB, et al. Infliximab treatment for refractory Kawasaki syndrome. J Pediatr 2005;146(5):662–7.

127. Raman V, Kim J, Sharkey A, et al. Response of refractory Kawasaki disease to pulse steroid and cyclosporine A therapy. Pediatr Infect Dis J 2001;20(6):635–7.

128. Ahn SY, Kim DS. Treatment of intravenous immunoglobulin-resistant Kawasaki disease with methotrexate. Scand J Rheumatol 2005;34(2):136–9.

129. Wallace CA, French JW, Kahn SJ, et al. Initial intravenous gammaglobulin treatment failure in Kawasaki disease. Pediatrics 2000;105:e78.

130. Inoue Y, Okada Y, Shinohara M, et al. A multicenter prospective randomized trial of corticosteroids in primary therapy for Kawasaki disease: clinical course and coronary artery outcome. J Pediatr 2006;149(3):336–41.

131. Newburger JW, Sleeper LA, McCrindle BW, et al. Randomized trial of pulsed corticosteroid therapy for primary treatment of Kawasaki disease. N Engl J Med 2007;356(7):663–75.

132. McCrindle BW. Kawasaki disease: a childhood disease with important consequences into adulthood. Circulation 2009;120:6–8.

133. Dhillon R, Clarkson P, Donald AE, et al. Endothelial dysfunction late after Kawasaki disease. Circulation 1996;94:2103–6.

134. Kavey RE, Allada V, Daniels SR, et al. Cardiovascular risk reduction in high-risk pediatric patients. Circulation 2006;114:2710–38.

135. Kato H, Ichinose E, Yoshioka F, et al. Fate of coronary aneurysms in Kawasaki disease: serial coronary angiography and long-term follow-up study. Am J Cardiol 1982;49:1758–66.

136. Sugimura T, Kato H, Inoue O, et al. Intravascular ultrasound of coronary arteries in children. Circulation 1994;89:258–65.

137. Yamakawa R, Ishii M, Sugimura T, et al. Coronary endothelial dysfunction after Kawasaki disease: evaluation by intracoronary injection of acetylcholine. J Am Coll Cardiol 1998;31:1074–80.

138. Fukushige J, Takahashi N, Ueda K, et al. Long-term outcome of coronary abnormalities in patients after Kawasaki disease. Pediatr Cardiol 1996;17:71–6.

139. Gidding SS. Late onset valvular dysfunction in Kawasaki disease. Prog Clin Biol Res 1987;250:305–9.

Autoinflammatory Syndromes

Philip J. Hashkes, MD, MSc[a,b,*], Ori Toker, MD[c]

KEYWORDS

- Autoinflammatory syndromes • Periodic fever • Interleukin-1

Autoinflammatory syndromes are defined as recurrent attacks of systemic inflammation that are often unprovoked (or triggered by a minor event) related to a lack of adequate regulation of the innate immune system. Unlike autoimmune diseases, there is a relative lack of autoantibodies or autoreactive T cells. In recent years there has been a substantial increase in the diseases classified (at least partially) as autoinflammatory because of better understanding of pathways of immune activation and regulation of the innate immune system (**Box 1**).[1] Much of this understanding was obtained from knowledge gained from rare autoinflammatory diseases with a genetic etiology (**Table 1**). Periodic fever syndromes, the former term for this group of diseases,[2] is not adequate because most syndromes are not truly periodic, and fever is not a necessary feature. This article includes those autoinflammatory syndromes (especially genetic) that do not fall into other diagnostic categories (eg, systemic juvenile idiopathic arthritis, vasculitis, and crystal disease).

These syndromes should be suspected in patients, mainly young children, with recurrent fever unexplained by infections and/or with episodic symptoms in various systems, especially the skin, gastrointestinal tract, chest, eyes, musculoskeletal, and central nervous system. These syndromes should also be suspected in patients with unexplained increased laboratory indices of inflammation even if the patient is asymptomatic. A family history of these syndromes is often but not always obtained, including a history of unexplained deafness, renal failure, or amyloidosis.

Most autoinflammatory syndromes have common clinical features including recurrent fevers, serositis, rashes, musculoskeletal manifestations, and increased laboratory markers of inflammation. However, a complete history and physical examination is

Financial disclosures: PJH has received speaker's bureau honoraria (<$5000) and research support for a clinical trial from Novartis, and has received free drug from Regeneron for a clinical trial. He was a consultant in 2010 (<$5000) and has received research support for a clinical trial from UrlPharma.

[a] Pediatric Rheumatology Unit, Department of Pediatrics, Shaare Zedek Medical Center, PO Box 3235, Jerusalem 91031, Israel; [b] Department of Rheumatology, Cleveland Clinic Lerner School of Medicine, 9500 Euclid Avenue, Cleveland, OH 44195, USA; [c] Allergy and Clinical Immunology Unit, Hadassah Medical Center, PO Box 3235, Jerusalem 91031, Israel
* Corresponding author. Pediatric Rheumatology Unit, Shaare Zedek Medical Center, PO Box 3235, Jerusalem 91031, Israel.
E-mail address: hashkesp@szmc.org.il

Pediatr Clin N Am 59 (2012) 447–470
doi:10.1016/j.pcl.2012.03.005
0031-3955/12/$ – see front matter © 2012 Elsevier Inc. All rights reserved.

Box 1
The expanding spectrum of the autoinflammatory diseases

Autosomal-recessive

Familial Mediterranean fever (FMF)

Mevalonate kinase deficiency: hyperimmunoglobulinemia D syndrome (HIDS)

Deficiency of the interleukin-1 receptor antagonist (DIRA)

Deficiency of the interleukin-36 receptor antagonist (DITRA): generalized familial pustular psoriasis

Majeed syndrome

Recurrent hydatidiform mole (NLRP7)

Autosomal-dominant

TNF-receptor–associated periodic syndrome (TRAPS)

Cryopyrin-associated periodic syndromes (CAPS, NLRP3)

    Familial cold-autoinflammatory syndrome (FCAS)

    Muckle-Wells syndrome (MWS)

    Neonatal-onset multisystem inflammatory disease (NOMID)

Pyogenic arthritis, pyoderma gangrenosum, acne syndrome (PAPA)

Familial cold-autoinflammatory syndrome 2 (FCAS2-NLRP12)

Cherubism (SH3BP2)

Granulomatous

Blau syndrome (autosomal-dominant)

Early onset sarcoidosis (autosomal-dominant)

Crohn disease (partially genetic)

Other, nongenetic

Periodic fever, aphthous stomatitis, pharyngitis, adenitis syndrome (PFAPA)

Systemic juvenile idiopathic arthritis

Behçet syndrome

Recurrent pericarditis

Chronic recurrent multifocal osteomyelitis (CRMO)

Schnitzler syndrome

Gout

Other, nongenetic, at least partially autoinflammatory

Spondyloarthropathies

Type II diabetes

Age-related macular degeneration

Fibrosing disorders

Hemolytic uremic syndrome

Atherosclerosis

Post–myocardial infarction muscle damage

Abbreviation: NLRP, nucleotide oligomerization domain–like receptor family, pyrin domain.

Table 1
Genetic characteristics of selected inherited autoinflammatory syndromes

Disease	Inheritance	Chromosome	Gene Defect	Protein Product	Common Mutations
FMF	Recessive	16p13	MEFV	Pyrin	M694V, M694I, M680I, V726A, E148Q[a]
HIDS	Recessive	12q24	MVK	Mevalonate Kinase	V377I, I268T
DIRA	Recessive	2q14	IL1RN	IL-1 receptor antagonist	175-kb deletion, 156_157delCA
DITRA	Recessive	2q13–14	IL36RN	IL-36 receptor antagonist	L27P, S113I
TRAPS	Dominant	12p13	TNFRSF1A	55-kDa TNF receptor	T50M, C52Y, R92Q,[a] P46L[a]
FCAS	Dominant	1q44	NLRP3	Cryopyrin	V198M,[a] R260W
MWS	Dominant	1q44	NLRP3	Cryopyrin	V198M,[a] L264 V, E311K, T348M, A439V
NOMID	Dominant/sporadic	1q44	NLRP3	Cryopyrin	L264F,H; D303H; V351M,L
PAPA	Dominant	15q	PSTPIP1	CD2 antigen-binding	A230T, E250Q,K
NLRP12	Dominant	19q13	NLRP12	NLR family, pyrin domain, containing 12	C850T

Abbreviations: DIRA, deficiency of the IL-1 receptor antagonist; DITRA, deficiency of the IL-36 receptor antagonist (generalized pustular psoriasis); FCAS, familial cold autoinflammatory syndrome; FMF, familial Mediterranean fever; HIDS, hyperimmunoglobulinemia D syndrome; MWS, Muckle-Wells syndrome; NLRP, nucleotide oligomerization domain–like receptor family, pyrin domain; NOMID, neonatal-onset multisystem inflammatory disorder; PAPA, pyogenic sterile arthritis, pyoderma gangrenosum, acne syndrome; TNF, tumor necrosis factor; TRAPS, TNF-receptor–associated periodic syndrome.

[a] Polymorphism, partial penetrance or mild phenotype mutation.

crucial and often the correct diagnosis can be attained before more genetic or sophisticated tests are used.[3] Syndromes can be differentiated by age of onset, ethnicity, attack triggers, duration of attacks, disease-free intervals between attacks, clinical manifestations, and the response to therapy (**Tables 2–4**). It is very useful to examine patients during an attack, or alternately to ask parents to record attacks carefully and take photos of relevant physical findings. It is also useful to obtain laboratory markers of inflammation during and between attacks, because in some syndromes attacks are only the "tip of the inflammatory iceberg" and patients consistently have increased inflammatory indices. These patients are at higher risk of developing Amyloid A (AA) amyloidosis, the major adverse outcome of the autoinflammatory syndromes.

THE INNATE IMMUNE SYSTEM AS IT RELATES TO THE PATHOGENESIS OF AUTOINFLAMMATORY SYNDROMES

The initial response to pathogens and damaged cells is mediated by the innate immune system (**Fig. 1**). The cells of the innate immune system, primarily epithelial, dendritic, polymorphonuclear, and macrophage cells, act not only as an immediate barrier, but also as effectors in the evolution of the inflammatory response. The innate immune system recognizes pathogen-associated molecular patterns and damage-associated molecular patterns by several complex mechanisms, involving cell-associated pattern recognition receptors and soluble recognition molecules. These receptors, such as toll-like receptors, are present on the surface of the cell. Nucleotide oligomerization domain–like receptors (NLRs) within the cell and other receptors further mediate intracellular innate immune system processes and development of the inflammatory response. NLRPs (NLRs with pyrin-domain–containing proteins) are a subfamily of the NLRs. NLRP3 assembles other proteins to form the inflammasome complex in response to cytoplasmatic pathogen-associated molecular patterns and damage-associated molecular patterns, which also triggers the expression of proinflammatory genes by transcription factors (eg, nuclear factor-κB). The inflammasome complex involving NLRP3 recruits and activates caspase 1, a protease that cleaves prointerleukin (IL)-1β and IL-18 to their active forms. The common pathogenic pathway of the autoinflammatory syndromes involves the excessive production and activity of these proinflammatory cytokines and molecules, not as a result of external stimuli but as a result of mutations in different proteins that regulate these pathways.[4]

FAMILIAL MEDITERRANEAN FEVER

Familial Mediterranean fever (FMF), described in 1945,[5] is the most common inherited autoinflammatory syndrome. Inherited in an autosomal-recessive manner, it results in recurrent attacks of fever, serositis, arthritis, and rash. Late complications of untreated FMF include the development of primarily renal AA amyloidosis leading to the nephrotic syndrome and renal failure.

The highest prevalence of FMF is in Sephardic Jews, Armenians, Arabs, and Turks. Because of the availability of genetic diagnosis FMF is now recognized more frequently among Ashkenazi Jews, Greeks, and Italians and even among Japanese, although the disease is usually milder in these groups.[6] It is estimated that there are between 100,000 and 120,000 FMF patients worldwide.[6] The carrier rate is as high as 1:3 to 1:5 among Armenians and North African Jews.

Etiology

The FMF gene (*MEFV*) is located on the short arm of chromosome 16.[7–9] The product of this gene is a 781–amino acid protein termed "pyrin" (marenostrin in Europe). There

Table 2
Clues that may assist in the diagnosis of autoinflammatory syndromes

Age of onset	
At birth	NOMID, DIRA, FCAS
Infancy and first year of life	HIDS, FCAS, NLRP12
Toddler	PFAPA
Late childhood	PAPA
Most common of autoinflammatory syndromes to have onset in adulthood	TRAPS, DITRA
Variable (mostly in childhood)	All others
Ethnicity and geography	
Armenians, Turks, Italian, Sephardic Jews	FMF
Arabs	FMF, DITRA (Arab Tunisian)
Dutch, French, German, Western Europe	HIDS, MWS, NLRP12
United States	FCAS
Can occur in blacks (West Africa origin)	TRAPS
Eastern Canada, Puerto Rico	DIRA
Worldwide	All others
Triggers	
Vaccines	HIDS
Cold exposure	FCAS, NLRP12
Stress, menses	FMF, TRAPS, MWS, PAPA, DITRA
Minor trauma	PAPA, MWS, TRAPS, HIDS
Exercise	FMF, TRAPS
Pregnancy	DITRA
Infections	All, especially DITRA
Attack duration	
<24 h	FCAS, FMF
1–3 d	FMF, MWS, DITRA (fever)
3–7 d	HIDS, PFAPA
>7 d	TRAPS, PAPA
Almost always "in attack"	NOMID, DIRA
Interval between attacks	
3–6 wk	PFAPA, HIDS
>6 wk	TRAPS
Mostly unpredictable	All others
Truly periodic	PFAPA, cyclic neutropenia
Useful laboratory tests	
Acute-phase reactants must be normal between attacks	PFAPA
Urine mevalonic acid in attack	HIDS
IgD >100 mg/dL	HIDS
Proteinuria (amyloidosis)	FMF, TRAPS, MWS, NOMID

(*continued on next page*)

Table 2 (continued)	
Response to therapy	
Corticosteroid dramatic	PFAPA
Corticosteroid partial	TRAPS, FCAS, MWS, NOMID, PAPA[a]
Colchicine	FMF, PFAPA (30% effective)
Cimetidine	PFAPA (30% effective)
Etanercept	TRAPS, FMF arthritis
Anti–IL-1 dramatic	DIRA (anakinra), FCAS, MWS, NOMID, PFAPA
Anti–IL-1 mostly	TRAPS, FMF
Anti–IL-1 partial	HIDS, PAPA

Abbreviations: DIRA, deficiency of the IL-1 receptor antagonist; DITRA, deficiency of the IL-36 receptor antagonist (generalized pustular psoriasis); FCAS, familial cold autoinflammatory syndrome; FMF, familial Mediterranean fever; HIDS, hyperimmunoglobulinemia D syndrome; IL, interleukin; MWS, Muckle-Wells syndrome; NLRP, nucleotide oligomerization domain–like receptor family, pyrin domain; NOMID, neonatal-onset multisystem inflammatory disorder; PAPA, pyogenic sterile arthritis, pyoderma gangrenosum, acne syndrome; PFAPA, periodic fever, aphthous stomatitis, pharyngitis, adenitis; TRAPS, tumor necrosis factor receptor–associated periodic syndrome.

[a] For intra-articular steroids.

may be a phenotype–genotype correlation with more severe disease and amyloidosis occurring in patients with the M694V, M694I, and M680I mutations.[10] In most series, at least 30% of patients diagnosed with definite FMF by clinical criteria lack one or even two mutations, especially patients from Western Europe or the United States; autosomal-dominant transmission has been demonstrated in some families.[11] Mutations or polymorphisms in genes other than *MEFV* gene may impact on the development of FMF or the severity of the disease, including the development of amyloidosis.[10]

Pathogenesis

The pyrin protein consists of three main domains: (1) the N-terminal 92–amino acid pyrin domain, (2) the B-box, and (3) the C-terminal B30.2 domain. Most disease-causing mutations occur in exon 10 of the *MEFV* gene encoding the B30.2 domain.[12] Pyrin directly interacts and binds to caspase 1, inhibiting its ability to cleave pro–IL-1β to IL-1β.[13] Mutations in the B30.2 region of pyrin, particularly those mutations considered more severe (positions 680 and 694) interfere in this binding process, thus contributing to increased levels of IL-1β and inflammation with and without exogenous stimulation.

Clinical Manifestations

Clinical signs of FMF develop by age 10 years in 80% of the patients and by age 20 years in 90%.[14] Attacks typically last 12 to 72 hours and are characterized by fever, serositis, monoarthritis of the knee or ankle, often accompanied by an erysipelas-like rash over the involved joint (**Fig. 2**). Severe abdominal pain (caused by peritonitis), often mimicking appendicitis, accompanies fever in nearly 90% of patients. Pleuritis occurs in 30% to 45% of patients, and patients occasionally develop pericarditis and scrotal swelling. Acute arthritis is seen in 50% to 75% of patients and is characterized by substantial effusions with polymorphonuclear predominance and usually

Table 3
System involvement of the main autoinflammatory syndromes

Disease	Serositis	Skin	Musculoskeletal	Eyes	Mucous Membranes	Reticuloendothelial	Neurologic
FMF	Peritonitis, pleuritis, pericarditis, scrotum	Erysipelas-like, vasculitis	Acute monoarthritis, 5%–10% chronic arthritis, exercise-related myalgia, prolonged febrile myalgia	No	Rare aphthous	Splenomegaly, adenopathy	Headaches
HIDS	Abdominal pain, vomiting, diarrhea	Maculo papular, mobiliform rash	Arthralgia, arthritis	No	Aphthous, vaginal sores	Cervical adenopathy	No
DIRA	None	Pustulosis	Bonyytic lesions, osteitis	No	No	No	No
DITRA	None	Pustular psoriasis, nail dystrophy	Arthralgia, arthritis	No	Tongue lesions (geographic)	No	No
TRAPS	Peritonitis, pleuritis pericarditis	Painful, migratory erythema, vasculitis	Myalgia, fasciitis, arthralgia, arthritis	Periorbital edema, conjunctival injection	Aphthous	Splenomegaly, adenopathy	Focal neuropathy
FCAS FCAS2/NLRP12	No	Urticaria-like	Arthralgia	Conjunctivitis	No	No	Headaches
MWS	No	Urticaria-like	Arthralgia	Conjunctivitis, episcleritis, uveitis	No	No	Hearing loss, headaches
NOMID	No	Urticaria-like	Epiphyseal overgrowth with deformities, cartilage defect, arthritis	Conjunctivitis, uveitis, papillitis	No	Adenopathy	Chronic meningitis, mental retardation, headaches
PAPA	No	Pyoderma gangrenosum, acne	Destructive 'pyogenic' large joint arthritis	No	No	No	No
PFAPA	No	No	Arthralgia	No	Aphthous, pharyngitis	Cervical lymphadenopathy	No

Abbreviations: DIRA, deficiency of the IL-1 receptor antagonist; DITRA, deficiency of the IL-36 receptor antagonist (generalized pustular psoriasis); FCAS, familial cold autoinflammatory syndrome; FMF, familial Mediterranean fever; HIDS, hyperimmunoglobulinemia D syndrome; MWS, Muckle-Wells syndrome; NLRP, nucleotide oligomerization domain–like receptor family, pyrin domain; NOMID, neonatal-onset multisystem inflammatory disorder; PAPA, pyogenic sterile arthritis, pyoderma gangrenosum, acne syndrome; PFAPA, periodic fever, aphthous stomatitis, pharyngitis, adenitis; TRAPS, tumor necrosis factor receptor–associated periodic syndrome.

Adapted from Hashkes PJ. Autoinflammatory Disorders. In: Rudolph CD, Rudolph AM, Lister GE, et al, editors. Rudolph's pediatrics. 22nd edition. New York: McGraw-Hill, 2011; p. 833; with permission.

Table 4
Effective treatments and strength of proof of the main autoinflammatory syndromes

Disease	Colchicine	Corticosteroids	TNF Inhibitors	IL-1 Inhibitors	Other
FMF	[a]Multiple controlled studies	Effective only in prolonged febrile myalgia, vasculitis	Effective for arthropathy, case reports/series	Controlled study (two-thirds of patients), case series	
HIDS	No	No	Case reports	About 40%, case series	Simvastatin shortens attacks
DIRA	No	No	Unknown	[a]Anakinra, case series	
DITRA	No	No	Case reports	Case reports	Oral retinoids cyclosporin
TRAPS	No	Yes, but loses effect over time	Case reports, [b]etanercept only, not in all cases, often loss of effect over time	Case series	Anti-IL-6, case report
FCAS	No	No	Unknown	[a]Two controlled studies	
MWS	No	No	Unknown	[a]Two controlled studies	
NOMID	No	No	Unknown, case reports	[a]Open study	
FCAS2/NLRP12	Unknown	Unknown	Unknown	No (case reports)	
PAPA	No	No	Case reports (partial)	Case reports	
PFAPA	30%–40%, case series	[a]Yes, may shorten intervals between attacks	Unknown	Case series	[a]Tonsillectomy, controlled studies; cimetidine (30%–40%), case series

Abbreviations: DIRA, deficiency of the IL-1 receptor antagonist; DITRA, deficiency of the IL-36 receptor antagonist (generalized pustular psoriasis); FCAS, familial cold autoinflammatory syndrome; FMF, familial Mediterranean fever; HIDS, hyperimmunoglobulinemia D syndrome; IL, interleukin; MWS, Muckle-Wells syndrome; NOMID, neonatal-onset multisystem inflammatory disorder; PAPA, pyogenic sterile arthritis, pyoderma gangrenosum, acne syndrome; PFAPA, periodic fever, aphthous stomatitis, pharyngitis, adenitis; TNF, tumor necrosis factor; TRAPS, TNF-receptor–associated periodic syndrome.

[a] Highly effective.
[b] Infliximab contraindicated.

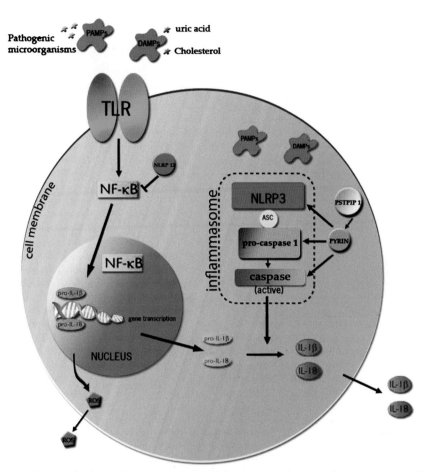

Fig. 1. Schema of selected innate immune inflammatory pathways related to the autoinflammatory syndromes. The schema demonstrates the effect of external stimuli on the development of inflammation and the relationship of several regulatory proteins (pyrin, NLRP3, NLRP12, and PSTPIP1) that when mutated result in the development of autoinflammatory diseases. DAMP, damage-associated molecular patterns; IL, interleukin; NF-κB, nuclear factor-κB; NLR, nucleotide oligomerization domain–like receptors; NLRPs, NLRs with pyrin-domain-containing proteins; PAMP, pathogen-associated molecular patterns; PSTPIP, proline-serine-threonine phosphatase-interacting protein; ROS, reactive oxygen species; TLR, toll-like receptors.

lasts up to 1 week. Chronic arthritis develops in 5% to 10%, especially in the hip and sacroiliac joint. Headaches related to aseptic meningitis may occur.

Since the discovery of the genetic cause of FMF more phenotype presentations have been recognized. These include exercise-induced myalgia, recurrent abdominal pain, and recurrent arthritis without fever in appropriate ethnic groups.[3]

Other less common manifestations include prolonged febrile myalgia and vasculitis, especially Henoch-Schönlein purpura and polyarteritis nodosa, and glomerulonephritis. Children with frequent attacks often have growth delay and short stature. Splenomegaly is common. In children younger than 5 years recurrent fever may be the sole feature.[15]

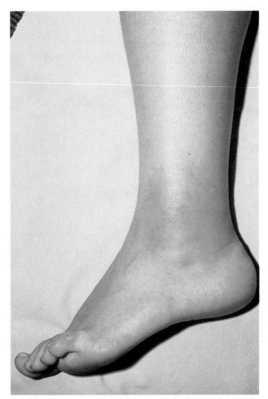

Fig. 2. Erysipelas-like rash in familial Mediterranean fever.

Amyloidosis

Amyloidosis was the major cause of morbidity and mortality before the discovery in 1972 of colchicine as an effective therapy for FMF. Renal amyloidosis usually starts with proteinuria and progresses to the nephrotic syndrome and renal failure within 3 to 5 years. FMF can rarely present with amyloidosis (type II phenotype). Later, patients develop gastrointestinal amyloidosis resulting in abdominal pain, diarrhea, malabsorption, and weight loss. Other manifestations may include cardiomyopathy, hepatosplenomegaly, macroglossia, joint stiffness, peripheral neuropathy, and bleeding disorders.

The most important risk factor for the development of amyloidosis in FMF is the geographic residence of the patient (with less amyloidosis in the United States). Other risk factors include the 694 and 680 mutations, family history of amyloidosis, male gender, the serum amyloid A genotype with an odds ratio of 7 for patients with an α/α genotype, and poor compliance with treatment.[16]

Amyloidosis is suspected by detecting proteinuria during routine urinalysis screening. Diagnostic methods less invasive than renal biopsy include subcutaneous abdominal fat aspiration, rectal biopsy, and nuclear ^{123}I-labeled scan for serum amyloid P-component. The latter can be used to monitor the total body load of amyloid.[17]

Diagnosis

The diagnosis of FMF is based on clinical criteria and not genetic testing. Two major criteria have been described. The 1997 Tel-Hashomer criteria are based on clinical manifestations, family history, and response to colchicine.[18] Pediatric criteria proposed in 2009 require at least three attacks with the presence of two of five features, including fever lasting between 12 and 72 hours, abdominal pain, chest pain, arthritis, and positive family history.[19] There is debate on the specificity of these criteria, across pediatric populations or varied ethnicities. Laboratory tests are nonspecific and reflect elevated acute-phase reactants, mainly during attacks but also frequently between attacks. Serum amyloid A levels may be especially helpful in monitoring treatment efficacy.[20] Unanswered questions remain on how to manage asymptomatic patients with homozygote genetic mutations and which asymptomatic relatives of patients with genetically proved FMF should be tested for mutations (eg, if there is a family history of amyloidosis).

Treatment

Treatment with colchicine (1–2 mg/d [Colcrys]) is effective in preventing amyloidosis in nearly all patients and in preventing attacks in 60% to 70% of patients.[21–23] However, 20% to 30% of patients respond only partially to maximal tolerated doses of colchicine and 5% of patients are nonresponders. These patients usually include those with more severe genetic mutations or those with modifying genes that may inhibit the intracellular accumulation of colchicine, such as polymorphisms in MDR-1 P-glycoprotein pump transporter genes.[24] Many attacks occur as a result of noncompliance; in some patients missing even one dose can precipitate an attack.

Colchicine is generally well tolerated. The most common adverse effects include abdominal pain and diarrhea, especially in those receiving higher doses of colchicine and in patients with lactose intolerance.[25] These effects are usually transient and respond to gradual dose changes, dividing the daily dose, lactose avoidance, and antidiarrheal and antibloating agents. Other rare adverse effects include myalgia and myositis, peripheral neuropathy, and bone marrow suppression. Medications that inhibit the cytochrome P-450 (CYP[3]A[4]) and P-glycoprotein pathways may increase colchicine toxicity, particularly erythromycin, clarithromycin, statins, cyclosporin, and grapefruit juice. Colchicine does not affect growth and development and seems to be safe for use in pregnancy.[26]

IL-1 inhibitors may be effective in nonresponders or patients who do not tolerate colchicine.[27,28] A recent controlled study has found that rilonacept (Arcalyst), an IL-1–soluble fusion protein receptor, significantly decreases the frequency of attacks among most patients, particularly children.[29] Corticosteroids are effective only for prolonged febrile myalgia and FMF-related vasculitis but not the acute febrile episodes.

HYPERIMMUNOGLOBULINEMIA D WITH PERIODIC FEVER SYNDROME

This autosomal-recessive disease, also known as mevalonic kinase deficiency, was first described in 1984 in six Dutch patients.[30] The mean age of onset is 6 months, with more than 70% of patients having the first episode before 12 months of age. It is seen mainly in patients from the Netherlands and Western Europe.

Etiology and Pathogenesis

Hyperimmunoglobulinemia D syndrome (HIDS) is a metabolic disease with mutations in the *MVK* gene of the long arm of chromosome 12, encoding mevalonate kinase[31,32] resulting in partial absence of mevalonate kinase activity. The disease mevalonic aciduria is a result of complete absence in mevalonate kinase, and includes severe neurologic manifestations in addition to febrile episodes. In HIDS, most patients have mutations in the V377I (founder gene) and I268 T positions. Mutations result in an unstable enzyme, which is even less active when patients are febrile, hence attacks are often precipitated by pyrogenic infection and vaccines.[33] It seems that a deficiency of geranylgeranyl and other isoprenoid substrates resulting from the lack of mevalonate kinase is responsible for affecting inflammation, rather than excessive mevalonate.[34] One theory is that this deficiency affects IL-1β processing through the effect on R-type GTPase, dependent on prenylation.

Clinical Manifestations

Attacks, often triggered by vaccines or infection, typically occur every 3 to 6 weeks and last 3 to 7 days.[35] Besides fever, patients develop abdominal pain with vomiting and diarrhea; a polymorphic rash (**Fig. 3**); cervical lymphadenopathy; oral and genital ulceration; and arthralgia or arthritis.

Diagnosis

IgD levels are usually, but not always markedly elevated (>100 IU/mL). Patients younger than 3 years may have normal IgD levels. IgA is elevated in most patients. Urine level of mevalonic acid is elevated, mainly during attacks. Homozygous genetic mutations are present in 75% of patients. The term "variant HIDS" is used for patients who have clinical manifestations without genetic mutations when tested in commercial laboratories. If clinical suspicion is high, serum IgD and either *MVK* genetic testing or urinary mevalonic acid during an attack should be obtained.[3] False-positive causes of increased IgD levels (usually not to the degree seen in HIDS) may also be found in other autoinflammatory diseases, diabetes mellitus, smoking, and pregnancy.

Treatment and Outcome

Nonsteroidal anti-inflammatory drugs (NSAIDs) have some symptomatic benefit. Corticosteroids, colchicine, and thalidomide are generally ineffective. Simvastatin may reduce the number of febrile days but has no effect on the frequency of attacks. Etanercept (Enbrel), a soluble tumor necrosis factor (TNF) fusion protein receptor developed for the treatment of inflammatory arthritis, and anakinra (Kineret), a recombinant IL-1 receptor antagonist, may be effective in approximately 40% of cases in decreasing the frequency of attacks[35] or (anakinra) in shortening attacks.

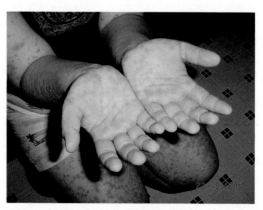

Fig. 3. Polymorphic rash on the hands, arms, and legs of a patient with hyperimmunoglobulinemia D syndrome (HIDS). (*From* Takada K, Aksentijevich I, Mahadevan V, et al. Favorable preliminary experience with etanercept in two patients with the hyperimmunoglobulinemia D and periodic fever syndrome. Arthritis Rheum 2003;48:2646; with permission.)

Attacks usually decrease in severity and frequency over time and amyloidosis is a rare complication (<3%).[35]

DEFICIENCY OF THE IL-1 RECEPTOR ANTAGONIST (DIRA)

This autosomal-recessive disease was described in 2009 in families from Newfoundland, Puerto Rico, Southern Netherlands, and Lebanon with onset in infancy.[36,37]

Etiology and Pathogenesis

The cause is a missense–nonsense mutation (or a 175-db deletion) in the *IL1RN* gene at the long arm of chromosome 2 that encodes the IL-1 receptor antagonist, leading to unopposed IL-1 stimulation.[36,37]

Clinical Manifestations

Affected infants present at birth or shortly after with a sterile pustular rash (localized or diffuse), multifocal osteomyelitis with lytic bone lesions, osteopenia, osteitis, arthritis, nail pits, respiratory distress with pneumonitis, oral ulcers, hepatosplenomegaly, and increased inflammatory indices. Of note, fever is absent.

Treatment and Outcome

Treatment with anakinra is remarkably effective in reversing clinical, laboratory, and imaging features. Before discovery of the cause and treatment of deficiency of the IL-1 receptor antagonist, infants succumbed to the disease with others suffering from skeletal deformities and failure to thrive.

DEFICIENCY OF IL-36 RECEPTOR ANTAGONIST (DITRA): FAMILIAL GENERALIZED PUSTULAR PSORIASIS

The discovery in 2011 of the genetic mutation that causes this rare autosomal-recessive disease is a recent discovery of a novel monogenetic autoinflammatory syndrome. The mutation has been reported in nine Tunisian families and five nonrelated European patients.[38,39]

Etiology and Pathogenesis

The cause is a missense–nonsense mutation in the *IL36RN* gene at the long arm of chromosome 2 (near the *IL1RN* gene) that encodes the IL-36 receptor antagonist, leading to unopposed IL-36 stimulation and the production of proinflammatory cytokines.[38,39] The IL-36 receptor antagonist is part of the IL-1 protein family and has many homologous regions to the IL-1 receptor antagonist.

Clinical Manifestations

The onset of disease can occur from infancy to mid-adulthood. Patients develop flares of high-grade fever with malaise lasting 1 to 3 days, and a generalized pustular rash, lasting days to weeks. Nail dystrophy and tongue (mainly geographic) lesions are common. About 30% of patients develop arthritis and about 30% develop a chronic course of psoriasis vulgaris.

Treatment and Outcome

Most commonly patients are treated with oral retinoids (aciterin). Immunosuppressive medications include corticosteroids, methotrexate, dapsone, and cyclosporine. Case reports on the efficacy of TNF-α and IL-1 inhibitors have been reported.[40] There is a high proportion of fatalities from sepsis related to the loss of the skin barrier from the widespread rash.

THE TNF-RECEPTOR–ASSOCIATED PERIODIC SYNDROME

First described in 1982 as familial Hibernian fever, the gene mutation for this autosomal-dominant disorder was discovered in 1999.[41,42] TNF-receptor–associated periodic syndrome (TRAPS) is the most common autosomal-dominant autoinflammatory disorder. Although initially described in patients of Irish or Scottish descent, TRAPS is found in all ethnic groups. TRAPS usually presents during the first decade of life (75%, median 3 years) but can present at any age and has the highest proportion of patients with adult onset among the genetic autoinflammatory diseases.

Etiology and Pathogenesis

The TRAPS gene (*TNFRSF1A*) has been localized to the short arm of chromosome 12.[42] The product of this gene is the 55-kDa TNF cell membrane receptor. There is a phenotype–genotype correlation with more severe disease and amyloidosis occurring in patients with protein structure altering cysteine residue mutations.[43] Certain mutations including R92Q and P46L are frequently seen in normal controls (up to 9% of the population), do not alter the protein structure, and may represent milder mutations of low penetrance.[4,44] Alternatively, these mutations may not be pathogenic by themselves but are polymorphisms that may contribute to a state of "increased" inflammation and nonspecific recurrent febrile syndromes.

The initial hypothesis to explain how the mutation results in clinical manifestations was that there is a decrease in the shedding of mutated membrane-bound TNF receptors when stimulated, leading to an increase of unopposed serum TNF.[45] However, it is clear that the pathogenesis of TRAPS is much more complicated and includes defects in intracellular trafficking (lack of internalization of receptors, protein misfolding, and intracellular aggregation of receptors in the cytoplasm instead of the Golgi apparatus) leading to defects in TNF-induced apoptosis and stimulation of intracellular inflammatory pathways, particularly reactive oxygen species.[4,46] There is also a decrease in the concentration of surface receptors.

Clinical Manifestations

Attacks typically last between 1 and 3 weeks (occasionally even up to 6 weeks), and occur two to six times per year.[43] Exercise is a common trigger of attacks. Besides fever patients develop serositis (abdominal, chest, and testicular pain); conjunctivitis; arthralgia; and myalgia. Two unique features are periorbital edema and a painful, distally migrating, erythematous rash (**Fig. 4**). This rash represents a mononuclear perivascular infiltrate of the subcutaneous fascia with occasional panniculitis. Patients with certain mutations, particularly R92Q, may develop a shorter and milder attack, with involvement of the pharynx and oral ulcerations, often resembling the periodic fever, aphthous-stomatitis, pharyngitis, and adenitis (PFAPA) syndrome.[44] Less common manifestations include recurrent pericarditis and central and focal neurologic abnormalities. Amyloidosis develops in 14% to 25% of patients, particularly those with cysteine mutations and a positive family history.

Diagnosis

The diagnosis of TRAPS is based on finding a genetic mutation in the *TNFRSF1A* gene, unlike other autoinflammatory diseases in which genetic mutations are only

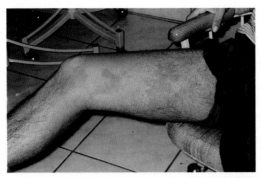

Fig. 4. Migratory erythematous rash of a patient with the tumor necrosis factor receptor–associated periodic syndrome (TRAPS). The rash is painful and migrates distally. (*From* Hashkes PJ. Autoinflammatory Disorders. In Rudolph CD, Rudolph AM, Lister GE, et al. editors. Rudolph's pediatrics. 22nd edition. New York: McGraw-Hill, 2011, p. 845; with permission.)

supporting evidence. Acute-phase reactants are persistently elevated, further increasing during attacks.

Treatment

NSAIDs may be effective for mild attacks. Corticosteroids are often beneficial for severe attacks but frequently patients need increasing doses with a decrease in efficacy in subsequent attacks. Colchicine is not effective.

Initial case reports showed that etanercept is beneficial.[45] However, recent literature has indicated that etanercept is not effective in all patients and in others may become less effective over time. Infliximab (Remicade), a TNF antibody, may worsen symptoms and should be avoided. IL-1 inhibitors may be effective in most etanercept-resistant patients.[47] A case of the efficacy of tocilizumab (Actemra), an antibody to the IL-6 receptor, was recently reported in a patient who failed etanercept and anakinra.[48] In general, aggressive therapy should be reserved for patients with severe disease, cysteine mutations, or a family history of amyloidosis.

THE CRYOPYRIN-ASSOCIATED PERIODIC SYNDROMES
Etiology and Pathogenesis

Three autosomal-dominant syndromes constitute cryopyrin-associated periodic syndromes (CAPS): (1) familial cold autoinflammatory syndrome (FCAS), (2) Muckle-Wells syndrome (MWS), and (3) neonatal-onset multisystem inflammatory disease (NOMID). They are considered variants of the same process that vary by severity of symptoms, systems involved, and outcome and all respond dramatically to IL-1 inhibitors. They are caused by single base mutations on the *NLRP3* gene located on the long arm of chromosome 1 encoding the protein cryopyrin.[49,50] Mutations may be specific or overlap among the three syndromes. No *NLRP3* mutations are found in about 50% of patients with NOMID and 25% to 33% of patients with MWS; these patients have a similar phenotype and response to treatment as mutation-positive patients.[51] Recently, it was found that nearly 70% of NOMID patients with a "negative" mutation have somatic mosaicism mutations in 4.2% to 35.8% of the cells.[52]

The cryopyrin protein has an important role in regulation of the assembly of the inflammasome (see **Fig. 1**). The mutated cryopyrin protein probably increases the rate of the inflammasome assembly independently of the usual stimuli needed in wild-type protein.[53]

Familial Cold Autoinflammatory Syndrome

FCAS (previously called familial cold urticaria) is the mildest form of CAPS. The first description was in 1940 and the genetic mutation was discovered in 2001. Almost all patients have a genetic mutation in the *NLRP3* gene and live in the United States. FCAS often presents at birth and is apparent in 95% of the patients by 6 months.

Clinical manifestations
Attacks usually start 2 to 3 hours after generalized (not by direct contact) cold exposure. Patients develop an urticaria-like rash, low-grade fever, arthralgia, conjunctivitis, nausea, extreme thirst, sweating, and headaches that peaks at 6 to 8 hours and lasts up to 24 hours. The attack frequency is variable but is often debilitating. The pathology of the rash is a perivascular polymorphonuclear cellular infiltrate in the dermis rather than mast cells as in true urticaria. Amyloidosis is rare, occurring in 2% to 4% of patients.

Treatment
IL-1 inhibitors are very effective in alleviating symptoms. Rilonacept and canakinumab (specific humanized antibody to IL-1β [Ilaris]) have been shown to be highly effective in controlled trials.[54,55] NSAIDs and antihistamines are not effective. High doses of corticosteroids can alleviate symptoms but are associated with many adverse effects.

Muckle-Wells Syndrome

MWS, the intermediate severity CAPS, was described in 1962 and the genetic mutation was also discovered in 2001. MWS can appear at any age and usually starts later in life than FCAS with most described cases coming from Europe.

Clinical manifestations and treatment
A typical attack lasts up to 3 days and includes fever, a more persistent urticaria-like rash than FCAS (**Fig. 5**), arthralgia, arthritis, myalgia, headaches, conjunctivitis, episcleritis, and uveitis. There are usually no triggers for attacks. Often starting in adolescence, 50% to 70% of patients develop sensorineural hearing loss, usually starting in high-frequency sounds. Amyloidosis develops in 25% of the patients. MWS also responds dramatically to IL-1 inhibitors.[54,55] However, existing hearing loss is

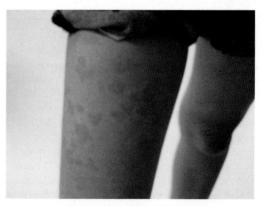

Fig. 5. Urticaria-like rash in a patient with Muckle-Wells syndrome.

reversible in only about one-third of cases.[56,57] In a 2-year follow-up of canakinumab use for MWS, nearly 25% of children needed dose increases or increased frequency of administration to sustain the effect.[57] Overall more than 70% retained complete, relapse-free remission throughout the study.

Neonatal-Onset Multisystem Inflammatory Disease

NOMID, the most severe of the CAPS, was first described in 1981 and the association with the *NLRP3* gene was found in 2002. In Europe NOMID is called "chronic infantile neurologic, cutaneous, articular syndrome."

Clinical manifestations

Patients present at birth or shortly after with urticaria-like rash and fever, often occurring daily with chronic aseptic meningitis.[58] Up to 50% of the infants are born prematurely. Symptoms associated with meningitis include headaches, irritability, and vomiting. Late complications include hydrocephalus, developmental delay, mental retardation, and hearing loss. Ocular findings include conjunctivitis, uveitis, and papillitis of the optic nerve resulting in visual loss. About 50% of NOMID patients develop a severe arthropathy (nonsynovial) by age 2 years, with cartilage growth abnormalities leading to substantial pain, bony overgrowth, ossification irregularities, deformities, and disabilities. Patients have characteristic morphologic abnormalities of short stature; frontal bossing; macrocephaly; saddle nose; short, thick extremities with clubbing of fingers; and wrinkled skin. Before modern therapy about 20% succumbed by age 20 years and others developed amyloidosis.

Treatment

Anakinra has dramatic effect on the rash, fever, and meningitis of NOMID with normalization of acute-phase reactants.[59] Existing hearing loss, neurologic, and joint manifestations are reversible only in a minority of patients.[56,57] Early recognition and treatment is crucial in preventing long-term damage and disability. Anti-inflammatory medications other than IL-1 inhibitors are of marginal effect.

FAMILIAL COLD AUTOINFLAMMATORY SYNDROME II RELATED TO MUTATIONS IN THE *NALP12* GENE

This autosomal-dominant disease with a clinical phenotype between FCAS and MWS was reported in several families, particularly from Guadeloupe, as a result of mutations in the *NALP12* gene that is an important regulator of nuclear factor-κB.[60] Usually triggered by generalized cold exposure patients develop from the first year of life frequent attacks of fever, urticaria-like rashes, arthralgia, myalgia, and headache lasting 2 to 15 days.[61] Many patients develop sensorineural hearing loss. Unlike CAPS-related FCAS, IL-1 inhibition was only transiently effective.[62]

PYOGENIC STERILE ARTHRITIS, PYODERMA GANGRENOSUM, ACNE SYNDROME

PAPA, a very rare syndrome, was first described in 1997[63] and is the result of mutations in the *PSTPIP1* gene on the long-arm of chromosome 15 encoding the CD2 antigen-binding protein.[64] This cytoskeleton protein binds to pyrin, thus similar to FMF, which may affect IL-1 activity.[65]

Clinical Manifestations and Treatment

Attacks are often triggered by minor trauma and result in fever and sterile joint effusion in large joints with massive polymorphonuclear infiltrates.[63] Patients develop pyoderma gangrenosum, severe scarring acne mainly in adolescence, and often develop diabetes mellitus and depression. Intra-articular corticosteroid injections can alleviate the acute inflammatory arthritis. Anti-TNF and anakinra therapy have been reported to be effective for the pyoderma gangrenosum.

PERIODIC FEVER, APHTHOUS STOMATITIS, PHARYNGITIS, ADENITIS SYNDROME

PFAPA is the most common autoinflammatory syndrome in childhood and was initially described in 1987.[66] The etiology is unknown but increased gene expression related to IL-1β, interferon, complement, and Th1 chemokines are found during attacks.[67] Although no specific genetic mutations have been found, familial cases of PFAPA are known and many Middle Eastern patients have heterozygous FMF mutations.[68] The latter patients may have a milder disease course.[69]

Clinical Manifestations

The onset of PFAPA is almost always before 5 years (mode 2–3 years); however, rare adult-onset cases have been reported.[68,70] This syndrome is truly periodic (parents can often predict the day of the attack) with attacks occurring usually every 21 to 28 days and fever lasting 4 to 7 days. Patients usually report an aura of "glazed" eyes or feeling unwell several hours before the start of an attack. Pharyngitis and cervical adenopathy are present is 80% to 100% of patients and aphthous stomatitis in 60% to 70%. Patients frequently complain of abdominal pain, nausea or vomiting, arthralgia, and headaches.

Diagnosis

Diagnostic criteria have been defined for children with typical clinical features with the exclusion of cyclic neutropenia.[71] For correct diagnosis, it is crucial that patients are completely asymptomatic (with normal acute-phase reactants) between attacks and exhibit normal growth and development. Other autoinflammatory syndromes, particularly TRAPS or HIDS, need to be considered in patients with nontypical features or who are not completely well between attacks.[44,72] Application of the Gaslini diagnostic score (http://www.printo.it/periodicfever/index.asp) can help differentiate patients with PFAPA from other hereditary autoinflammatory syndromes.[3,72]

Treatment

A single dose of prednisone (0.6–2 mg/kg) at the onset of symptoms usually aborts that attack.[68,70–72] However, the intervals between attacks may shorten. In about one-third of the patients cimetidine (Tagamet) may be effective as a prophylactic agent (40 mg/kg/d, in two divided doses).[73] Colchicine is effective in preventing attacks in few patients, particularly those with MEFV mutations.[67] Anakinra administration at the start of attacks may shorten or abort attacks without the effect of shortening intervals between attacks.[70] Recent controlled studies have shown that tonsillectomy (with or without adenoidectomy) is curative in most patients with a meta-analysis showing complete resolution in 83% (95% confidence interval, 77%–89%)[74] and may be an option for those with frequent need for corticosteroids or with marked effect on quality of life.

Outcome

Patients do not develop amyloidosis. The frequency and severity of attacks decrease with time and tend to resolve during the second decade of life.[68,70,71] However, a recent study has indicated than approximately 15% of patients continued to have attacks for at least 18 years.[75]

CHRONIC RECURRENT MULTIFOCAL OSTEOMYELITIS

Chronic recurrent multifocal osteomyelitis (CRMO), first described by Giedion and colleagues[76] in 1972, is usually sporadic with an unknown cause. However, up to 25% of patients have a positive family history for either psoriasis or inflammatory bowel disease. There are several rare genetic autoinflammatory bone disorders resembling CRMO including deficiency in IL-1 receptor antagonist; Majeed syndrome (CRMO with congenital dyserythropoietic anemia); cherubism (bone degradation of the jaws); and a mouse model of CRMO with mutations in the *pstpip2* gene.

Clinical Manifestations

Patients with CRMO develop recurrent episodes of bone pain with or without fever with sterile osteolytic lesions surrounded by sclerotic bone,[77] especially in the metaphysis of long bones. Other bones can be involved, particularly the clavicle, vertebral bodies, and ribs. Often asymptomatic lesions are found by technetium nuclear bone scans or whole-body MRI scans. Associated clinical findings may include synovitis, acne, pustulosis, hyperostosis, and osteitis (SAPHO syndrome); isolated palmoplantar pustolosis; psoriasis; sacroiliitis; inflammatory bowel disease; and pyoderma gangrenosum. Patients have spontaneous remissions with healing of lesions and relapses. Chronic disease may develop in approximately 50% of patients with long-term bone sequela, leg length inequality, and disability.

Treatment

Most patients respond to NSAIDs with occasional need for corticosteroids. Bisphosphonates have been reported to be effective in several case series.[78] Other treatments described in case reports include methotrexate, sulfasalazine, azithromycin, interferon, anakinra, and the anti-TNF agents infliximab and etanercept.[78]

THE OUTCOME OF PATIENTS WITH UNDIAGNOSED NONINFECTIOUS RECURRENT FEVER

Despite the major advances in the autoinflammatory syndromes in the last decade more than 60% of children with recurrent fever still go undiagnosed at tertiary centers (personal observation). Most of these children do well, with resolution of their febrile episodes or decrease in the frequency and severity.[79,80] Only a small minority later develop a recognizable autoinflammatory or rheumatic disease.[80]

SUMMARY

Several authors have offered stepwise pathways to the clinical and genetic diagnosis of the expanding spectrum of the autoinflammatory diseases.[3,81–83] A thorough history and physical examination often leads to a diagnosis. It is crucial to see the child during an attack or ask the family to take photographs of findings. Genetic testing should be performed in a logical manner and be reserved to confirm the diagnosis and gather prognostic information while recognizing limitations. A simple interactive tool available on the Internet (http://www.printo.it/periodicfever/index.asp) based on an Italian cohort of 228 patients with recurrent fever[3] can help differentiate patients with a high risk of a genetic autoinflammatory disease, realizing the limitation that this score may not fully apply to cohorts of differing ethnicities. Families of those patients who remain undiagnosed after a thorough investigation should be reassured of a general good prognosis.

ACKNOWLEDGMENTS

The authors thank Keren Dror for her illustration of **Fig. 1**.

REFERENCES

1. McGonagle D, Aziz A, Dickie LJ, et al. An integrated classification of pediatric inflammatory diseases, based on the concepts of autoinflammation and the immunological disease continuum. Pediatr Res 2009;65:38R–45R.
2. Padeh S. Periodic fever syndromes. Pediatr Clin North Am 2005;52:577–609.
3. Gattorno M, Sormani MP, D'Osualdo A, et al. A diagnostic score for molecular analysis of hereditary autoinflammatory syndromes with periodic fever in children. Arthritis Rheum 2008;58:1823–32.
4. Masters SL, Simon A, Aksentijevich I, et al. Horror Autoinflammaticus: the molecular pathophysiology of autoinflammatory disease. Annu Rev Immunol 2009;27:621–68.
5. Siegal S. Benign paroxysmal peritonitis. Ann Intern Med 1945;22:1–21.
6. Ben-Chetrit E, Touitou I. Familial Mediterranean fever in the world. Arthritis Rheum 2009;61:1447–53.
7. Pras E, Aksentijevich I, Gruberg L, et al. Mapping of a gene causing familial Mediterranean fever to the short arm of chromosome 16. N Engl J Med 1992;291:932–44.
8. The International FMF Consortium. Ancient missense mutations in a new member of the RoRet gene family are likely to cause familial Mediterranean fever. Cell 1997;90:797–807.
9. The French FMF Consortium. A candidate gene for familial Mediterranean fever. Nat Genet 1997;17:25–31.
10. Gershoni-Baruch R, Brik R, Zacks N, et al. The contribution of genotypes at the MEFV and SAA1 loci to amyloidosis and disease severity in patients with familial Mediterranean fever. Arthritis Rheum 2003;48:1149–55.
11. Tchernitchko D, Moutereau S, Legrendre M, et al. MEFV analysis is of particularly weak diagnostic value for recurrent fevers in Western European Caucasian patients. Arthritis Rheum 2005;52:3603–5.
12. Infevers. Available at: http://fmf.igh.cnrs.fr/ISSAID/infevers/. Accessed September 21, 2011.
13. Chae JJ, Wood G, Masters SL, et al. The B30.2 domain of pyrin, the familial Mediterranean fever protein, interacts directly with caspase-1 to modulate IL-1beta production. Proc Natl Acad Sci U S A 2006;103:9982–7.
14. Samuels J, Aksenitjevich I, Yelizaveta T, et al. Familial Mediterranean fever at the millennium: clinical spectrum, ancient mutations, and a survey of 100 American referrals to the National Institutes of Health. Medicine (Baltimore) 1998;77:268–97.
15. Padeh S, Livneh A, Pras E, et al. Familial Mediterranean fever in children presenting with attacks of fever alone. J Rheumatol 2010;37:865–9.
16. Touitou I, Sarkisian T, Medlej-Hashim M, et al. Country as the primary risk factor for renal amyloidosis in familial Mediterranean fever. Arthritis Rheum 2007;56:1706–12.
17. Hawkins PN, Lavender JP, Pepys MB. Evaluation of systemic amyloidosis by scintigraphy with 123I-labeled serum amyloid P component. N Engl J Med 1990;323:508–13.
18. Livneh A, Langevitz P, Zemer D, et al. Criteria for the diagnosis of familial Mediterranean fever. Arthritis Rheum 1997;40:1879–85.

19. Yalçinkaya F, Ozen S, Ozçakar ZB, et al. A new set of criteria for the diagnosis of familial Mediterranean fever in childhood. Rheumatology (Oxford) 2009;48: 395–8.
20. Berkun Y, Padeh S, Reichman B, et al. A single testing of serum amyloid A levels as a tool for diagnosis and treatment dilemmas in familial Mediterranean fever. Semin Arthritis Rheum 2007;37:182–8.
21. Goldfinger SE. Colchicine for familial Mediterranean fever. N Engl J Med 1972; 287:1302.
22. Zemer D, Revach M, Pras M, et al. A controlled trial of colchicine in preventing attacks of familial Mediterranean fever. N Engl J Med 1974;291:932–4.
23. Zemer D, Pras M, Sohar E, et al. Colchicine in the prevention and treatment of the amyloidosis of familial Mediterranean fever. N Engl J Med 1986;314:1001–5.
24. Lidar M, Scherrmann JM, Shinar Y, et al. Colchicine nonresponsiveness in familial Mediterranean fever: clinical, genetic, pharmacokinetic, and socioeconomic characterization. Semin Arthritis Rheum 2004;33:273–82.
25. Kallinich T, Haffner D, Nichues T, et al. Colchicine use in children and adolescents with familial Mediterranean fever: literature review and consensus statement. Pediatrics 2007;119:e474–83.
26. Ben-Chetrit E, Ben-Chetrit A, Berkun Y, et al. Pregnancy outcomes in women with familial Mediterranean fever receiving colchicine: is amniocentesis justified? Arthritis Care Res (Hoboken) 2010;62:143–8.
27. Meinzer U, Quartier P, Alexandra JF, et al. Interleukin-1 targeting drugs in familial Mediterranean fever: a case series and a review of the literature. Semin Arthritis Rheum 2011;41(2):265–71.
28. Ozen S, Bilginer Y, Aktay Ayaz N, et al. Anti-interleukin 1 treatment for patients with familial Mediterranean fever resistant to colchicine. J Rheumatol 2011;38: 516–8.
29. Hashkes PJ, Spalding SJ, Giannini EH, et al. Rilonacept (interleukin-1 trap) for treatment of colchicine resistant familial Mediterranean fever: a randomized, multicenter double-blinded, alternating treatment phase II trial. Arthritis Rheum 2011;63(Suppl):S952.
30. van der Meer JW, Vossen JM, Radl J, et al. Hyperimmunoglobulinaemia D and periodic fever: a new syndrome. Lancet 1984;1:1087–90.
31. Houton SM, Kuis W, Duran M, et al. Mutations in MVK, encoding mevalonate kinase, cause hyperimmunoglobulinaemia D and periodic fever syndrome. Nat Genet 1999;22:175–7.
32. Drenth JP, Cuisset L, Grateau G, et al. Mutations in the gene encoding mevalonate kinase cause hyper-IgD and periodic fever syndrome. Nat Genet 1999;22: 178–81.
33. Houten SM, Frenkel J, Rijkers GT, et al. Temperature dependence of mutant mevalonate kinase activity as pathogenic factor in hyper-IgD and periodic fever syndrome. Hum Mol Genet 2002;11:3115–24.
34. Frenkel J, Rijkers GT, Mandey SH, et al. Lack of isoprenoid products raises ex vivo interleukin-1 beta secretion in hyperimmunoglobulinemia D and periodic fever syndrome. Arthritis Rheum 2002;46:2794–803.
35. Simon A, International HIDS Study Group. Long-term follow-up, clinical features, and quality of life in a series of 103 patients with hyperimmunoglobulinemia D syndrome. Medicine (Baltimore) 2008;87:301–10.
36. Aksentijevich I, Masters SL, Ferguson PJ, et al. An autoinflammatory disease with deficiency of the interleukin-1-receptor antagonist. N Engl J Med 2009;360: 2426–37.

37. Reddy S, Jia S, Geoffrey R, et al. An autoinflammatory disease due to homozygous deletion of the IL1RN locus. N Engl J Med 2009;360:2438–44.

38. Marrakchi S, Guigue P, Renshaw BR, et al. Interleukin-36-receptor antagonist deficiency and generalized pustular psoriasis. N Engl J Med 2011;365:620–8.

39. Onoufriadis A, Simpson MA, Pink AE, et al. Mutations in IL36RN/IL1F5 are associated with the severe episodic inflammatory skin disease known as generalized pustular psoriasis. Am J Hum Genet 2011;89:432–7.

40. Viguier M, Guigue P, Pagès C, et al. Successful treatment of generalized pustular psoriasis with the interleukin-1-receptor antagonist anakinra: lack of correlation with IL1RN mutations. Ann Intern Med 2010;153:66–7.

41. Williamson LM, Hull D, Mehta R, et al. Familial Hibernian fever. Q J Med 1982;51:469–80.

42. McDermott MF, Aksentijevich I, Galon J, et al. Germline mutation in the extracellular domains of the 55 kDa TNF receptor, TNFR1, define a family of dominantly inherited autoinflammatory syndromes. Cell 1999;97:133–44.

43. Aganna E, Hammond L, Hawkins P, et al. Heterogeneity among patients with tumor necrosis factor-associated periodic syndrome phenotypes. Arthritis Rheum 2003;48:2632–44.

44. Pelagatti MA, Meini A, Caorsi R, et al. Long-term clinical profile of children with the low-penetrance R92Q mutation of the TNFRSF1A gene. Arthritis Rheum 2011;63:1141–50.

45. Arkwright PD, McDermott MF, Houton SM, et al. Hyper IgD syndrome (HIDS) associated with in vitro evidence of defective monocyte TNFRSF1A shedding and partial response to TNF receptor blockade with etanercept. Clin Exp Immunol 2002;130:484–8.

46. Bulua AC, Simon A, Maddipati R, et al. Mitochondrial reactive oxygen species promote production of proinflammatory cytokines and are elevated in TNFR1-associated periodic syndrome (TRAPS). J Exp Med 2011;208:519–33.

47. Gattorno M, Pelagatti MA, Meini A, et al. Persistent efficacy of anakinra in patients with tumor necrosis factor receptor-associated periodic syndrome. Arthritis Rheum 2008;58:1516–20.

48. Vaitla PM, Radford PM, Tighe PJ, et al. Role of interleukin-6 in a patient with tumor necrosis factor receptor-associated periodic syndrome: assessment of outcomes following treatment with the anti-interleukin-6 receptor monoclonal antibody tocilizumab. Arthritis Rheum 2011;63:1151–5.

49. Hoffman H, Mueller J, Brodie D, et al. Mutation of a new gene encoding a putative pyrin-like protein causes familial cold autoinflammatory syndrome and Muckle-Wells syndrome. Nat Genet 2001;29:301–5.

50. Feldmann J, Prieur AM, Quartier P, et al. Chronic infantile neurological cutaneous and articular syndrome is caused by mutations in CIAS1, a gene highly expressed in polymorphonuclear cells and chondrocytes. Am J Hum Genet 2002;71:198–203.

51. Aksentijevich I, Putnam CD, Remmers EF, et al. The clinical continuum of cryopyrinopathies: novel CIAS1 mutations in North American patients and a new cryopyrin model. Arthritis Rheum 2007;56:1273–85.

52. Tanaka N, Izawa K, Saito MK, et al. High incidence of NLRP3 somatic mosaicism in chronic infantile neurological cutaneous and articular syndrome patients: the results of an international multicenter collaborative study. Arthritis Rheum 2011;63:3625–32.

53. Gattorno M, Tassi S, Carta S, et al. Pattern of IL-1β secretion on response to lipopolysaccharide and ATP before and after IL-1 blockade in patients with CIAS1 mutations. Arthritis Rheum 2007;56:3138–48.

54. Hoffman HM, Throne ML, Amar NJ, et al. Efficacy and safety of rilonacept (inter-leukin-1 trap) in patients with cryopyrin-associated periodic syndromes. Arthritis Rheum 2008;58:2443–5.
55. Lachmann HJ, Kone-Paut I, Kuemmerle-Deschner JB, et al, Canakinumab in CAPS Study Group. Use of canakinumab in the cryopyrin-associated periodic syndrome. N Engl J Med 2009;360:2416–25.
56. Neven B, Marvillet I, Terrada C, et al. Long-term efficacy of the interleukin-1 receptor antagonist anakinra in ten patients with neonatal-onset multisystem inflammatory disease/chronic infantile neurologic, cutaneous, articular syndrome. Arthritis Rheum 2010;62:258–67.
57. Kuemmerle-Deschner JB, Hachulla E, Cartwright R, et al. Two-year results from an open-label, multicentre, phase III study evaluating the safety and efficacy of canakinumab in patients with cryopyrin-associated periodic syndrome across different severity phenotypes. Ann Rheum Dis 2011;70:2093–102.
58. Aksentijevich I, Nowak M, Mallah M, et al. De novo CIAS1 mutations, cytokine acti-vation, and evidence for genetic heterogeneity in patients with neonatal-onset multi-system inflammatory disease (NOMID): a new member of the expanding family of pyrin-associated autoinflammatory diseases. Arthritis Rheum 2002;46:3340–8.
59. Goldbach-Mansky R, Dailey NJ, Canna SW, et al. Neonatal-onset multisystem inflammatory disease responsive to interleukin-1β inhibition. N Engl J Med 2006;355:581–92.
60. Jeru I, Duquesnoy P, Fernandes-Alnemri T, et al. Mutations in NALP12 cause hereditary periodic fever syndromes. Proc Natl Acad Sci U S A 2008;105:1614–9.
61. Borghini S, Tassi S, Chiesa S, et al. Clinical presentation and pathogenesis of cold-induced autoinflammatory disease in a family with recurrence of an NLRP12 mutation. Arthritis Rheum 2011;63:830–9.
62. Jéru I, Hentgen V, Normand S, et al. Role of interleukin-1β in NLRP12-associated autoinflammatory disorders and resistance to anti-interleukin-1 therapy. Arthritis Rheum 2011;63:2142–8.
63. Lindor NM, Arsenault TM, Solomon H, et al. A new autosomal dominant disorder of pyogenic sterile arthritis, pyoderma gangrenosum and acne: PAPA syndrome. Mayo Clin Proc 1997;72:611–5.
64. Wise CA, Gillum JD, Seidman CE, et al. Mutations in CD2BP1 disrupt binding to PTP PEST and are responsible for PAPA syndrome, an autoinflammatory disorder. Hum Mol Genet 2002;11:961–9.
65. Shoham NG, Centola M, Mansfield E, et al. Pyrin binds the PSTPIP1/CD2BP1 protein, defining familial Mediterranean fever and PAPA as disorders in the same pathway. Proc Natl Acad Sci U S A 2003;100:13501–6.
66. Marshall GS, Edwards KM, Butler J, et al. Syndrome of periodic fever, pharyn-gitis, and aphthous stomatitis. J Pediatr 1987;110:43–6.
67. Stojanov S, Lapidus S, Chitkara P, et al. Periodic fever, aphthous stomatitis, phar-yngitis, and adenitis (PFAPA) is a disorder of innate immunity and Th1 activation responsive to IL-1 blockade. Proc Natl Acad Sci U S A 2011;108:7148–53.
68. Padeh S, Brezniak N, Zemer D, et al. Periodic fever, aphthous stomatitis, pharyn-gitis, and adenopathy syndrome: clinical characteristics and outcome. J Pediatr 1999;135:98–101.
69. Berkun Y, Levy R, Hurwitz A, et al. The familial Mediterranean fever gene as a modifier of periodic fever, aphthous stomatitis, pharyngitis, and adenopathy syndrome. Semin Arthritis Rheum 2011;40:467–72.
70. Tasher D, Somekh E, Dalal I. PFAPA syndrome: new clinical aspects revealed. Arch Dis Child 2006;91:981–4.

71. Thomas KT, Feder HM Jr, Lawton AR, et al. Periodic fever syndrome in children. J Pediatr 1999;135:15–21.
72. Gattorno M, Caorsi R, Meini A, et al. Differentiating PFAPA syndrome from monogenic periodic fevers. Pediatrics 2009;124:e721–8.
73. Feder HM Jr. Cimetidine treatment for periodic fever associated with aphthous stomatitis, pharyngitis and cervical adenitis. Pediatr Infect Dis J 1992;11:318–21.
74. Garavello W, Pignataro L, Gaini L, et al. Tonsillectomy in children with periodic fever with aphthous stomatitis, pharyngitis, and adenitis syndrome. J Pediatr 2011;159(1):138–42.
75. Wurster VM, Carlucci JG, Feder HM Jr, et al. Long-term follow-up of children with periodic fever, aphthous stomatitis, pharyngitis, and cervical adenitis syndrome. J Pediatr 2011;159:958–64.
76. Giedion A, Holthusen W, Masel LF, et al. Subacute and chronic "symmetrical" osteomyelitis. Ann Radiol 1972;15:329–42.
77. Laxer RM, Shore AD, Manson D, et al. Chronic recurrent multifocal osteomyelitis and psoriasis: a report of a new association and review of related disorders. Semin Arthritis Rheum 1988;17:260–70.
78. Twilt M, Laxer RM. Clinical care of children with sterile bone inflammation. Curr Opin Rheumatol 2011;23:424–31.
79. John C, Gilsdorf J. Recurrent fever in children. Pediatr Infect Dis J 2002;21: 1071–7.
80. Long SS. Distinguishing among prolonged, recurrent, and periodic fever syndromes: approach of a pediatric infectious diseases subspecialist. Pediatr Clin North Am 2005;52:811–35.
81. Grateau G. Clinical and genetic aspects of the hereditary periodic fever syndromes. Rheumatology 2004;43:410–5.
82. Federici L, Rittore-Domingo C, Kone-Paut I, et al. A decision tree for genetic diagnosis of hereditary periodic fevers in unselected patients. Ann Rheum Dis 2006; 65:1427–32.
83. Simon A, van der Meer JW, Vesely R, et al. Approach to genetic analysis in the diagnosis of hereditary autoinflammatory syndromes. Rheumatology (Oxford) 2006;45:269–73.

Approach to the Patient with Noninflammatory Musculoskeletal Pain

Peter Weiser, MD

KEYWORDS

- Musculoskeletal pain • Hypermobility syndrome
- Overuse syndrome • Pain amplification syndromes

Musculoskeletal pain is one of the most common presenting symptoms at the pediatrician's office. Etiology ranges from benign conditions to serious ones requiring prompt attention. This article discusses entities presenting as musculoskeletal pain while not being associated with arthritis, the latter being dealt with in detail in other articles in this issue. The most common nonarthritic conditions are benign limb pain of childhood (growing pains), hypermobility, overuse syndromes with or without skeletal abnormalities, malignancies, and pain amplification syndromes. **Fig. 1** shows the possible initial decision process regarding evaluation, after ruling out trauma and infection.

BENIGN LIMB PAIN OF CHILDHOOD
When to Consider

Benign limb pain is a chronic, intermittent, paroxysmal nighttime shin pain without daytime symptoms or limitation.

Background

Benign limb pain is also known as growing pains; a clear misnomer because it usually occurs outside of major growth spurt periods between ages 3 to 5 and 8 to 12 years. Children are characterized by recurrent lower extremity pain, mostly bilateral,[1] occurring at night or in the evenings. The prevalence is variable, between 4% and 37% of studied children, depending on the targeted age groups.[2,3] Diagnostic criteria were suggested by Naish and Apley[3] in 1951 (**Box 1**). Their cohort included 721 children attending school clinics, recognizing the existence of 3 groups: (1) children with "ill-defined pains," vaguely distributed symptoms both daytime and nighttime; (2) the largest group of children, with "diurnal fatigue pains," whose pain was associated with "emotional disturbance" and postural defects including flat feet, pain being brought on by activities; and (3) the true "paroxysmal nocturnal pains" group, without

Division of Pediatric Rheumatology, Department of Pediatrics, Children's of Alabama, University of Alabama at Birmingham, Birmingham, AL 35233, USA
E-mail address: ideirj@gmail.com

Pediatr Clin N Am 59 (2012) 471–492
doi:10.1016/j.pcl.2012.03.012
0031-3955/12/$ – see front matter © 2012 Elsevier Inc. All rights reserved.

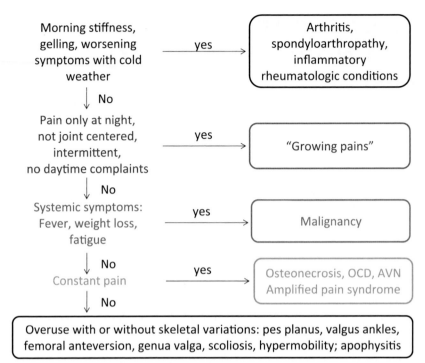

Fig. 1. Musculoskeletal pain decision tree. AVN, avascular necrosis; OCD, osteochondrosis dissecans.

association with daily activities but with the presence of similar symptoms in 20% of parents, and without any obvious etiology.

To this day, the etiology remains unknown. A link with restless leg syndrome has been suggested by Rajaram and colleagues,[4] but the concomitant diagnosis of growing pains differed slightly from the criteria by Naish and Appley, the sample size was low (10 children), and some of the children listed had daytime symptoms as well. Limb pain seemed to get better on moving the extremities, which is characteristic for restless leg syndrome but not for growing pains. Hashkes and colleagues[5] showed no association with vascular perfusion changes in affected areas, but there

---

Box 1
Criteria for the diagnosis of growing pains (based on Naish and Apley[3])

1. At least a 3-month history of pain

2. Intermittent pain with symptom-free intervals of days, weeks, or months

3. Pain late in day or awakening child at night

4. Pain not specifically related to joints

5. Pain of significant severity to interrupt such normal activity as sleep

6. Normal physical examination, laboratory data, and roentgenograms

seemed to be decreased bone speed of sound,[6] suggesting a local overuse syndrome. However, this does not explain the paroxysmal character of nighttime appearance only. Interestingly enough, children with this type of pain have decreased pain thresholds, which would suggest that this entity is a form of pain amplification syndrome.[7]

How to Diagnose

The term benign limb pain of childhood likely should be used for children belonging to the third group of Naish and Apley. Episodes are heralded by occurrence at night and wake the child (and subsequently the whole family) from sleep. It is described as very intense pain of mostly the shins with peak intensity of 10 to 15 minutes that slowly regresses over the following hour. It is not joint centered, but young children might not be capable of proper localization. There are no changes of the affected area when examined, such as redness, rashes, or swelling. Massaging might help or at least provide comfort, and nonsteroidal anti-inflammatory drugs (NSAIDs) also seem to provide relief albeit it might be coincidental, considering the time of onset of action of medication and natural resolution of symptoms. Children are well during the day, have no limitations, and there are asymptomatic periods between the episodes lasting from days to weeks.[8,9]

Upper extremity or joint pain, daytime complaints, limping, systemic symptoms including fevers, weight loss, and decreased energy/activity are not part of the presentation and require further workup. Pain presentation later in the day and in the evening, especially associated with increased activities, suggests overuse syndromes, and common skeletal variations such as femoral anteversion, genua valga, flat feet, and hypermobility need to be assessed. Again, children should be asymptomatic during the day, with normal physical examination. Otherwise, radiographic imaging and, if indicated, complete blood count (CBC) and erythrocyte sedimentation rate (ESR) should be performed to look for other entities. **Table 1** lists findings that suggest benign limb pain.

How to Treat

Initially reassurance is important, although parents might find it unsatisfactory. Massaging and NSAIDs can provide help. Considering the asymptomatic intervals, daily prophylactic NSAID administration might be more harmful than beneficial in the long run.

What to Expect

There are few studies addressing long-term evolution of this condition. Five-year follow-up suggests resolution of symptoms in half of the patients, but the remainder seem to have persistent complaints even in adulthood.[10]

Table 1
Findings suggesting benign limb pain

Likely Benign Limb Pain	Unlikely Benign Limb Pain
Shin pain	Joint pain
Paroxysmal night time occurrence	Daytime
Episodic with asymptomatic periods	Constant/fluctuating
Well otherwise	Systemic symptoms
Normal physical examination	Findings on physical examination

MALIGNANCY
When to Consider

It is paramount to consider an underlying malignancy when there is daytime and nighttime joint pain, arthritis without morning stiffness, systemic symptoms including fever, weight loss, and night sweats. Infections and systemic inflammatory conditions should also be part of the differential diagnosis.

Background

Fewer than 1% of patients presenting with musculoskeletal complaints will end up being diagnosed with malignancy whereby leukemia, lymphoma, Ewing sarcoma, and neuroblastoma are the most common entities (**Table 2**).[11–13] Although a rare event, symptoms can overlap with those of juvenile idiopathic arthritis (JIA), overuse syndrome, or the previously mentioned benign limb pain of childhood, which can lead to a delay in the diagnosis. Symptoms are due to either local tissue destruction or the paraneoplastic effect.

How to Diagnose

Clinical evaluation

The most common presentation is monoarthritis of the large joints, musculoskeletal pain, night sweats, and fevers. Malignancy as an underlying diagnosis should be considered every time systemic symptoms or an atypical presentation of a diagnosis is present (solitary elbow arthritis without morning stiffness diagnosed as JIA). Possible red flags appearing during workup are summarized in **Table 3**. The physical examination may be noncontributory besides the overall chronically ill appearance. However, bony tenderness, decreased strength, hepatosplenomegaly, and lymphadenopathy are clear indications for further workup.

Laboratory evaluation

Laboratory indicators can be normal (see **Table 2**).[11–15] Nevertheless, CBC (leukopenia or leukocytosis, anemia, thrombocytopenia), and elevated ESR, C-reactive protein (CRP), uric acid, lactate dehydrogenase (LDH), and urine vanillylmandelic acid (especially in a young child with back pain) can be helpful. Diseases with systemic inflammation such as systemic lupus erythematosus (SLE) or systemic JIA might present with similar findings. Cytopenias with elevated ESR and normal CRP can occur in SLE; leukocytosis with anemia may occur in systemic JIA, polyarteritis nodosa, and Kawasaki disease, although in the latter 2, thrombocytosis rather than thrombocytopenia is more usual. Elevated uric acid can occur in kidney diseases but primary gout is almost unheard of in childhood. A high LDH seems to be the best predictor for leukemia,[14] but it also can be elevated in hemolysis and myositis. Nevertheless, Coombs negative anemia with thrombocytopenia, and elevated ESR, CRP, LDH, and uric acid should lead to imaging and bone marrow biopsy.

Imaging

Localized constant bone pain, especially if not joint centered, warrants imaging. Unfortunately, positive findings including metaphyseal growth arrest lines on radiographic studies occur late during the disease process and are often nonspecific. Hepatosplenomegaly, lymphadenopathy, systemic symptoms, and elevated uric acid and LDH should prompt computed tomography scans of the chest, abdomen, and pelvis. Multiple sites of involvement can be assessed by whole-body tri-phase bone scan, but this is nonspecific as is magnetic resonance imaging, because misinterpretation of the image as osteomyelitis can delay diagnosis.[11]

Table 2 Malignancies in 3 patient cohorts			
	Cabral and Tucker,[13] 1999	Trapani et al,[11] 2000	Gonçalves et al,[12] 2005
Total number of patients	Approximately 8400	1254	3528
Patients with malignancies (%)	29 (0.35)	10 (0.8)	9 (0.25)
Most common	Leukemia, lymphoma, neuroblastoma, Ewing sarcoma	Ewing sarcoma	Leukemia, Ewing sarcoma, lymphoma
Presentation (%)			
Musculoskeletal pain	82	80	88
Fever	54	80	100
Fatigue	50	50	22
Weight loss	42	20	33
Hepatosplenomegaly	29	30	—
Lymphadenopathy	18	30	—
Arthritis	25	50	55
Night sweats	14	30	—
Bruising	14	—	—
Laboratory findings (%)			
Abnormal CBC	31	20–80	11–66
Abnormal WBC	—	20	11
Anemia	—	80	66
Abnormal platelets	—	70	50
Elevated ESR	26	80	75
Elevated LDH	24	10	50

Numbers represent percentage of patients.
Abbreviations: CBC, complete blood count; ESR, erythrocyte sedimentation rate; LDH, lactate dehydrogenase; WBC, white blood cell count.

Table 3
Red flags suggesting malignancy (after excluding infections)

Pain	Disproportionate to physical examination
	Not joint centered
	Migratory
	Night time pain (except for growing pains)
Arthritis	No morning stiffness
	Atypical onset: elbow, back
Systemic symptoms	Night sweats
	Weight loss
	Fever

In summary, being a relatively rare entity, the presentation of childhood malignancy can be misleading. In the study by Gonçalves and colleagues,[12] all 9 affected patients had relief from pain either spontaneously or with massage and analgesics, and 2 had benign laboratory findings.

HYPERMOBILITY SYNDROMES
When to Consider

Hypermobility syndromes need to be considered when there is mostly lower extremity joint pain toward the afternoon or end of the day, pain is worse with activities, and resting helps. Also, it should be suspected in children with repeated joint subluxations, loose skin, and capillary fragility because it can be part of complex genetic syndromes (**Table 4**).

Background

Range of motion of the joints is variable; it is increased in childhood and decreases with aging.[16] There are syndromes in which molecular defects of connective tissue such as collagen disorder in Ehlers-Danlos or fibrillin mutations in Marfan syndrome have been proved, but in the majority of cases one cannot identify the biochemical defect. Prevalence varies between various races but, in general, 1 of 5 girls and 1 of 10 boys are hypermobile and up to 75% of these children present with musculoskeletal pain.[17] Increased range of motion of ankles or knees can result in repeated microtrauma of the tendons, asymmetric or abnormal muscle involvement, and even frequent clumsiness. Impaired proprioception is seen in those with knee hypermobility[18,19] but not in those with hypermobility of the shoulder girdle.[20] Recurrent joint subluxations, loose skin, increased capillary fragility, thin scars, or lens abnormalities

Table 4
Select syndromes associated with hypermobility

Syndrome	Notable Associated Pathology
Marfan	MVP, aortic dilatation, dissection
Ehlers-Danlos	MVP, aortic dilatation, dissection
Stickler	Myopia, glaucoma, cataract, hearing loss
Williams	Supravalvular aortic stenosis
Osteogenesis imperfecta	Recurrent fractures, blue sclerae
Trisomy 21	VSD

Abbreviations: MVP, mitral valve prolapse; VSD, ventricular septal defect.

should alert for further workup, especially considering the various cardiac abnormalities that can be associated with these symptoms.[21–24]

How to Diagnose

There have been multiple attempts to classify abnormal range of motion, and one of the most commonly used methods is the Beighton scale (**Table 5**).[25] Nevertheless, cutoff values for positivity (4–6 of 9), the choice of joints tested, and validity and reproducibility of the testing are still undergoing scrutiny.[26,27]

For everyday practice, however, the important questions to ask are:

1. Can presenting symptoms be attributed to increased range of motion of joints?
2. Is it a benign condition affecting only the joints, or should one be concerned about other organ involvement?
3. Is there a possibility of a genetic syndrome that would require further workup and referral?
4. Are there any limitations that one should promote in a child regarding choice of sports or activities?

How to Treat

Physical therapy with isometric exercises, proprioception training, and minimizing stretching is the most common first step. Exercise tolerance might be lower than in children without hypermobility but is thought to be due to deconditioning,[28] and an inactive lifestyle should be discouraged. Lower extremity joint pain due to valgus ankles can benefit from proper arch support. Recurrent subluxation limited to 1 or 2 joints might eventually benefit from surgical correction, but true collagen disorder (Ehlers-Danlos syndrome) comes with a limited success rate, as tightened ligaments and capsules tend to loosen up over time. For children actively participating in sports, protective soft bracing of the ankles and knees can be beneficial.

What to Expect

Hypermobility of the lower extremities can predispose individuals to frequent injuries when participating in sports such as soccer, rugby, or lacrosse[29] whereas in other sports, such as gymnastics, it might provide an advantage.[30] Increased joint laxity per se does not seem to be associated with scoliosis and does not seem to increase the prevalence of joint dislocation during the early teens.[31] In general, quality of life seems to be lower in these children because of frequent pain,[32] and hypermobility

Table 5
Beighton scale of hypermobility

Movement Assessed	Score
Passive apposition of the thumb to the flexor side of the forearm	1 for each side
Passive dorsiflexion of the little finger >90°	1 for each side
Passive hyperextension of the elbow >10°	1 for each side
Passive hyperextension of the knee >10°	1 for each side
Forward flexion of the trunk with straight knees and palms resting on the floor	1

Total score is 9; variably, scores 4–6 out of 9 define hypermobility.

Data from Beighton P, Solomon L, Soskolne CL. Articular mobility in an African population. Ann Rheum Dis 1973;32:413–8; and Juul-Kristensen B, Røgind H, Jensen DV, et al. Interexaminer reproducibility of tests and criteria for generalized hypermobility and benign joint hypermobility syndrome. Rheumatology 2007;46:1835–41.

is almost twice as common among adult women with fibromyalgia.[33] In addition to joint symptoms, in comparison with the general population, 5 times more boys with hypermobility have constipation (twice as many have soiling) and urinary incontinence, and urinary infections are more common in girls.[34]

OVERUSE SYNDROMES (OSTEOCHONDROSES) AND SKELETAL DEFECTS
When to Consider

One should suspect overuse syndromes in the setting of repetitive movement causing localized pain, mostly during or after sports but also in games and daily activities. In the case of skeletal defects, there is localized constant bone pain or deformity without systemic symptoms.

Background

Overuse syndromes occur as a result of increased stress to areas of growth (osteochondrosis involving epiphysitis, secondary ossification centers in apophysitis, epicondylitis) during mechanical-skeletal maturation. In addition to classic sports, one should think of recently emerging entities associated with repetitive usage causing "nintendinitis," texting tendinitis, or "Wiitis."[35–39] Skeletal defects including those attributable to bone necrosis or avascular necrosis should be considered.

How to Diagnose

Overuse syndromes are generally diagnosed clinically when localized pain and tenderness are exacerbated with certain repetitive movements, and improve with rest. In the case of apophysitis, imaging is seldom necessary unless avulsion of bony fragments is suspected. On the other hand, skeletal defects such as osteochondrosis and osteonecrosis are characterized by localized pain without change in intensity, and diagnosis is established with imaging. The physical examination should evaluate the affected area and look for structural defects in the bones, ligaments, and cartilage. **Fig. 2** and **Table 6** show the most common osteochondroses, and **Table 7** lists skeletal defects.[40–45] When assessing knee pain the hip should be carefully examined because

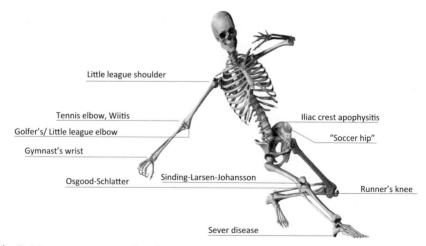

Fig. 2. Most common osteochondroses.

Table 6
Most common osteochondroses

Disease	Age (Years)	Activity	Pathology
Little league shoulder	11–16	Pitching curveballs and sliders Baseball	Traction on the proximal physis of the humerus
Little league elbow (golfer's elbow)	8–12	Throwing Baseball, golf	Lateral epicondylitis
Tennis elbow/Wiitis	Any	"Backhand" Tennis, Wii	Lateral epicondylitis
Gymnast's wrist	12–14 (girls)	Tumbling, vaulting	Radial epiphysitis
Iliac crest apophysitis	<15, but up to 25	Gymnastics, sprinting	Iliac crest apophysitis; avulsion can occur
Anterior superior iliac spine	Up to late teens	Kicking, "soccer hip"	Anterior superior iliac spine apophysitis
Sinding-Larsen-Johansson	10–12	Running, cutting, jumping Soccer, basketball, ballet	Apophysitis of the Inferior pole of patella
Osgood-Schlatter	10–15 (boys) 8–13 (girls)	Cutting and jumping Soccer, basketball, volleyball	Tibial tuber apophysitis
Sever disease	7–10	Jumping, running Basketball, soccer, track	Calcaneal apophysitis

Table 7
Selected skeletal defects

Disease	Age (Years)	Presentation	Pathology
Panner disease	4–10	Lateral elbow pain	Abnormal ossification and necrosis of capitellum humeri
SCFE	12 (obese boys)	Limp, hip, groin, and knee pain (referred)	Displacement of proximal femoral epiphysis
Legg-Calvé-Perthes	4–9 (boys > girls)	Hip pain, 10% bilateral, 25% painless limp	Avascular necrosis of femoral head
Meyer dysplasia	<5	Hip pain mimics Legg-Calvé-Perthes on radiograph	Dysplasia epiphysis, capitis femoris
Patellofemoral syndrome (runner's knee)	Adolescents	Pain with keeping knees flexed, squatting, going upstairs	Lateral tracking of the patella, chondromalacia patellae
Osteochondritis dissecans	Adolescents	Persistent knee pain 20%–30% bilateral	Osteonecrosis of lateral aspect of the medial condyle
Köhler disease	2–8 (boys > girls)	Midfoot pain and limp	Navicular osteonecrosis
Freiberg disease	Adolescents	Painful forefoot in dancers	Ossification disorder of the second metatarsal head
Spondylolysis/spondylolisthesis	Adolescents	Back pain Sports with hyperextension, runners, gymnasts, ballet, dance, martial arts, weight lifters	Pars interarticularis defect L4–5
Scheuermann disease	10–12	Back pain and deformity "humpback"	Anterior vertebral body wedging, end-plate irregularity

of the possibility of referred pain. Radiographic imaging is indicated in the case of constant pain or lack of improvement over time.[41]

How to Treat

In general, overuse syndromes are treated with NSAIDs and discontinuation of the repetitive stress-causing activity. If there is any suspicion about loose bone fragments or if skeletal defects are found on imaging, referral to orthopedics is warranted. Most entities, including patellofemoral syndrome, respond well to physical therapy.

AMPLIFIED MUSCULOSKELETAL PAIN SYNDROMES

Amplified musculoskeletal pain syndromes (AMPS) represent the most challenging, but at the same time most rewarding disease entity of the noninflammatory musculo-skeletal pain syndromes.

When to Consider

Musculoskeletal pain of fluctuating intensity without complete remission even for a short time should lead one to suspect an amplified pain syndrome; there might be newly onset physical limitations or disability, dystonic position of extremities, change in mood, social dysfunction, and lack of sleep hygiene. There are no systemic symptoms including fever, weight loss, or laboratory signs of inflammation or infection.

Background

The prevalence of chronic musculoskeletal pain is variable. One-third of school-age children reported pain lasting longer than 6 months, more than half of which was described as musculoskeletal.[46] In a Dutch study the highest prevalence was in young teen girls,[47] and across all ages girls are more commonly affected.[48,49] Although this could be a true biological difference, one should consider a gender bias in social expectations for pain reporting. Pain seems to be more prevalent with older age[50] as well. In general there is an inciting event that results in pain, and multiple other factors chime in to perpetuate it. The pain might start as an injury or illness, but also seems to be related to emotional stress such as loss of a family member, friend, or pet, or moving house. After onset, the pain either stays localized or spreads diffusely. There is gradual increase of hypervigilance toward the affected part, which is focused on by the patient to the extent that he or she fears increased pain even by touching. As a result, the patient starts to protect the area, and can develop increased tone in certain muscle groups while becoming deconditioned in others. This process can lead to profound disability such as being on crutches or in a wheelchair, being unable to function even to the point of needing help with basic activities of daily living, social withdrawal, and isolation.

There are 2 major forms of this condition: localized AMPS and diffuse AMPS, between which overlap is possible.

Localized AMPS

Localized AMPS is also known as reflex neuropathic (or sympathetic) dystrophy or complex regional pain syndrome (CRPS). Both names carry a descriptive property in that it is a pain syndrome affecting certain areas of the body, most commonly the extremities, with complex presentation including sensory, autonomic, and motor changes heralded by dysfunction of the sympathetic nervous system (**Box 2**).[51]

Box 2
Diagnostic criteria of complex regional pain syndrome

Regional pain and 2 of each	
Neuropathic descriptor	*Autonomic dysfunction*
Burning	Cyanosis
Dysesthesia	Mottling
Paresthesia	Hyperhidrosis
Allodynia	Coolness (by at least 3°C)
Cold hyperalgesia	Edema

Data from Wilder RT, Berde CB, Wolohan M, et al. Reflex sympathetic dystrophy in children. Clinical characteristics and follow-up of seventy patients. J Bone Joint Surg Am 1992;74:910–9.

Pathogenesis is somewhat complex. More recent publications show disorganization in the sensory cortex corresponding to the affected body part that can revert back to normal once the condition is treated, maladaptive neuronal plasticity leading to distortion of mental image of the limb, reduction of descending inhibition, and augmentation of descending facilitation resulting in hyperalgesia.[52–56]

Diffuse AMPS

The diffuse form is characterized by widespread pain of high intensity, and is also known as juvenile primary fibromyalgia syndrome. The prevalence is around 6% of children.[57] There are no validated diagnostic criteria for children, and the ones for adult fibromyalgia or those by Yunus and Masi[58] are often used (**Table 8**). Patients present with diffuse, widespread pain, multiple areas of allodynia (pain to touch) with changing borders, sleep disturbances, fatigue, and functional impairment. Diffuse AMPS is many times accompanied by other functional disorders such as irritable bowel syndrome, migraines, chronic abdominal pain, and chronic fatigue. Conversion symptoms are not uncommon. Pathogenesis is also complex, and likely related to abnormal pain processing and central amplification.[59]

How to Diagnose

Amplified pain is a complex entity and therefore multiple areas need to be assessed, especially the 4 Ps: pain, presentation, patient, and parent (**Box 3**). Each patient with

---

Table 8
Yunus and Masi criteria for diffuse AMPS: fibromyalgia

Pain at least in 3 areas lasting more than 3 months without underlying cause and with normal laboratory tests	
More than 5 of 18 typical tender points	
Three of 10 minor criteria:	
Fatigue	Poor sleep
Headaches	Chronic anxiety or tension
Irritable bowel syndrome	Pain affected by weather
Subjective soft tissue swelling	Pain affected by anxiety and stress
Paresthesia	Pain affected by activities

Data from Yunus MB, Masi AT. Juvenile primary fibromyalgia syndrome: a clinical study of thirty-three patients and matched normal controls. Arthritis Rheum 1985;28:138–45.

Box 3
The 4 Ps of AMPS assessment

Pain:

Onset, localization, quality, radiation, intensity (0–10 visual analog scale,[60,61] Wong-Baker face scale[62]; factors exacerbating and relieving pain (activities, rest, medications). Is there pain to soft touch? Patients usually report lack of response to pain medications: "take the edge off," even in the case of opiates. The latter usually help the patient to fall asleep rather than provide true pain relief.

Presentation:

Consider associated symptoms; ruling out trauma, infectious conditions (septic arthritis, osteomyelitis), malignancy. Any stressful event at onset or currently? (Death in the family, friends, pet. Moving: new school, lack of friends. Interaction with siblings, peers, bullying/cyber bullying).

Patient:

Are there any changes of daily routine, sleep hygiene? (What time in bed, out of bed, feels rested? Taking naps during the day? Activities before going to sleep: television, texting, computer, instant messaging, Internet. Is the television on at night? If sleep disturbance, what do you do to fall asleep again?) How is school attendance? Patient's view of change in environment if occurred; interaction with friends and pursuing or stopping prior hobbies. Activities: exercise routine. Patient's approach to symptoms: fighting or giving in. Assessing possible mood or personality changes. Looking for signs of sexual-orientation confusion in teens.

Parent (caregiver):

Parental support and family structure. How is their interaction with the child; how do they view complaints: dismissing or driving them? Presence of pain syndromes or pain disorders in the immediate family. What is their opinion about the symptoms? If they bring up the word "fibromyalgia," what do they understand by it and what is their attitude toward it?

---

pain is somewhat different, but there are some screening clues that help direct the provider (**Fig. 3**).

1. La belle indifference: incongruent affect

On a pain scale of 1 to 10, pain is reported as very high, 7 to 10; sometimes even 10 of 10, even in the office while the patient seems to be not in much discomfort and even being jovial.

2. High pain tolerance

High pain tolerance is a quality very often reported by the parent, and makes all members of the family think that there must be something very seriously wrong going on. High pain tolerance leads to multiple and various provider visits, laboratory and imaging tests, and therapeutic trials.

3. Enmeshment

The parent and patient seem to be one personality. At the extreme, they might even arrive dressed the same, the parent refers to the pain as "our pain," and a sentence started by one is finished by the other.

4. Lack of sleep hygiene

The patient reports staying up late while engaged on the computer, television, or Internet, then gets up late being unable to go to school. Many times the television is

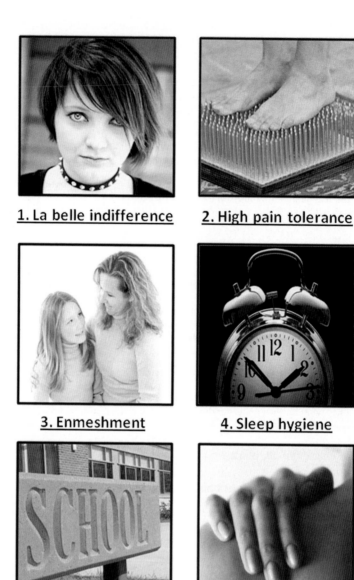

Fig. 3. Screening clues for AMPS.

on all night long, preventing the patient from reaching appropriate cycles of deep sleep. Frequent napping is common.

5. Missed school days

The majority of these children miss a disproportionate amount of school because of pain, inability to concentrate, fatigue, or a host of other complaints such as abdominal pain or visual problems.

6. Allodynia

Allodynia, or pain to light touch, can be present in both the localized in diffuse forms of amplified pain. Some patients report pain with wind, showering, and wearing tight clothes. The area of allodynia can be localized or generalized, and the borders of increased sensitivity may move when reassessed shortly afterward. The area of increased pain frequently crosses dermatomes.

The physical examination is slightly different between groups. Localized AMPS patients have limitations on movement of the extremity, holding it many times in a contorted position. By contrast, one can hardly find any positive pathological factors in diffuse AMPS patients. Fibromyalgia tender points that are widely used in adults can be present in children as well, but as there are contradicting reports about their validity, the diagnosis should not rely on them. Adolescents seem to have more positive tender points than adults, 15 of 18 rather than more than 5 (**Table 9**).[63] Back pain should be thoroughly assessed, including single-leg hyperextension and testing for Waddell signs of nonorganic back pain (**Table 10**).[64]

Differential Diagnosis

Apart from the already mentioned benign musculoskeletal syndromes, there are 2 other entities that should be considered. The first is malignancy presenting as musculoskeletal pain. Diffuse body pain and migratory joint pain with systemic symptoms, especially in a young child, should raise suspicion for an organic cause because AMPS is extremely rare in children younger than 7 years.[65] The other entity is spondyloarthritis. As mentioned, some of the arthritic conditions can result in the development of chronic pain syndromes. On the other hand, enthesitis, tenderness, and inflammation of the attachments of the tendons can be confused with the fibromyalgia tender points. Therefore, morning stiffness gelling in a patient with diffuse body ache should prompt an evaluation for an underlying spondyloarthropathy.

Table 9 Fibromyalgia tender points	
Occiput	Suboccipital muscle insertions
Low cervical	Anterior aspects of the intertransverse spaces at C5–C7
Trapezius	Midpoint of the upper border
Supraspinatus	Above the scapula spine near the medial border
Second rib	Second costochondral junctions, just lateral to the junctions on upper surfaces
Lateral epicondyle	2 cm distal to the epicondyles
Gluteal	Upper outer quadrants of buttocks in anterior fold of muscle
Greater trochanter	Posterior to the trochanteric prominence
Knee	Medial fat pad proximal to the joint line

Nine areas each side, total of 18. Patient has to report area as painful and not just tender, approximate pressure of 8 to 9 lb (4 kg).

Data from Wolfe F, Smythe HA, Yunus MB, et al. The American College of Rheumatology 1990 criteria for the classification of fibromyalgia: report of the multicenter criteria committee. Arthritis Rheum 1990;33:160–72.

Table 10	
Assessment of back pain in AMPS	
"Stork" test	Patient standing, single leg elevated. Low back pain increases with back being hyperextended. Positive test indicates spondylolysis
Waddell nonorganic back pain signs: if positive, likely AMPS or malingering:	
Passive rotation	Patient standing, examiner rotates patient at ankles and knees with back fixed. Back pain should not be due to organic cause, as back is not moving during this maneuver
Axial loading test	Patient standing straight, examiner pushes downward on the top of the head. Test is positive if patient reports low back pain. Neck pain is possible
Distracted straight leg raise	Test is positive if patient reports pain when straight leg raised while being supine, but not when flexed knee is extended in sitting position

How to Treat

Treatment is somewhat complex and should address all parts of the etiology. The initial focus is not only on pain control but also on regaining function and returning to regular daily activities. There are several practice points that one should keep in mind:

1. Explanation of symptoms and reassurance. Labeling the diagnosis as an amplified pain syndrome is much more preferable to using the term fibromyalgia,[66] the latter being a double-edged sword. On the one hand, most people know about it and can relate to it. On the other hand, it is considered to be "not a real diagnosis" by many parents; the term being used by physicians "when they cannot find anything else." Also, most reports on fibromyalgia list it as a lifelong condition with minimal response to therapy, which is not the case in children.
2. Acknowledge the patient's pain. Providers are often tempted to disprove the pain by checking vital signs (pulse rate, blood pressure) while examining the patient. Acute pain comes with increased heart rate and blood pressure, but chronic pain is associated with normal levels. Through the course of workup most, if not all, patients will come across disbelief regarding their condition. One of the most common complaints of the patients is that nobody believes them. There are very few patients who malinger.
3. Avoid saying "it's only in your head." If patients have already heard it, explain that it is true, but only because the brain is in the head and that this condition is due to a disorganization of certain parts of the brain. Patients need to hear that you believe them.
4. Explain what pain is, that is, a danger signal to the brain. One may compare it with the check-engine light on a car's dashboard. Sometimes it signals malfunction of the car itself, but if after fixing the error one does not reboot the system, it will stay on. And sometimes it stays on for many months without affecting the function of the car. It becomes annoying, but does not signal major trouble. Once the patient realizes that the pain is not associated with any damage, he or she will be much more likely to follow the therapeutic plan.
5. Try to address all aspects of the syndrome (see the action plan for patients in **Fig. 4**).
6. Assess the parent. Is he or she an ally or not? Consider that some of this presentation has a genetic component. The type-A personality patient frequently has one

Fix ALL the planks on your boat

Pain
Do not talk about it but once a day. "My pain level is 0-10." It will increase initially with exercise but then it will get better. It might take some time to get rid of all of it.

Life
Keep going to school, restart hobbies and hang out with friends. Your brain needs the routine of the day, a schedule it can hold onto.

Sleep
Plan 9-10 hrs of night sleep. In bed/out of bed same time every day, weekend/weekday. No sleeping in. No TV/computer/texting/phone starting 30 minutes prior to going to sleep. No screen on at night.

Exercise
40-50 min daily aerobic activities. Running, biking, cardio fitness.

Physical therapy
Focusing on fixing limitations, stretching, strengthening and generalized conditioning. The more actively you do it, the sooner you will get better.

Desensitization
Touch and rub where it hurts. Use lotion, towel several times a day. Have others draw shapes, numbers and letters with their fingers on it. The "picture" of the touch information in your brain will overrule the perception of the pain of that place

Counseling – stress management
Do not underestimate this step. Look at stressors in your life, learn how to handle them so they do not win again.

Fig. 4. Action plan for patients.

or both parents driving his or her expectations, and careful "unscheduling" might be necessary. If the parent himself or herself is battling adult fibromyalgia, it is useful to know how he or she handles it and treats it.

7. Sleep hygiene. Sleep is often underestimated, despite the multitude of publications on association of sleep quality and adjustment to pain and stress.[67–70] If they cannot fall asleep and toss and turn in bed, patients should rather get out of the bed, sit in a chair until feeling drowsy, then return to bed. In this way the brain associates being in bed with sleeping, rather than with the forced effort of trying to get to sleep. Once an intensive exercise program is started, there are very few patients who have difficulties falling asleep. Patients should avoid taking naps. Breaking up the normal wake/sleep cycle is very counterproductive, and patients should rather find some activities to do.

8. Exercise, physical therapy, and occupational therapy. This triad is the mainstay of management, focusing on pain relief but also on regaining function. Exercise has been reported to affect epigenetic brain-derived neurotropic factor (BDNF) gene transcription, altering brain function and plasticity[71]; it decreases pain ratings in

adult fibromyalgia patients[72] and even in people with spinal cord injury.[73] A Cochrane review suggests gold-level evidence of aerobic exercise having a positive impact on adult-type fibromyalgia.[74] It is important to discuss the plan with the physical therapist, whose role is to push beyond pain rather than stop at discomfort as in other cases of rehabilitation. Desensitization is part of rehabilitation, as listed in the patient action plan. In CRPS, mirror-box therapy regularly used in phantom limb pain has been shown to be beneficial.[75]

9. Counseling. This is one of the toughest selling points. Most patients resent the idea; they perceive counseling as being stigmatized. Do tell them that success will not be reached unless all items of the list are followed through. Counselors should assess for presence of mood disorders and possible family or peer conflicts, and teach stress management techniques. It is necessary to ask about suicidal ideations. The patient population affected by this condition is not homogeneous and there are some who, after prolonged pain, cannot see improvement and have no hope. The author has diagnosed AMPS in a patient brought to the emergency department by her mother who found her farewell letter. Living in pain without a hope for improvement during an already emotionally labile period can drive teenagers to desperate measures. There are some suggestions of underlying mood disorders affecting not only generalized AMPS but even development of the localized form,[76] although there are other reports refuting this.

10. Daily routine. Patients need a structured day with a schedule and goals to follow through. For this reason, changing from regular school to home-bound instruction is generally not beneficial, with only rare exceptions.

11. Pharmacotherapy. This is a controversial issue, and opinions vary. At the time of writing (October 2011) there are 3 medications approved by the Food and Drug Administration for use in adult fibromyalgia: pregabalin (Lyrica), duloxetine (Cymbalta), and milnacipran (Savella). All of these agents had trials showing a beneficial effect, but this effect was somewhat modest and did not help every patient. Pediatric usage is not well studied, and there might be unpredictable side effects associated with the immature and developing brain. The nonpharmacologic complex rehabilitation approach, as discussed earlier, has been shown to be very successful and might be superior. Analgesic medications do not help, and patients should discontinue their use. Trigger-point injection and sympathetic blockade are temporary solutions only, and should be avoided. Vitamin C can decrease the chances of CRPS development after fractures in adults.[77] There is insufficient evidence for use of NSAIDs, opioids, oral muscle relaxants, and botulinum toxin A for CRPS.[77]

Additional information can be found online (**Box 4**).

What to Expect: Prognosis

Children with amplified pain syndromes go through tremendous suffering and disability. The long-term prognosis reports differ because of the variable treatment

---

Box 4
Additional online resources

www.childhoodrnd.org

www.noigroup.com

www.rsds.org

approaches. CRPS seems to respond better and faster. In general, the diffuse form of AMPS is considered to have a more chronic course,[58] but improvement has been reported.[78] The complex approach with intensive exercise therapy as discussed here seems to be the most effective.[79] In a cohort of 103 children with CRPS, 92% become symptom-free after initial therapy and 88% were symptom-free after 5 years of follow-up, albeit one-third of those had short recurrence of symptoms, most of them in the first 6 months.[79] None required pharmacotherapy.

REFERENCES

1. Pabone V, Lionetti E, Gargano V, et al. Growing pains: A study of 30 cases and review of the literature. J Pediatr Orthop 2011;31:606–9.
2. Evans AM, Scutter SD. Prevalence of "growing pains" in young children. J Pediatr 2004;145:255–8.
3. Naish JM, Apley J. "Growing pains": a clinical study of non-arthritic limb pains in children. Arch Dis Child 1951;26:134–40.
4. Rajaram SS, Walters AS, England SJ, et al. Some children with growing pains may actually have restless legs syndrome. Sleep 2004;27:767–73.
5. Hashkes PJ, Gorenberg M, Oren V, et al. "Growing pains" in children are not associated with changes in vascular perfusion patterns in painful regions. Clin Rheumatol 2005;24:342–5.
6. Friedland O, Hashkes PJ, Jaber L, et al. Decreased bone speed of sound in children with growing pains measured by quantitative ultrasound. J Rheumatol 2005; 32:1354–7.
7. Hashkes PJ, Friedland O, Jaber L, et al. Decreased pain threshold in children with growing pains. J Rheumatol 2004;31:610–3.
8. Uziel J, Hashkes PJ. Growing pains in children. Pediatr Rheumatol Online J 2007; 5:5.
9. Lowe RM, Hashkes PJ. Growing pains: a noninflammatory pain syndrome of early childhood. Nat Clin Pract Rheumatol 2008;4:542–9.
10. Uziel J, Chapnick G, Jaber L, et al. Five-year outcome of children with "growing pains", correlations with pain threshold. J Pediatr 2010;156:838–40.
11. Trapani S, Grisolia F, Simonini G, et al. Incidence of occult cancer in children presenting with musculoskeletal symptoms: a 10-year survey in a pediatric rheumatology unit. Semin Arthritis Rheum 2000;29:348–59.
12. Gonçalves M, Terreri MT, Barbosa CM, et al. Diagnosis of malignancies in children with musculoskeletal complaints. Sao Paulo Med J 2005;123:21–3.
13. Cabral DA, Tucker LB. Malignancies in children who initially present with rheumatic complaints. J Pediatr 1999;134:53–7.
14. Wallendal M, Stork L, Hollister JR. The discriminating value of serum lactate dehydrogenase levels in children with malignant neoplasms presenting as joint pain. Arch Pediatr Adolesc Med 1996;150:70–3.
15. Murray MJ, Tang T, Ryder C, et al. Childhood leukaemia masquerading as juvenile idiopathic arthritis. BMJ 2004;329:959–61.
16. Seow CC, Chow PK, Khong KS. A study of joint mobility in a normal population. Ann Acad Med Singapore 1999;28:231–6.
17. Woo P, Laxer RM, Sherry DD. Noninflammatory mechanical pain syndrome. In: Pediatric rheumatology in clinical practice. London: Springer-Verlag; 2007. p. 145–55.
18. Fatoye F, Palmer S, Macmillan F, et al. Proprioception and muscle torque deficits in children with hypermobility syndrome. Rheumatology 2009;48:152–7.

19. Rombaut L, De Paepe A, Malfait F, et al. Joint position sense and vibratory perception sense in patients with Ehlers-Danlos syndrome type III (hypermobility type). Clin Rheumatol 2010;29:289–95.

20. Jeremiah HM, Alexander CM. Do hypermobile subjects without pain have alteration to the feedback mechanism controlling the shoulder girdle? Musculoskeletal Care 2010;8:157–63.

21. Beighton P, De Paepe A, Steinmann B, et al. Ehlers-Danlos syndromes: revised nosology, Villefranche. Am J Med Genet 1998;77:31–7.

22. De Paepe A, Devereux RB, Dietz HC, et al. Revised diagnostic criteria for the Marfan syndrome. Am J Med Genet 1996;62:417–26.

23. Wenkert D. Primary disorders of bone and connective tissues. In: Cassidy JT, Laxer RM, Petty RE, et al, editors. Textbook of pediatric rheumatology. 6th edition. Elsevier Inc; 2011. p. 750–4.

24. Adib N, Davies K, Grahame R, et al. Joint hypermobility syndrome in childhood. A not so benign multisystem disorder? Rheumatology (Oxford) 2005;44:744–50.

25. Beighton P, Solomon L, Soskolne CL. Articular mobility in an African population. Ann Rheum Dis 1973;32:413–8.

26. Juul-Kristensen B, Røgind H, Jensen DV, et al. Inter-examiner reproducibility of tests and criteria for generalized hypermobility and benign joint hypermobility syndrome. Rheumatology 2007;46:1835–41.

27. Remvig L, Jensen DV, Ward RC. Are diagnostic criteria for general joint hypermobility and benign joint hypermobility syndrome based on reproducible and valid test? A review of the literature. J Rheumatol 2007;34:798–803.

28. Engerlbert RH, Van Bergen M, Henneken T, et al. Exercise tolerance in children and adolescents with musculoskeletal pain in joint hypermobility and joint hypermobility syndrome. Pediatrics 2006;118:e690–6.

29. Wolf JM, Cameron KL, Owens BD. Impact of joint laxity and hypermobility on the musculoskeletal system. J Am Acad Orthop Surg 2011;19:463–71.

30. Grahame R, Jenkins JM. Joint hypermobility—asset or liability? A study of joint mobility in ballet dancers. Ann Rheum Dis 1972;31:109–11.

31. Remvig L, Jensen DV, Ward RC. Epidemiology of general joint hypermobility and basis for the proposed criteria for benign joint hypermobility syndrome: review of the literature. J Rheumatol 2007;34:804–9.

32. Fatoye F, Pamer S, Macmillan F, et al. Pain intensity and quality of life perception in children with hypermobility syndrome. Rheumatol Int 2011. [Epub ahead of print].

33. Sendur OF, Gurer G, Bozbas GT. The frequency of hypermobility and its relationship with clinical findings of fibromyalgia patients. Clin Rheumatol 2007;25:291–3.

34. Engelbert RH, Bank RA, Sakkers RJ, et al. Pediatric generalized joint hypermobility with and without musculoskeletal complaints: a localized or systemic disorder? Pediatrics 2003;111:e248–54.

35. Brasington R. Nintendinitis. N Engl J Med 1990;322:1473–4.

36. Macgregor DM. Nintendonitis? A case report of repetitive strain injury in a child as a result of playing computer games. Scott Med J 2000;45:150.

37. Menz RJ. "Texting" tendinitis. Med J Aust 2005;182:308.

38. Karim SA. Playstation thumb—a new epidemic in children. S Afr Med J 2005;95:412.

39. Bonis J. Acute Wiitis. N Engl J Med 2007;356:2431–2.

40. Atanda A, Shah SA, O'Brien K. Osteochondrosis: common causes of pain in growing bones. Am Fam Physician 2011;83:258–91.

41. Cassas KJ, Cassettari-Wayhs A. Childhood and adolescent sports-related overuse injuries. Am Fam Physician 2006;73:1014–22.

42. Biber R, Gregory A. Overuse injuries in youth sports: is there such a thing as too much sports? Pediatr Ann 2010;39:286–92.
43. Arnaiz J, Piedra T, de Lucas EM, et al. Imaging findings of lower limb apophysitis. AJR Am J Roentgenol 2011;196:W316–25.
44. Dwek JR, Cardoso F, Chung CB. MR imaging of overuse injuries in the skeletally immature gymnast: spectrum of soft tissue and osseous lesions in the hand and wrist. Pediatr Radiol 2009;39:1310–6.
45. McMahon PJ, Kaplan LD. Sports Medicine. In: Skinner HB, editor. Current Diagnosis & Treatment in Orthopedics. 4th edition. New York: McGraw-Hill; 2006. Chapter 4. Available at: http://www.accessmedicine.com/content.aspx?aID=2318624. Accessed March 28, 2012.
46. Roth-Isigkeit A. Pain among children and adolescents: restrictions in daily living and triggering factors. Pediatrics 2005;115:152–62.
47. Perquin CW, Hazebroek-Kampschreur AA, Hunfeld JA, et al. Pain in children and adolescents: a common experience. Pain 2000;87:51–8.
48. Lamber L. Girls' and boys' differing response to pain starts early in their lives. JAMA 1998;280:1035–6.
49. Balague F, Dutoit G, Waldburger M. Low back pain in school-children. Scand J Rehabil Med 1988;20:175–9.
50. Sherry DD, McGuire T, Mellins E, et al. Psychosomatic musculoskeletal pain in childhood: clinical and psychological analyses of 100 children. Pediatrics 1991;88:1093–9.
51. Wilder RT, Berde CB, Wolohan M, et al. Reflex sympathetic dystrophy in children. Clinical characteristics and follow-up of seventy patients. J Bone Joint Surg Am 1992;74:910–9.
52. Lebel A, Becerra L, Wallin D, et al. fMRI reveals distinct CNS processing during symptomatic and recovered complex regional pain syndrome in children. Brain 2008;131:1854–79.
53. Marinus J, Moseley GL, Birklein FB, et al. Clinical features and pathophysiology of complex regional pain syndrome. Lancet Neurol 2011;10:637–48.
54. Maihöfner C, Forster C, Briklein F, et al. Brain processing during mechanical hyperalgesia in complex regional pain syndrome: a functional MRI study. Pain 2005;114:93–103.
55. Maihöfner C, Handwerker HO, Neundörfer B, et al. Patterns of cortical reorganization in complex regional pain syndrome. Neurology 2003;61:1707–15.
56. Maihöfner C, Handwerker HO, Neundörfer B, et al. Cortical reorganization during recovery from complex regional pain syndrome. Neurology 2004;63:693–701.
57. Anthony KK, Schanberg LE. Juvenile primary fibromyalgia syndrome. Curr Rheumatol Rep 2001;3:165–71.
58. Yunus MB, Masi AT. Juvenile primary fibromyalgia syndrome: a clinical study of thirty-three patients and matched normal controls. Arthritis Rheum 1985;28:138–45.
59. Petersel D, Dror V, Cheung R. Central amplification and fibromyalgia: disorder of pain processing. J Neurosci Res 2011;89:29–34.
60. Varni JW, Thompson KL, Hanson V. The Varni/Thompson pediatric pain questionnaire. I. Chronic musculoskeletal pain in juvenile rheumatoid arthritis. Pain 1987;28:27–38.
61. Schanberg LE, Sandstrom MJ. Causes of pain in children with arthritis. Rheum Dis Clin North Am 1999;25:31–53.
62. Wong DL, Baker CM. Pain in children: comparison of assessment scales. Pediatr Nurs 1988;14:9–17.

63. Swain NF, Kashikar-Zuck S, Graham TB, et al. Tender point assessment in juvenile primary fibromyalgia syndrome. Arthritis Rheum 2005;53:785–7.
64. Wolfe F, Smythe HA, Yunus MB, et al. The American College of Rheumatology 1990 criteria for the classification of fibromyalgia: report of the multicenter criteria committee. Arthritis Rheum 1990;33:160–72.
65. Sherry DD. Fibromyalgia in children. In: Wallace DJ, Clauw DJ, editors. Fibromyalgia and other central pain syndromes. 1st edition. Philadelphia: Lippincott Wolliams & Wilkins; 2005. p. 177–85.
66. Sherry DD. Amplified musculoskeletal pain: treatment approach and outcomes. J Pediatr Gastroenterol Nutr 2008;47:693–5.
67. Hamilton NA, Catley D, Karlson C. Sleep and the affective response to stress and pain. Health Psychol 2007;26:288–95.
68. Bromberg MH, Gil KM, Schanberg LE. Daily sleep quality and mood as predictors of pain in children with juvenile polyarticular arthritis. Health Psychol 2012; 31(2):202–9. DOI: 10.1037/a0025075 Advance online publication.
69. Karlson C, Luxton D, Preacher K, et al. Fibromyalgia: the role of sleep in affect and in negative event reactivity and recovery. Health Psychol 2008;27:490–4.
70. O'Brien EM, Waxenberg LB, Atchison JW, et al. Intraindividual variability in daily sleep and pain ratings among chronic pain patients: bidirectional association and the role of negative mood. Clin J Pain 2011;27:425–33.
71. Gomez-Pinilla F, Zhuang Y, Feng J, et al. Exercise impacts brain-derived neurotrophic factor plasticity by engaging mechanisms of epigenetic regulation. Eur J Neurosci 2011;33:383–90.
72. McLoughlin MJ, Stegner AJ, Cook DB. The relationship between physical activity and brain responses to pain in fibromyalgia. J Pain 2011;12(6):640–51.
73. Ginis KA, Latimer AE, McKechnie K, et al. Using exercise to enhance subjective well-being among people with spinal cord injury: the mediating influences of stress and pain. Rehabil Psychol 2003;48:157–64.
74. Busch AJ, Barber KA, Overend TJ, et al. Exercise for treating fibromyalgia syndrome. Cochrane Database Syst Rev 2007;4:CD003786.
75. Bultitude JH, Rafal RD. Derangement of body representation in complex regional pain syndrome: a report of a case treated with mirror and prisms. Exp Brain Res 2010;204:409–18.
76. Dilek B, Yemez B, Kizil R, et al. Anxious personality is a risk factor for developing complex regional pain syndrome type I. Rheumatol Int 2011. [Epub ahead of print].
77. Perez RS, Zollinger PE, Dijksrta PU, et al. Evidence based guidelines for complex regional pain syndrome type I. BMC Neurol 2010;10:20.
78. Siegel DM, Janeway D, Baum J. Fibromyalgia syndrome in children and adolescents: clinical features at presentation and follow-up. Pediatrics 1998;101: 377–82.
79. Sherry DD, Wallace CA, Claudia K, et al. Short- and long-term outcomes of children with complex regional pain syndrome type I treated with exercise therapy. Clin J Pain 1999;15(3):218–23.

Immunodeficiency Diseases with Rheumatic Manifestations

Troy R. Torgerson, MD, PhD[a,b,*]

KEYWORDS

- Immunodeficiency • Autoimmunity • Immune dysregulation
- Lupus • Arthritis • Vasculitis

Primary immunodeficiencies have traditionally been described in patients with recurrent, severe, or unusual infections. Before the broad availability of effective antibiotics and ready access to safe, plentiful immunoglobulin preparations, patients often succumbed to infections at an early age. As patients began to survive longer, the conundrum of autoimmunity associated with immunodeficiency became apparent; that is, why would an immune system that is incapable of effective responses to foreign antigens seemingly be capable of responding to host antigens and causing autoimmunity? Over time, more of the molecular and cellular mechanisms that underlie this autoimmunity have come to be understood, but many questions remain. As new genetic defects have been identified in association with immunodeficiency, it has become clear that autoimmunity or autoinflammation is the primary clinical manifestation of some disorders.

PREVALENCE OF PRIMARY IMMUNODEFICIENCY DISORDERS

In the absence of uniform, population-based programs that screen for all types of immunodeficiency, the actual incidence and prevalence of primary immunodeficiency disorders (PIDDs) is not clear. A recent randomized survey of 10,000 US households, however, estimated the prevalence of diagnosed PIDDs at approximately 1:1200 individuals.[1] Blood bank studies evaluating donors for the most common immunodeficiency, selective IgA deficiency, have estimated an even higher prevalence (1:333

[a] Division of Immunology, Department of Pediatrics, University of Washington and Seattle Children's Hospital, 4800 Sandpoint Way NE, Seattle, WA 98105, USA; [b] Division of Rheumatology, Department of Pediatrics, University of Washington and Seattle Children's Hospital, Seattle, WA, USA
* Corresponding author. Seattle Children's Research Institute, 1900 9th Avenue, C9S-7, Seattle, WA 98101-1304.
E-mail address: troy.torgerson@seattlechildrens.org

Pediatr Clin N Am 59 (2012) 493–507
doi:10.1016/j.pcl.2012.03.010
0031-3955/12/$ – see front matter © 2012 Published by Elsevier Inc.

individuals among US donors).[2] Many of these are asymptomatic from the standpoint of recurrent or severe infections, but there is significant evidence that patients with selective IgA deficiency are at increased risk for autoimmunity.[3–5]

THE 4 MAJOR COMPARTMENTS OF THE IMMUNE SYSTEM

The body's natural defenses against pathogens include a network of physical barriers (eg, skin and mucosal surfaces), immune cells (eg, lymphocytes and phagocytes), and soluble mediators (eg, complement, antibodies, and cytokines). Trying to remember and consider all these pieces can be daunting to busy clinicians so there is value in using a framework of 4 major compartments when thinking about and evaluating patients. The 4 major compartments are complement, phagocytes, B cells, and T cells (**Fig. 1**). The Complement and phagocyte compartments together make up the majority of the immune system that is referred to as *innate*. The innate immune system mounts rapid responses to infectious organisms by recognizing patterns of molecules or groups of molecules that are present on pathogens but typically not on human cells. Each time a particular pathogen is encountered, the components of the innate immune system respond but do so in the same way each time because they are unable to adapt or improve their response. In contrast, the B-cell and T-cell compartments make up the *adaptive* portion of the immune system. The adaptive immune system has the ability to adapt and change each time it encounters a pathogen. This adaptability makes it possible to generate memory responses. Because of the time required to modify the response to each individual pathogen, the adaptive system typically takes on a major role in fighting pathogens after the innate system has already begun its response.

Together, the innate and adaptive systems work to maintain normal host function and resistance to infection. Disruption of any part of this intricate network can result in increased numbers of infections, susceptibility to specific pathogens, or autoimmunity. The pattern of infections, clinical symptoms, and laboratory abnormalities differs depending on which part of the immune system is affected and can provide important clues to the diagnosis in each individual case. Because some deficiencies can be rapidly fatal whereas others are mild, making a timely and accurate diagnosis is critical

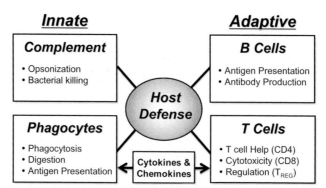

Fig. 1. The 4 major compartments of the immune system and their most important functions. The complement and phagocytes compartments constitute much of the innate portion of the immune response whereas the B-cell and T-cell compartments constitute most of the adaptive parts of the immune response. All of the compartments function together to create the host defense. In addition to direct cell-cell interactions, cytokines and chemokines play a critical role in communication of one compartment with another.

to providing appropriate clinical care. Clinical manifestations that are typical of immunodeficiencies in each of the immune compartments are described in **Table 1**.

IMMUNODEFICIENCIES BY COMPARTMENT
Disorders of the Complement Compartment

Overview
The complement system consists of a series of more than 20 plasma proteins that are activated on encountering immune complexes or pathogens. Activation of the complement system initiates a cascade of protein cleavage events that produce active complement protein fragments that opsonize bacteria, attract immune cells, increase blood flow, and initiate formation of the membrane attack complex (consisting of the terminal complement components, C5, C6, C7, C8, and C9) on the surface of target cells (**Fig. 2**). The complement cascade is activated via 3 major pathways: the classical pathway, initiated by antigen/antibody complexes; the alternative pathway, activated directly by bacterial cell wall components; and the lectin pathway, activated by mannose residues on the surface of pathogens. Under normal conditions, complement is continually activated at a low level in response to pathogens or fragments of pathogens encountered in the environment. Were it not for a group of complement regulatory proteins (factor H, factor I, and membrane cofactor protein [MCP]) that restrain complement activation at the level of C3, there would be rampant, continual activation of complement.

Complement deficiencies make up only a fraction (approximately 2%) of al primary immunodeficiencies but absence or dysfunction of only 1 of the more than 20 complement proteins can cause defective activation of the entire complement cascade. The proteins most often affected are C2, C3, and C4. **Table 2**[6] summarizes key clinical features of various complement defects but, in general, deficiencies of early complement components (C1–C4) in the classical pathway are associated with recurrent, invasive infections with encapsulated organisms (in particular, sepsis with organisms, such as *Streptococcus pneumoniae*). Patients with defects in late complement components involved in formation of the membrane attack complex (C5–C9) typically present with neisserial infections.[7] Defects of complement regulatory proteins are generally associated with familial hemolytic uremic syndrome (HUS) and age-related macular degeneration.[8] The clinical symptoms of major complement disorders are outlined in **Table 2**.

Rheumatologic disease associated with defects in the complement compartment
Systemic lupus erythematosus In addition to infection, patients with deficiency of early components of the classical complement pathway often present with symptoms of systemic lupus erythematosus (SLE) or a lupus-like glomerulonephritis. The reported prevalence of SLE is 93% with C1q deficiency, 57% with C1r/s deficiency, 75% with C4 deficiency, 32% to 33% with C2 deficiency, and 10% with C3 deficiency.[9,10] Among these, C2 deficiency is most common, with an estimated incidence of 1 in 20,000. The mechanism behind the association between SLE and complement deficiency is thought to relate to the role that complement (in particular C1q) plays in binding to apoptotic cells and clearing them from the body. In the absence of C1q binding, dead and dying cells take longer to be cleared, thereby inducing inflammation that leads to the generation of autoantibodies such as anti-double-stranded DNA antibodies.[11]

Screening for complement deficiency in the classical pathway typically involves performing a 50% complement hemolytic activity test (CH50) as well as evaluating the levels of specific complement components, including C2, C3, and C4. The CH50 is

Table 1
Summary of PIDD clinical features in each of the 4 immune compartments

Complement	Phagocytes	B Cell	T Cell
Infections			
• (C1–C4) Recurrent invasive infections (sepsis, etc) with encapsulated organisms (*S pneumonia*, etc) • (C5–C9) Recurrent, invasive neisserial infections	• Recurrent skin and soft tissue infections, including abscesses and boils • Recurrent infections with catalase (+) organisms • Omphalitis, delayed shedding of umbilical cord	• Recurrent bacterial sinopulmonary infections (sinusitis, otitis, bronchitis, pneumonia) • Recurrent infectious enteritis (*Cryptosporidium*, *Giardia*, enterovirus, etc)	• Recurrent, severe viral infections (CMV, EBV, herpes simplex virus, adenovirus, respiratory syncytial virus, etc) • Recurrent, severe fungal infections (*Pneumocystis jirovecii* pneumonia, candidiasis, etc)
Autoimmunity			
• Systemic SLE • Glomerulonephritis (lupus like)	• Discoid lupus (carriers of X-CGD)	• AIHA, autoimmune thrombocytopenia • Interstitial lung disease • Inflammatory bowel disease	• AIHA, autoimmune thrombocytopenia • Diarrhea, enteropathy • Dermatitis, severe eczema
Screening tests			
Numbers: C2, C3, C4 levels Function: CH50	Numbers: CBC with differential, absolute neutrophil count Function: CD18 expression, neutrophil oxidative burst	Numbers: CBC with differential, absolute lymphocyte count, T/B/NK-cell counts, quantitative IgG, IgM, and IgA Function: vaccine titers (tetanus, diphtheria, pneumococcal)	Numbers: CBC with differential, absolute lymphocyte count, T/B/NK-cell counts Function: T-cell proliferative responses to mitogens and antigens

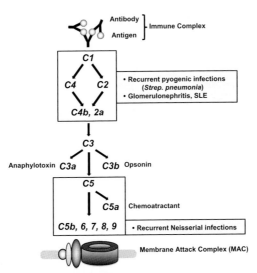

Fig. 2. The classical pathway of complement activation. Immune complexes initiate the activation of complement via this pathway. During activation, split products of complement proteins play important roles in opsonization of bacteria, increasing blood flow, attracting other immune cells, and directly destroying pathogens. Deficiency of early complement components leads to recurrent infections with encapsulated organisms or to autoimmunity (glomerulonephritis and SLE) whereas deficiency of late complement components leads to recurrent neisserial infections.

often moderately low in patients with active lupus of various causes; however, in patients with true complement deficiency, the CH50 is typically near zero.

Hemolytic uremic syndrome Atypical HUS has now been linked to several defects in complement components, in particular those involved in regulation of complement activation, including factor H, factor I, and MCP. The recommended screening approach in patients with atypical HUS is to measure the levels of C3, C4, factor H, factor I, and MCP. This testing can be followed by gene sequencing to identify the specific genetic defect.

Disorders of the Phagocyte Compartment

Overview

One of the major roles of phagocytic cells (neutrophils, macrophages, and dendritic cells) is to continuously survey the body for infection. Infectious organisms in the tissues induce expression of adhesion molecules on the surface of nearby vascular endothelial cells. These adhesion receptors stop neutrophils that are rolling down the wall of the vessel, causing them to migrate out into the tissues toward the site of the infection where they begin to ingest both opsonized and nonopsonized pathogens and debris. The ingested material is degraded and fragments of digested proteins are loaded into MHC class II molecules that are presented at the cell surface where they can be recognized by cells of the adaptive immune system. In addition to destroying pathogens, phagocytes play a major role in clearing cellular debris, including dead and dying cells, from the body. As a result, patients with phagocyte deficiencies often exhibit poor wound healing.

Table 2
Major defects in the complement compartment

Deficiency	Clinical Presentation	Testing
C1–C4 (early)	• Recurrent/severe invasive infections with encapsulated organisms (*S pneumoniae*, etc) • SLE or SLE-like glomerulonephritis	• CH50 • C1, C2, C3, C4 levels
C5–C9 (late)	• Recurrent infections with neisserial species	• CH50 • C5, C6, C7, C8, C9 levels
Factor H Factor I MCP	• Recurrent/severe invasive infections with encapsulated organisms • Familial HUS • Age-related macular degeneration	• Sequencing of *CFH*, *CFI*, and *MCP* genes

Phagocyte disorders can be classified in 3 different groups: (1) absence of particular phagocyte subsets (congenital neutropenia or monocytopenia), (2) defective phagocyte migration (leukocyte adhesion deficiency), and (3) inability of phagocytes to process or degrade organisms that have been ingested. In general, symptoms of phagocytic disorders include recurrent skin or soft tissue abscesses, lymphadenitis, pneumonia, hepatic abscesses, inflammatory bowel disease, and gingivitis. The clinical symptoms of major phagocytic disorders are outlined in **Table 3**.

Table 3
Major defects in the phagocyte compartment

Disorder	Clinical Presentation	Testing
Congenital neutropenia	• Recurrent/severe invasive bacterial infections • Gingivostomatitis • Osteopenia and osteoporosis • Myelodysplastic syndrome and leukemia	• ANC (low)
Congenital monocytopenia (*GATA2*)	• Invasive nontuberculous mycobacterial infections • Monocyte and B-cell deficiency • Myelodysplasia and acute myeloid leukemia • Lymphedema	• Monocyte count • B-cell count • *GATA2* sequencing
LAD	• Recurrent skin/soft tissue abscesses but no puss formation • Omphalitis • Leukocytosis	• ANC (high) • CD18 expression and sequencing
CGD	• Recurrent skin/soft tissue abscesses • Lymphadenitis • Pneumonia • Inflammatory colitis (bloody diarrhea)	• ANC • Neutrophil oxidative burst

Abbreviations: ANC, absolute neutrophil count; LAD, leukocyte adhesion deficiency.

Rheumatologic disease associated with defects in the phagocyte compartment
Discoid lupus erythematosus Discoid lupus erythematosus (DLE) has been described in girls and women who carry the gene for the X-linked form of chronic granulomatous disease (X-CGD). In a US registry study, 9% of kindreds with X-CGD
reported at least one female carrier with DLE.[12] Other case series have reported
a prevalence of DLE in X-CGD carriers of 30% to 31% (DLE-like lesions in carriers
of X-CGD).[13,14] A recent small study of 19 female carriers of X-CGD suggests that
in addition to frank DLE, the incidence of cutaneous manifestations is high in this
population, including photosensitive skin rashes (58%), mouth ulcers (42%), and
joint pains not attributable to other causes (37%).[15] Not all patients with DLE had
a positive antinuclear antibody test and biopsies of the DLE lesions were sometimes
described as atypical, which raises the question of whether the lesions observed in
X-CGD carriers are DLE or an entity unique to this disorder.[14] Because there is no
apparent selective advantage conferred by mutation of gp91 Phox, the gene that
causes X-CGD, the neutrophils in female carriers demonstrate random X chromosome lionization. Patients, therefore, have a mixed population of neutrophils, with
some that use the normal X chromosome and have a normal oxidative burst and
others that use the mutant X chromosome and demonstrate a lack of oxidative burst
activity. Given that DLE is not described in patients with X-CGD, the intriguing possibility is raised that development of disease is dependent on the presence of both
mutant and wild-type neutrophils. One study suggests that X-CGD neutrophils
exhibit an atypical pattern of apoptosis and that clearance of apoptotic cells is
delayed in X-CGD, which is consistent with the known function of neutrophils in
removing cellular debris.[16]

Diagnosis of CGD is dependent on demonstrating an abnormal neutrophil oxidative
burst. The flow cytometry–based dihydrorhodamine 123 assay to assess neutrophil
oxidative burst activity holds many advantages over the traditional nitroblue tetrazo-
lium test in that it can differentiate between X-CGD and the autosomal recessive
form of CGD as well as assess the degree of X chromosome lionization in X-CGD
female carriers. Genetic testing to identify the specific gene defect is also valuable.

Inflammatory bowel disease Inflammatory bowel disease occurs in approximately
30% of patients with CGD. It is more common among patients with X-CGD (43%)
than among those with autosomal recessive CGD (11%) but can occur in either
form.[17] The presentation is typically one of hemorrhagic inflammatory colitis that is
often characterized by the presence of noncaseating granulomas histologically in the
bowel biopsies. Onset of colitis is typically before age 10 and it may be the presenting
symptom in some patients.

Disorders of the B-Cell Compartment

Overview
The predominant role of B cells in the immune system is to produce antibodies.
Although they can also play an important role as antigen presenting cells, patients
who lack B cells altogether (eg, those with X-linked agammaglobulinemia [XLA]) do
well clinically with only IgG supplementation. To make an effective antibody response,
T cells must provide help through specific costimulatory interactions with B cells. Deficits in either cell type have the ability to adversely affect antibody production.

Antibody production defects account for approximately 50% of all primary immunodeficiencies.[18–20] In general, patients with antibody deficiency present with recurring
sinopulmonary infections (sinusitis, otitis media, bronchitis, and pneumonia) caused
by encapsulated bacteria and with gastrointestinal infections caused by pathogens,

such as *Giardia lamblia* and *Cryptosporidium*. The clinical symptoms of major B cell disorders are outlined in **Table 4.**

Rheumatologic disease associated with defects in the B-cell compartment

Autoimmune hematologic disease Autoimmune hemolytic anemia (AIHA) and idiopathic thrombocytopenic purpura (ITP) are among the most common autoimmune disorders that occur in patients with primary immunodeficiency diseases. Among patients with common variable immundeficiency (CVID) and selective IgA deficiency, AIHA occurs in 2% to 7% of patients and ITP occurs in 2% to 14% of patients.[21–23] The mechanism is thought related to dysregulation of B cell development and tolerance checkpoints that allow them to produce autoantibodies to self-antigen even though they are unable to make adequate protective antibody responses to foreign antigen.

The diagnosis of CVID revolves around documenting that immunoglobulin levels are less than 2 standard deviations below the mean for age and that patients are unable to generate productive antibody responses to vaccination. Other causes of hypogammaglobulinemia should be excluded. Selective IgA deficiency has the highest prevalence of any PIDD (1:333 blood donors). Most patients are asymptomatic and undiagnosed.[2] Unlike patients with CVID, patients with selective IgA deficiency typically have normal IgG responses to vaccination but low quantitative IgA levels.[19]

Organ-specific autoimmunity Patients with CVID have a high rate of inflammatory/autoimmune complications affecting specific organs, including the lung (lymphocytic interstitial pneumonitis), the bowel (lymphonodular hyperplasia and lymphocytic colitis), the liver (autoimmune hepatitis), endocrine organs (thyroiditis and diabetes), and skin (psoriasis and vitiligo). Together, these have been shown to affect between one-third and two-thirds of patients with CVID. In addition, recent data derived from the long-term follow-up of a large cohort of CVID patients over 40 years demonstrate that in patients with certain inflammatory or autoimmune complications, survival is significantly compromised, decreasing to 42% in those patients with complications versus 95% survival among CVID patients who only had infections over the same time period.[23]

Despite their underlying immunodeficiency, CVID patients with inflammatory or autoimmune complications sometimes require aggressive immunosuppression to

Table 4
Major defects in the B-cell compartment

Disorder	Clinical Presentation	Testing
XLA (*BTK*)	• Recurrent bacterial sinopulmonary infections • Enteritis—*Giardia*, enterovirus, etc • Low immunoglobulin levels • Few or absent B cells	• B-cell count • IgG, IgM, IgA levels • *BTK* sequence
CVID	• Recurrent bacterial sinopulmonary infections • Autoimmunity—AIHA, ITP, lymphocytic colitis, lymphocytic interstitial pneumonitis, endocrinopathies, psoriasis, etc • Low immunoglobulin levels	• IgG, IgM, IgA levels • Vaccine titers
sIgAD	• Most patients are asymptomatic • Recurrent bacterial sinopulmonary infections	• IgG, IgM, IgA levels • Vaccine titers

Abbreviation: sIgAD, selective IgA deficiency.

control these complications. This increases their risk of other infections and requires optimization of supplemental immunoglobulin therapy and antibiotics as well as close follow-up to optimize outcomes. Although bone marrow transplantation has been used successfully in a small number of CVID cases with complications, there is significant disagreement about its role in CVID and little is published about its use.

Arthritis/arthropathy Arthritis is the most common rheumatologic manifestation in boys with XLA. It is reported in 15% to 20% of patients and typically affects the large joints of the lower extremities. Although destructive infectious arthritis caused by organisms, such as mycoplasma, has been reported in XLA, the majority of the arthritis observed in patients is aseptic and is not particularly inflammatory or destructive. In many of these cases, the arthritis resolves with administration of adequate immunoglobulin replacement therapy, leading to the hypothesis that the arthritis may be the result of an intra-articular infection, although organisms are rarely identified in joint fluid.[24]

XLA is typically diagnosed by demonstrating markedly reduced immunoglobulin levels (IgG, IgM, and IgA) combined with absent or reduced circulating B-cell numbers. The diagnosis can be confirmed by demonstrating the absence of BTK protein expression in platelets or monocytes by flow cytometry or by sequencing of the *BTK* gene.

Disorders of the T-Cell Compartment

Overview

T cells play several essential roles in the immune system. CD4+ helper T cells direct the immune response by interacting with B cells to facilitate immunoglobulin class switching and antibody production, and absence of helper T cells causes an inability to make productive antibody responses to most protein antigens. CD8+ cytotoxic T cells play a key role in detecting and eradicating intracellular pathogens, including viruses and fungal organisms, such as *Pneumocystis jirovecii*, and absence of cytotoxic T cells leads to recurrent and severe viral and fungal infections. Regulatory T cells (T_{REG}), in particular CD4 + CD25 + FOXP3 + T_{REG}, play a critical role in mediating immune tolerance in the periphery, and absence of T_{REG} leads to severe, fatal, early-onset autoimmunity.

Patients with cellular or combined immune defects have abnormal T-cell function and as a result are susceptible to serious viral infections (eg, cytomegalovirus [CMV], Epstein-Barr virus [EBV], and adenovirus) and fungal infections (eg, *Pneumocystis jirovecii* pneumonia). These primary cellular deficiency disorders are generally more severe than antibody deficiencies but often have antibody deficiency as a component because of dysfunctional helper T cells. In addition to disseminated infections, patients tend to present early in life with failure to thrive and, at times, autoimmunity.[25]

In addition to the cellular disorders that are characterized by the susceptibility to infections, a new subset of cellular disorders characterized by severe autoimmunity as a result of absence or dysfunction of T-cell–mediated tolerance mechanisms has been defined over the past decade. These include the IPEX (immune dysregulation, polyendocrinopathy, enteropathy, X-linked) syndrome, characterized by the absence of CD4 + CD25 + FOXP3 + T_{REG} cells; APECED (autoimmune polyendocrinopathy, candidiasis, ectodermal dystrophy) syndrome, characterized by absence of functional thymic medullary epithelial cells capable of effectively selecting against autoreactive T-cell clones in the thymus; and autoimmune lymphoproliferative syndrome (ALPS), characterized by the presence of disease-inducing double-negative (CD4−CD8−) T cells that are resistant to apoptosis due to defects in Fas or Fas ligand. The clinical symptoms of major T-cell disorders are outlined in **Table 5**.

Table 5
Major defects in the T-cell compartment

Disorder	Clinical Presentation	Testing
SCID (*21 genes*)	• Recurrent/severe viral infections (CMV, EBV, adenovirus, RSV, etc) • Invasive fungal infections, including *Pneumocystic jirovecii* pneumonia • Autoimmunity—AIHA, ITP, etc	• Lymphocyte count • T/B/NK-cell count • TREC levels
DiGeorge syndrome (*del 22q11*)	• Congenital heart defects • Hypocalcemia—parathyroid hypoplasia • Recurrent bacterial and viral infections • T-cell deficiency—thymic hypoplasia	• T-cell count • 22q11 FISH
WAS (*WAS*)	• Bruising/bleeding with thrombocytopenia and small platelets • Recurrent/invasive bacterial infections • Eczema • *Pneumocystis jirovecii* pneumonia	• Platelet count and size • *WAS* sequencing
X-HIM (*CD40L*)	• Recurrent/invasive bacterial sinopulmonary infections • *Pneumocystis jirovecii* pneumonia in first 5 years of life • High IgM, low IgG and IgA • Tumors of the gastrointestinal tract (liver, biliary tree, pancreas, etc)	• IgG, IgM, IgA levels • *CD40L* sequencing
IPEX (*FOXP3*)	• Severe autoimmune enteropathy • Endocrinopathies (type 1 diabetes mellitus and thyroiditis) • Eczematous dermatitis • Other autoimmunity—hematologic, hepatic, renal, etc • Absence of CD4 + CD25 + T_{REG}	• T_{REG} cell numbers • *FOXP3* sequencing
APECED (*AIRE-1*)	• Autoimmune hypoparathyroidism • Adrenal insufficiency (autoimmune) • Chronic mucocutaneous candidiasis • Other autoimmunity—bowel, endocrine organs, etc	• *AIRE-1* sequencing
ALPS (*FAS, FAS-L*)	• Recurrent AIHA and thrombocytopenia • Massive hepatosplenomegaly and lymphadenopathy • Abnormal lymphocyte apoptosis • Increased circulating DN (CD4−CD8−) T cells	• $\alpha\beta$ TCR DN T cells • *FAS* sequencing
Ataxia telangiectasia	• Ataxia—onset typically below 5 years of age • Telangiectasias—typically on corners of eyes, cheeks, or ears • Malignancy—in particular lymphomas/leukemias • Recurrent/invasive bacterial sinopulmonary infections • Autoimmunity	• AFP level • Radiation sensitivity testing

Abbreviations: AFP, α-fetoprotein; DN, double-negative; FISH, fluorescence in situ hybridization; RSV, respiratory syncytial virus; TREC, T-cell receptor excision circles.

Rheumatologic disease associated with defects in the T-cell compartment

Autoimmune hematologic disease Among the defects in the T cell compartment, recurrent episodes of AIHA and ITP are particularly characteristic of ALPS. In addition, patients typically have massive hepatosplenomegaly and lymphadenopathy with an increased percentage (usually more than approximately 2.5%) of double-negative (CD4−CD8−) T cells within the CD3 + αβ T-cell receptor (TCR) + T-cell population. A diagnosis of ALPS can be made by evaluating the percentage of CD3 + double-negative T cells in the peripheral blood. Additional testing that supports a diagnosis of ALPS includes elevated plasma interleukin (IL)-10, elevated plasma IL-18, and elevated serum or plasma vitamin B_{12} levels.[26] Sequencing the FAS and FAS ligand genes can confirm the diagnosis.

In addition to ALPS, other disorders of the T-cell compartment that frequently present with AIHA and ITP include certain types of severe combined immunodeficiency (SCID) and Wiskott-Aldrich syndrome (WAS). In the case of WAS, all patients have thrombocytopenia. This is due in part to the platelets being small and dysfunctional but there is also a significant component of the thrombocytopenia that is thought to be autoimmune mediated.

Autoimmune enteropathy Autoimmune enteropathy is a common feature of several defects in the T cell compartment. The most consistent among these is IPEX syndrome, which is caused by mutations in the *FOXP3* gene, resulting in the absence of CD4 + CD25 + T_{REG}. Virtually 100% of patients with IPEX develop severe, autoimmune enteropathy that leads to malnutrition and failure to thrive.[27] T_{REG} cells are thought particularly important in the bowel where the mucosa is perpetually in contact with bacteria, Toll-like receptor ligands, and other proinflammatory molecules.

In addition to IPEX, other immunodeficiencies in the T-cell compartment can present with autoimmune enteropathy. Among these, APECED syndrome is one of the more common, in which approximately 25% of patients have gastrointestinal complaints.[28] In approximately 10% of patients, gastrointestinal disease is the presenting clinical manifestation.[29,30] Some patients develop autoantibodies to intrinsic factor and develop pernicious anemia as a feature of their disease. A diagnosis of APECED syndrome is considered in patients who have clinical features of APECED syndrome, including hypoparathyroidism, adrenal insufficiency, and mucocutaneous candidiasis, but the diagnosis is confirmed by sequencing of the *AIRE-1* gene.

Despite their underlying immunodeficiency, CVID patients with inflammatory or autoimmune complications sometimes require aggressive immunosuppression to control these complications. This increases their risk of other infections and requires optimization of supplemental immunoglobulin therapy and antibiotics as well as close follow-up to obtain the best outcomes. Although bone marrow transplantation has been used successfully in a small number of CVID cases with complications, there is significant disagreement about its role in CVID and there is little published about its use.

Arthritis/arthropathy The incidence of inflammatory arthritis/juvenile idiopathic arthritis has been reported to be high among patients with a variety of immunodeficiencies that affect the T-cell compartment, including WAS (20%), ALPS (4%), X-linked hyper-IgM syndrome [X-HIM] (11%), and DiGeorge syndrome, in which juvenile idiopathic arthritis is approximately 20 times more common than in the normal population.[12,31–35] The mechanisms by which these defects in the T-cell compartment allow or promote development of joint inflammation is not well understood but is of significant interest.

Other organ-specific autoimmunity The incidence of organ-specific autoimmunity is high in defects of the T-cell compartment. In addition to enteropathy, autoimmunity directed toward the skin, endocrine organs (pancreas and thyroid), liver, and kidneys is common in IPEX.[27] In APECED syndrome, autoimmunity is often directed toward endocrine organs (parathyroids, adrenals, pancreas, and gonads), liver, bowel, and lungs.[29,30] In WAS, autoimmunity is directed toward blood vessels (vasculitis), bowel, and kidneys,[31] and in X-HIM, autoimmune hepatitis is common, sometimes driven by *Cryptosporidium* bowel infection.[36,37]

Management of organ-specific autoimmunity is critical in these disorders to prevent end-organ damage. This becomes complicated, however, when considering aggressive immunosuppression in patients who have severe, underlying cellular immunodeficiencies and typically is best done in consultation with a clinical immunologist.

OVERALL DIAGNOSTIC APPROACH TO IMMUNODEFICIENCY DISORDERS

The hallmarks of PIDD are recurrent infections, unusual infections, and autoimmunity. Some of the infections may be persistent whereas others may be due to unusual microorganisms that normally do not cause problems in healthy individuals. Because most of these conditions are lifelong, it is important to perform a detailed diagnostic evaluation before initiating therapy.

Sometimes the signs and symptoms of PIDD are so severe or so characteristic that it is easy for a diagnosis to be made. In most cases, however, it is not as clear because PIDDs often present as a series of treatable, ordinary infections or autoimmune features that are not suspected to be an immunodeficiency until the patient has "too many." To complicate matters, some illnesses and certain medications can produce a temporary immunodeficiency state that should be considered.

History and Physical Examination

When a pattern of frequent infections or autoimmunity suggests an immunodeficiency, the physician should conduct a thorough patient history. Questions should include the type and length of infection, response to therapy, severity of infection, and frequency of infection. A thorough family history should include questions about other family members with similar clinical symptoms, other family members with severe or recurrent infections, early deaths in the family (particularly male), and consanguinity.

A thorough physical examination should then be performed, looking particularly for findings that may suggest immunodeficiency. Suggestive findings may include the following: head, ears, eyes, nose, and throat—microcephaly (Nijmegen breakage syndrome, cernunnos, or ligase IV deficiency), scarred tympanic membranes that may suggest recurrent infections and frequent rupture (antibody deficiency), gingivitis (neutrophil defects), or absence of tonsils (XLA); cardiovascular—murmur or cyanosis that may suggest a congenital heart defect (DiGeorge syndrome); lungs—rhonchi or rales that may suggest chronic lung disease or bronchiectasis as a result of frequent infections (antibody deficiency, CGD, or hyper-IgE syndrome); abdomen—splenomegaly (CVID or autoimmune lymphoproliferative syndrome); lymph nodes—absent lymph nodes (XLA or SCID), disseminated lymphadenopathy (CVID, Omenn syndrome, autoimmune lymphoproliferative syndrome, or autosomal recessive hyper-IgM syndrome); skin—eczema (WAS, Omenn syndrome, IPEX syndrome, or Netherton syndrome), petechiae (WAS), boils/soft tissue abscesses (CGD, hyper-IgE syndrome, or leukocyte adhesion deficiency), or telangiectasia (ataxia telangiectasia or ataxia telangiectasia–like disorder).

Laboratory Testing

When a PIDD is suspected, laboratory screening should start with a few diagnostic tests that screen for defects in each of the 4 major compartments of the immune system (see **Table 1**). A complete blood cell count (CBC) with differential can determine whether the hematocrit and platelet counts (WAS) are normal and can demonstrate that a normal number of neutrophils (neutropenia) and lymphocytes (SCID) is present. Lymphocyte subset analysis can be obtained to determine if patients have T cells, B cells, and natural killer (NK) cells, an effective method to screen for various forms of SCID and for XLA. A neutrophil oxidative burst assay is a rapid and economical method to screen patients for CGD, the most common phagocyte deficiency. Quantitative immunoglobulin testing (IgG, IgM, and IgA) combined with measurement of specific antibody levels to evaluate vaccine responses (tetanus and Pneumovax) is an effective method to evaluate patients for antibody deficiency. Lastly, a CH50 test efficiently screens the entire classical complement pathway for defects. Additional testing, such as specific gene sequencing or immunophenotyping, may be necessary.

Caution should be used when assessing immunologic function in a newborn because the normal values for many immunologic parameters, including lymphocyte counts and immunoglobulin levels, are substantially different from those of adults.[38] When a diagnosis is uncertain or further guidance is needed regarding the work-up or treatment options, a primary care physician or pediatrician should consult a clinical immunologist. If SCID is suspected, a clinical immunologist should be consulted immediately.

SUMMARY

Understanding that primary immunodeficiency diseases may present with inflammatory complications and autoimmunity as well as severe, recurrent, or unusual infections is critical in caring for patients with this group of disorders. Recognizing and appropriately managing autoimmune complications in patients with underlying immunodeficiencies is particularly challenging and requires an understanding of which compartment of the immune system is most affected by a patient's particular disorder. Expanded understanding of basic mechanisms of autoimmunity will continue to grow as new genetic defects are identified that present with dysregulated immune tolerance. Hopefully these will inform both the search for the underlying causes of common autoimmune disorders and potential pathways that may be targeted therapeutically to modulate immunity.

REFERENCES

1. Boyle JM, Buckley RH. Population prevalence of diagnosed primary immunodeficiency diseases in the United States. J Clin Immunol 2007;27:497–502.
2. Clark JA, Callicoat PA, Brenner NA, et al. Selective IgA deficiency in blood donors. Am J Clin Pathol 1983;80:210–3.
3. Cunningham-Rundles C, Brandeis WE, Pudifin DJ, et al. Autoimmunity in selective IgA deficiency: relationship to anti-bovine protein antibodies, circulating immune complexes and clinical disease. Clin Exp Immunol 1981;45:299–304.
4. Edwards E, Razvi S, Cunningham-Rundles C. IgA deficiency: clinical correlates and responses to pneumococcal vaccine. Clin Immunol 2004;111:93–7.
5. Jacob CM, Pastorino AC, Fahl K, et al. Autoimmunity in IgA deficiency: revisiting the role of IgA as a silent housekeeper. J Clin Immunol 2008;28(Suppl 1):S56–61.
6. Smith S, Sweetser MT, Wilson CB. The immunocompromised host. Pediatr Rev 1996;17:435–40.
7. Frank MM. Complement deficiencies. Pediatr Clin North Am 2000;47:1339–54.

8. Roumenina LT, Loirat C, Dragon-Durey MA, et al. Alternative complement pathway assessment in patients with atypical HUS. J Immunol Methods 2011; 365:8–26.

9. Pickering MC, Botto M, Taylor PR, et al. Systemic lupus erythematosus, complement deficiency, and apoptosis. Adv Immunol 2000;76:227–324.

10. Sullivan KE. Complement deficiency and autoimmunity. Curr Opin Pediatr 1998; 10:600–6.

11. Schulze C, Munoz LE, Franz S, et al. Clearance deficiency—a potential link between infections and autoimmunity. Autoimmun Rev 2008;8:5–8.

12. Winkelstein JA, Marino MC, Johnston RB Jr, et al. Chronic granulomatous disease. Report on a national registry of 368 patients. Medicine (Baltimore) 2000;79:155–69.

13. Kragballe K, Borregaard N, Brandrup F, et al. Relation of monocyte and neutrophil oxidative metabolism to skin and oral lesions in carriers of chronic granulomatous disease. Clin Exp Immunol 1981;43:390–8.

14. Sillevis Smitt JH, Weening RS, Krieg SR, et al. Discoid lupus erythematosus-like lesions in carriers of X-linked chronic granulomatous disease. Br J Dermatol 1990;122:643–50.

15. Cale CM, Morton L, Goldblatt D. Cutaneous and other lupus-like symptoms in carriers of X-linked chronic granulomatous disease: incidence and autoimmune serology. Clin Exp Immunol 2007;148:79–84.

16. Sanford AN, Suriano AR, Herche D, et al. Abnormal apoptosis in chronic granulomatous disease and autoantibody production characteristic of lupus. Rheumatology (Oxford) 2006;45:178–81.

17. Marciano BE, Rosenzweig SD, Kleiner DE, et al. Gastrointestinal involvement in chronic granulomatous disease. Pediatrics 2004;114:462–8.

18. Ballow M. Primary immunodeficiency disorders: antibody deficiency. J Allergy Clin Immunol 2002;109:581–91.

19. Cooper MA, Pommering TL, Koranyi K. Primary immunodeficiencies. Am Fam Physician 2003;68:2001–8.

20. Woroniecka M, Ballow M. Office evaluation of children with recurrent infection. Pediatr Clin North Am 2000;47:1211–24.

21. Agarwal S, Cunningham-Rundles C. Autoimmunity in common variable immunodeficiency. Curr Allergy Asthma Rep 2009;9:347–52.

22. Quinti I, Soresina A, Spadaro G, et al. Long-term follow-up and outcome of a large cohort of patients with common variable immunodeficiency. J Clin Immunol 2007; 27:308–16.

23. Resnick ES, Moshier EL, Godbold JH, et al. Morbidity and mortality in common variable immune deficiency over 4 decades. Blood 2012;119(7):1650–7. [Epub 2011 Dec 16].

24. Lee AH, Levinson AI, Schumacher HR Jr. Hypogammaglobulinemia and rheumatic disease. Semin Arthritis Rheum 1993;22:252–64.

25. Buckley RH. Primary cellular immunodeficiencies. J Allergy Clin Immunol 2002; 109:747–57.

26. Oliveira JB, Bleesing JJ, Dianzani U, et al. Revised diagnostic criteria and classification for the autoimmune lymphoproliferative syndrome (ALPS): report from the 2009 NIH International Workshop. Blood 2010;116:e35–40.

27. Gambineri E, Torgerson TR. Genetic disorders with immune dysregulation. Cell Mol Life Sci 2012;69:49–58.

28. Ekwall O, Hedstrand H, Grimelius L, et al. Identification of tryptophan hydroxylase as an intestinal autoantigen. Lancet 1998;352:279–83.

29. Ahonen P, Myllarniemi S, Sipila I, et al. Clinical variation of autoimmune polyendocrinopathy-candidiasis-ectodermal dystrophy (APECED) in a series of 68 patients. N Engl J Med 1990;322:1829–36.

30. Betterle C, Greggio NA, Volpato M. Clinical review 93: autoimmune polyglandular syndrome type 1. J Clin Endocrinol Metab 1998;83:1049–55.

31. Dupuis-Girod S, Medioni J, Haddad E, et al. Autoimmunity in Wiskott-Aldrich syndrome: risk factors, clinical features, and outcome in a single-center cohort of 55 patients. Pediatrics 2003;111:e622–7.

32. Keenan GF, Sullivan KE, McDonald-McGinn DM, et al. Arthritis associated with deletion of 22q11.2: more common than previously suspected. Am J Med Genet 1997;71:488.

33. Levy J, Espanol-Boren T, Thomas C, et al. Clinical spectrum of X-linked hyper-IgM syndrome. J Pediatr 1997;131:47–54.

34. Sneller MC, Dale JK, Straus SE. Autoimmune lymphoproliferative syndrome. Curr Opin Rheumatol 2003;15:417–21.

35. Sullivan KE, McDonald-McGinn DM, Driscoll DA, et al. Juvenile rheumatoid arthritis-like polyarthritis in chromosome 22q11.2 deletion syndrome (DiGeorge anomalad/velocardiofacial syndrome/conotruncal anomaly face syndrome). Arthritis Rheum 1997;40:430–6.

36. Stephens J, Cosyns M, Jones M, et al. Liver and bile duct pathology following Cryptosporidium parvum infection of immunodeficient mice. Hepatology 1999;30:27–35.

37. Wolska-Kusnierz B, Bajer A, Caccio S, et al. Cryptosporidium infection in patients with primary immunodeficiencies. J Pediatr Gastroenterol Nutr 2007;45:458–64.

38. Muller SM, Ege M, Pottharst A, et al. Transplacentally acquired maternal T lymphocytes in severe combined immunodeficiency: a study of 121 patients. Blood 2001;98:1847–51.

Index

Note: Page numbers of article titles are in **boldface** type.

A

Abatacept, for JIA, 311, 319
Abdominal pain
   in JIIM, 368–369
   in SLE, 353
Acne syndrome, 277–278, 463
Activated partial thromboplastin time, 271–272
Acute phase reactants, 265–266
   in cytokine storm syndromes, 330
   in Kawasaki disease, 430
Acute respiratory distress syndrome, in antiphospholipid syndrome, 294–295
Adalimumab, for JIA, 311, 318
Adaptive immunity
   description of, 225–226
   in inflammatory response, 234–241
Adaptor apoptosis-associated specklike protein containing a caspase activation and
   recruitment domain (ASC), 231
Agammaglobulinemia, X-linked, 500–501
Alanine aminotransferase, measurement of, 273
Aldolase, measurement of, 273
Allergens, cytokine storm syndromes due to, 337
Alopecia, in SLE, 346–347
American College of Rheumatology, SLE criteria of, 346
American Heart Association, Kawasaki disease recommendations of, 434
Amplified musculoskeletal pain syndromes, 481–489
   diagnosis of, 482–485
   differential diagnosis of, 485
   diffuse, 482
   localized, 481–482
   prevalence of, 481
   prognosis for, 488–489
   treatment of, 486–488
Amyloidosis, 456
Anakinra
   for hyperimmunoglobulinemia D, 458
   for interleukin-1 receptor antagonist deficiency, 459
   for JIA, 311, 318
   for macrophage activation syndrome, 340
   for neonatal-onset multisystem inflammatory disorder, 463
Anaphylatoxins, in immune response, 233
Anemia, 263–264
   in JIA, 303

doi:10.1016/S0031-3955(12)00038-7

Moving?

Make sure your subscription moves with you!

To notify us of your new address, find your **Clinics Account Number** (located on your mailing label above your name), and contact customer service at:

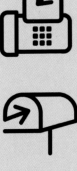

Email: **journalscustomerservice-usa@elsevier.com**

800-654-2452 (subscribers in the U.S. & Canada)
314-447-8871 (subscribers outside of the U.S. & Canada)

Fax number: **314-447-8029**

Elsevier Health Sciences Division
Subscription Customer Service
3251 Riverport Lane
Maryland Heights, MO 63043

*To ensure uninterrupted delivery of your subscription, please notify us at least 4 weeks in advance of move.